Nutrition Optimization for Health and Longevity

Herbert Zeng, Ph.D.

iUniverse, Inc.
New York   Bloomington

Nutrition Optimization for Health and Longevity

The information, ideas, and suggestions in this book are not intended as a substitute for professional medical advice. Before following any suggestions contained in this book, you should consult your personal physician. Neither the author nor the publisher shall be liable or responsible for any loss or damage allegedly arising as a consequence of your use or application of any information or suggestions in this book.

iUniverse books may be ordered through booksellers or by contacting:

iUniverse
1663 Liberty Drive
Bloomington, IN 47403
www.iuniverse.com
1-800-Authors (1-800-288-4677)

Because of the dynamic nature of the Internet, any Web addresses or links contained in this book may have changed since publication and may no longer be valid. The views expressed in this work are solely those of the author and do not necessarily reflect the views of the publisher, and the publisher hereby disclaims any responsibility for them.

ISBN: 978-1-4401-9697-3 (sc)
ISBN: 978-1-4401-9699-7 (dj)
ISBN: 978-1-4401-9698-0 (ebk)

Library of Congress Control Number: 2009913771

Printed in the United States of America

iUniverse rev. date: 3/29/2010

To my loving wife, Lin, for her understanding and support, and our two daughters, Regina and Marina, and our son, Elbert.

Acknowledgments

With deep gratitude, I would like to thank my first daughter, Regina (Chuli) Zeng, my wonderful editor, who gave me the support needed during work on this book and the freedom to shape the content.

Also, I thank Kyle Randolph (Publishing Consultant), Kathi Wittkamper (Editorial Consultant), and Cory Hovious (Publishing Services Associate) at iUniverse for their kind assistance with the publication of this book.

Contents

List of Tables

Introduction

Life is in the blood, but our health is in the pH of the blood, and the pH of the blood is in what we breathe, drink, and eat. Therefore, optimizing your nutrition makes you healthier and helps you live longer.

Dr. Wright wrote in the Foreword of the book, *Total Wellness*: "If there's something wrong with our bodies, it's very likely that there's a problem with the molecules that make up our bodies—a lack of this, an excess of that, perhaps the presence of molecules that don't belong there at all. Germs and microorganisms don't cause disease all by their microscopic selves; they only take advantage of us when our bodies are weakened by nutrient-poor food or burdened by toxins that don't belong in our systems anyway. Healthy, vibrant plants, animals, and people don't 'catch' germs very often, if at all!" This indicates that providing nutrients (molecules) in right amounts and preventing toxins from entering our bodies can decrease disease, improve our health, and prolong our longevity.

This book teaches you how to optimize what you breathe, drink, and eat to achieve optimal amounts of the nutrients your body needs, rather than giving general recommendations to everyone about what you should eat and what you shouldn't eat. From the optimization point of view, you can eat any kinds of food, but they must be in the right amounts with the right combinations in the right time (age) in order to satisfy your daily energy and nutrition requirements.

I came to the topic, human nutrition optimization, when I worked at a nutritional company several years ago. I read many books and articles about how to eat balanced foods, how to take dietary supplements, and how to lose weight to achieve optimum health. However, none of them tells us how to optimize what we eat and drink in the right amounts to meet our bodies' daily energy and nutrition requirements. I have a wide academic and industrial background in the fields of chemistry, materials science, pharmaceutical science, and nutraceutical science, and have over ten years of experience in industries of materials, pharmaceutics and dietary supplements, specializing in the optimization of drug, nutritional, and material formulations. Hence, I was determined to write this book using my expertise about Nutrition Optimization for Health and Longevity five years ago.

Upon collecting data and reading articles and books from libraries and on the Internet in my spare time, I completed this book.

Chapter One presents data of human body elements and chemical compositions. You will learn what elements make up the human body, and what amount and biological functions each element has. Also, you will understand chemical compositions of various organs/tissues in a normal adult human body: water, fat, protein, carbohydrate, and minerals. We lose all of these compositions in different amounts every day, due to metabolism, which helps us understand why we need to supplement nutrition daily.

Chapter Two introduces macronutrients. You will learn that oxygen is considered the most important nutrient and that water is considered the second most important nutrient. In addition, you will familiarize yourself with the different biological functions of various macronutrients, which will help you recognize the vital significance of air and water quality to your health and longevity and understand the essence of eating protein, fat, carbohydrate, and fiber daily in certain amounts.

Chapters Three and Four introduce micronutrients. The functions, health benefits, and deficiency symptoms of various vitamins and minerals are summarized in detail. It is very helpful for you to recognize the significance of these nutrients.

Chapter Five discusses ORAC of foods and human health. ORAC, Oxygen Radical Absorption Capacity, is a measure of antioxidant capacities of different foods or dietary supplements. This chapter briefly introduces free-radical theory of aging and disease, and then calculates daily free-radical amounts produced in human body weights from 44 kg to 90 kg. It also lists ORAC values of 147 commonly consumed foods. And, it explains roles of food antioxidants in helping eliminate free radicals that contributes to or causes aging and disease.

Chapter Six discusses pH of blood and human health. The chapter introduces composition of blood and its normal pH range. It summarizes functions of blood and computes blood weights and volumes of different body weights from 44 kg to 90 kg. This chapter also introduces blood pH theory of disease and aging and explains how to balance the pH of blood in the human body. Finally, it stresses effects of common foods on balancing the pH of blood.

Chapter Seven explains human body daily energy and nutrition requirements. First, it discusses human body daily energy requirements and you will find out how to calculate your body mass index (BMI), through which you use to determine if your weight is normal, overweight, or obese. Then, it teaches you how to determine your physical activity level. This chapter shows you how to compute your daily energy requirements according to your age, weight, and physical level by following two different examples. This chapter also summarizes human body daily nutrition requirements in the form of tables, from which you can easily obtain the data of your dietary reference intakes for macronutrients and micronutrients. Lastly, Chapter Seven explains the difference between energy requirements and nutrition requirements.

Chapter Eight summarizes energy and nutrition values of 379 best foods, which are listed in Appendix A in terms of their categories: vegetables, fruits, legumes, cereal, grain, bread, dairy, egg, cheese, nuts and seeds, fish and shell-fish, meat and poultry, and oil. Also, this chapter separately lists 10 foods containing the various richest macronutrients and micronutrients. It is very helpful in order for you to familiarize yourself with the energy and nutrition values of these selected foods in Appendix A and to optimize your nutrition from the foods you eat.

Chapter Nine introduces human nutrition optimization in detail. You will first learn how to calculate daily human body requirements of oxygen and air amounts in accordance with body weights and understand the importance of optimizing outdoor and indoor air quality. Then, you will find out how many cups of water you need a day and how to drink water and beverages in the right amounts. In the optimization of air and water quality, the government's responsibility is emphasized. Lastly, you will learn how to optimize the foods you eat by following a step-by-step procedure instructed with two examples to meet your daily energy and nutrition requirements.

Chapter Ten briefly introduces dietary supplements and their energy and nutrition values. This chapter teaches you how to read the labels of dietary supplements in order to obtain the energy and nutrition values. Also, it shows you how to determine your daily requirements of dietary supplements after evaluating your nutrition status, if you cannot optimize your menus to satisfy your daily energy and nutrition requirements.

Chapter Eleven is about achieving optimum health and longevity through human nutrition optimization. First, this chapter describes human longevity: the average life expectancy today is around 80 years, but it has a full potential of 120 years. Then, it summarizes the factors affecting human longevity: genetics, exercise, spirituality, and nutrition. Next, it explains how to achieve optimum health and longevity through human nutrition optimization for different people. This chapter teaches people, especially people who are overweight or obese, how to design a reasonable weight loss and maintenance schedule by using an example, and how to optimize their menus to meet their daily energy and nutrition requirements during the period of weight loss and maintenance plan.

The summary summarizes the main points of this book. This summary helps you recall the main contents and valuable thoughts. And, it emphasizes that if we learn to optimize our nutrition, we will be able to solve the world-wide problem of over-nutrition and malnutrition and at the same time, we will be able to reduce medical expenditures.

Near the end of the book, Appendix A lists the energy and nutrition values of 379 best foods, which had been selected from more than the 7000 foods in the SR20 Search Database USDA, in terms of their categories: vegetables, fruits, legumes, cereal, grain, bread, dairy, egg, cheese, nuts and seeds, fish and shellfish, meat and poultry, and oil. The first table lists their amounts of energy, water, protein, fat, carbohydrate, fiber, sugar, saturated fat, trans-fat, cholesterol, and ORAC in 100g of weight. The second table lists their amounts of 12 minerals in 100 g of weight. The third table lists their amounts of 14 vitamins in 100 g of weight. The fourth table lists their amounts of 11 amino acids, eicosapentaenoic acid (EPA), docosahexaenoic acid (DHA), lutein and zeaxanthin in 100g of weight. These foods should satisfy the daily needs of our absolute majority.

This is a unique book. There are many books available that say that vitamins and minerals are vitally important to our health, but there are no books that treat oxygen as the most important nutrient. Many books tell you that you should eat a balanced diet in order to obtain enough nutrition for your body, but none exactly teaches you how to optimize what you eat at various physical levels and at different ages. Many books introduce ways to help you lose weight, but none explains how to design a reasonable weight loss and maintenance schedule and how to optimize the foods you eat to meet your energy and nutrition requirements at each stage. Many books tell you to take dietary supplements, but none proves by actual data through calculations that if you take too many supplements, it will actually harm your health.

This is a practicable book. This book shows you a step-by-step procedure of optimizing the foods you eat with two examples. For a normal adult, he/she only needs about three U.S. dollars a day to buy the optimized foods that will meet his/her daily energy and nutrition requirements. My family has two adults, one 14-year-old girl, one 7-year-old girl, and one 3 year-old boy, and it only costs us about thirteen U.S. dollars a day to buy the optimized foods. Nobody in my family takes any dietary supplements, and we all have a normal weight with optimal health. So, anyone who wants to save money and keep optimum health should read this book and practice optimizing the foods he/she eats.

This is a book for everyone. Government leaders should read this book, in which their responsibilities for optimizing air and water quality are emphasized, because both play a key role in our health and longevity. Normal weight people should read this book because it teaches them how to optimize the foods they eat in order to meet their energy and nutrition requirements at different ages and at different physical activity levels. Overweight or obese persons should read this book because it teaches them how to design a reasonable weight loss and maintenance schedule and how to optimize the foods they eat at each stage. People with diabetes should read this book because it tells them that they should optimize the foods they eat to keep the pH of their diets in the range of 7.0– 8.5, chromium in the daily range of 150–350 μm, and the energy from the sugar not more than 10 percent of the total energy, so they can control diabetes or even get rid of it. Also, people with Alzheimer's disease should read this book because it recommends that they should optimize the foods they eat to keep selenium in the daily range of 150–300 μm, so they will be able to control Alzheimer's disease.

The intent of this book is to help everyone understand why we need nutrition, what kinds and amounts of nutrients we require, how to obtain enough energy and nutrients from the foods we eat, and why nutrition optimization can help improve our health and prolong our longevity.

Chapter One
Human Body Elements and Chemical Compositions

1. Human Body Elements

Everything in the world is composed of chemical elements. Elements combine with one another in different proportions to form everything from the air that we breathe, to the food that we eat, to the wood that we use to build our homes, to the earth that we live, and even to our own bodies. Elements are the basic building blocks of our lives.

On the earth, 94 elements have been discovered, and in total, 117 elements have been observed as of 2007. In the human body, 59 elements have been found, while 99.4 percent of our bodies' mass is composed of just six elements: oxygen (61.43 percent), carbon (22.86 percent), hydrogen (10 percent), nitrogen (2.57 percent), calcium (1.43 percent), and phosphorus (1.11 percent). The other 53 elements only account for 0.6 percent of our bodies' weight. Percentage of each element in the human body is summarized in Table 1-1.

The Bible says that *the LORD GOD formed man from the dust of the ground* (Genesis 2:7). The 59 elements in the human body all come from the 94 elements on the earth, which demonstrates that man was created by GOD using the dust of the ground because up to date nobody can make a cell of the human body.

Of the 59 elements in the human body, almost 30 elements have been found to have a key function in helping us live and be healthy. Oxygen is the most abundant element in the human body, which combines with hydrogen to form water that makes up about 60% of an average adult's weight. Water is incredibly important for our bodies. It dissolves other life-supporting substances and transports them to fluids in and around our cells. It is also a place in which most reactions take place in our bodies. Many people consider water to be the "blood of life". In addition, it may seem obvious that people need to breathe oxygen to survive, but plants need this element too. Many people think plants "breathe" carbon dioxide and "exhale" oxygen. But in reality, plants also "breathe" oxygen at certain times. Without oxygen, plants could not survive. Without plants, we wouldn't have food to eat. Therefore, it becomes clear that this versatile element is the single most important substance to life.

Carbon is the second most abundant element in the human body, perhaps even the most essential element to life. The carbon atom is ideal for building big biological molecules. The carbon atom can be thought of as a basic building block. These building blocks can be attached to each other to form long chains, or they can be attached to other elements. This is a lot like the way the big molecules are made in the body. Without carbon, these big molecules could not be built, and every part of our bodies is made up of these big molecules. This is the reason we are known as "carbon-based life forms". Without carbon, our bodies would just be a big pile of loose atoms with no way of being built into a person.

It would be virtually impossible to understate the importance of hydrogen—the third richest element in our bodies. First of all, remember that water is a compound of hydrogen and oxygen. We can survive years, or at least months without getting most of the other elements that we need to survive. We can survive weeks without food, but we would die after only a few days without water. Chemically, water is a remarkable substance and its many unique attributes make life possible. Hydrogen is obviously a critical component of water and minute chemical bonds called "hydrogen bonds", which is what gives water many of its unique attributes. Also, hydrogen is practically always bound to the carbon that our bodies are constructed of. Without this arrangement, our bodies would be nothing more than a pile of atoms on the ground. Stomach acid is a compound of hydrogen and chlorine (hydrochloric acid, or HCl). Logically, hydrogen is extremely important because it allows us to digest our food properly and to absorb the many other elements that we need to survive. Finally, many chemical reactions that make life possible involve hydrogen ion. Without this unique element, we simply couldn't exist.

Nitrogen is another essential element—the fourth richest element in our bodies. It is a key constituent of all proteins and nucleic acids in our bodies. It plays an important role in digestion of food and growth. As you may know, 78% of the air we breathe is made up of nitrogen. But human beings cannot use the nitrogen in the air we breathe; that nitrogen is in the wrong form. We have to get nitrogen, but in a different form, from the food that we eat. Fortunately, there is plenty of nitrogen in food to nourish our bodies.

Calcium is the most abundant mineral element in our bodies, which accounts for 2 to 3 pounds of our total bodies' weight. Most of us know that calcium is important in building and maintaining strong bones and teeth, but it is also essential for many other things. It helps control things like muscle growth and the electrical impulses in your brain. This vital element is also necessary for maintaining proper blood pressure and making blood clot when you get cut. Calcium also enables other molecules to digest food and make energy for the body. Increasing calcium intake in our diet is believed to lower high blood pressure and prevent heart disease. It is also used to treat arthritis.

Phosphorus is the second richest mineral in the human body. This essential mineral is required for the healthy formation of bones and teeth, and is necessary for our bodies to process many of the foods that we eat. It is a part of the body's energy storage system, and helps the body maintain healthy blood sugar levels. Phosphorus is also found in substantial amounts in the nervous system. The regular contractions of the heart are dependant upon phosphorus, and so are normal cell growth and repair.

Besides the 6 main elements in the human body that make up 99.4% of our weights, the other 53 elements that only account for 0.6 percent of the human body weight also play some significant biological roles. Their key biological functions along with those of the 6 main elements are summarized in Table 1-1.

Table 1-1 Amount of each element in the human body and their biological functions

Element	Mass of element in a 70-kg person	Percentage	Biological Functions
Oxygen (O)	43 kg	61.43%	• Is a component of water that is more than 60% of our bodies' weights. • Is an integral component of all proteins, DNA (deoxyribonucleic acid) and RNA (ribonucleic acid)), carbohydrates, and fats. • Plays a key role in metabolism. • Is essential for respiration.
Carbon (C)	16 kg	22.86%	• Is an important component of all proteins, DNA and RNA, carbohydrates, and fats.
Hydrogen (H)	7 kg	10.00%	• Is a component of water. • Is an integral component of all proteins, DNA and RNA, carbohydrates, and fats.

Nitrogen (N)	1.8 kg	2.57%	• Is an important constituent of all proteins and DNA and RNA.
Calcium (Ca)	1.0 kg	1.43%	• See chapter four.
Phosphorus (P)	780 g	1.11%	• See chapter four.
Potassium (K)	140 g	0.20%	• See chapter four.
Sulfur (S)	140 g	0.20%	• Is a primary constituent of three amino acids: cystine, cystein, and methionine. • Is a minor constituent of fats, body fluids, and bones. • Increases blood circulation. • Detoxifies. • Reduces muscle cramping and back pain. • Removes inflammation. • Assists in the healing of muscles. • Helps liver produce choline. • Stimulates flow of bile. • Regulates heart and brain function. • Promotes healthy skin, nails, and hair. • Helps lubricate joints.
Sodium (Na)	100 g	0.14%	• See chapter four.
Chlorine (Cl)	95 g	0.14%	• See chapter four.
Magnesium (Mg)	19 g	0.03%	• See chapter four.
Iron (Fe)	4.2 g	0.006%	• See chapter four.
Fluorine (F)	2.6 g	0.004%	• See chapter four.
Zinc (Zn)	2.3 g	0.003%	• See chapter four.

Silicon (Si)	1.0 g	0.001%	• Along with calcium, silicon grows and maintains strong bones. • Is important to the formation of connective tissues, like ligaments and tendons. • Is important for the growth of hair, skin, and fingernails. • Is influential in preventing veins and arteries from getting hard and stiff. • Reduces the effectiveness of aluminum in the body.
Rubidium (Rb)	0.68 g	0.001%	• Has no known biological use.
Strontium (Sr)	0.32 g	0.0005%	• Has no known biological use.
Bromine (Br)	0.26 g	0.0004%	• Has no known biological use.
Lead (Pb)	0.12 g	0.0002%	• Has no known biological use.
Copper (Cu)	72 mg	0.0001%	• See chapter four.
Aluminum (Al)	60 mg	0.00009%	• Is now thought to be involved in the action of a small number of enzymes.
Cadmium (Cd)	50 mg	0.00007%	• Is believed to be a required trace element, although its need and use are not currently understood. • Is thought to be involved with metabolism.
Cerium (Ce)	40 mg	0.00006%	• Has no known biological use.
Barium (Ba)	22 mg	0.00003%	• Has no known biological use.
Iodine (I)	20 mg	0.00003%	• See chapter four.
Tin (Sn)	20 mg	0.00003%	• Has no known biological use.
Titanium (Ti)	20 mg	0.00003%	• Has no known biological use.

Boron (B)	18 mg	0.00003%	• Helps build muscle and bones and makes bones more flexible. • Is necessary for brain function, memory, and alertness. • Is necessary for the activation of vitamin D. • Assists and improves retention of calcium, magnesium, and phosphorus.
Nickel (Ni)	15 mg	0.00002%	• Interacts with iron in oxygen transport. • Stimulates the metabolism. • Is a key metal in several enzymes.
Selenium (Se)	15 mg	0.00002%	• See chapter four.
Chromium (Cr)	14 mg	0.00002%	• See chapter four.
Manganese (Mn)	12 mg	0.00002%	• See chapter four.
Arsenic (As)	7 mg	0.00001%	• Is necessary for the functioning of the nervous system.
Lithium (Li)	7 mg	0.00001%	• Has no known biological use.
Cesium (Cs)	6 mg	0.000009%	• Has no known biological use.
Mercury (Hg)	6 mg	0.000009%	• Has no known biological use.
Germanium (Ge)	5 mg	0.000007%	• Helps activate various organs to attract more oxygen. • Expels harmful pollutants and pathogens from the body. • Helps maintain a strong immune system by assisting in the production of killer cells and T-suppresser cells. • Assists in electron transmissions.
Molybdenum (Mo)	5 mg	0.000007%	• See chapter four.

Cobalt (Co)	3 mg	0.000004%	• Is a core constituent of vitamin B12 (cyanocobalamin). • Is essential for the normal function of all cells, particularly cells of bone marrow and nervous and gastrointestinal systems.
Antimony (Sb)	2 mg	0.000003%	• Has no known biological use.
Silver (Ag)	2 mg	0.000003%	• Has no known biological use.
Niobium (Nb)	1.5 mg	0.000002%	• Has no known biological use.
Zirconium (Zr)	1 mg	0.000001%	• Has no known biological use.
Lanthanum (La)	0.8 mg	0.000001%	• Has no known biological use.
Gallium (Ga)	0.7 mg	0.000001%	• Has no known biological use.
Tellurium (Te)	0.7 mg	0.000001%	• Has no known biological use.
Yttrium (Y)	0.6 mg	0.0000009%	• Has no known biological use.
Bismuth (Bi)	0.5 mg	0.0000007%	• Has no known biological use.
Thallium (Tl)	0.5 mg	0.0000007%	• Has no known biological use.
Indium (In)	0.4 mg	0.0000006%	• Has no known biological use.
Gold (Au)	0.2 mg	0.0000003%	• Has no known biological use.
Scandium (Sc)	0.2 mg	0.0000003%	• Has no known biological use.
Tantalum (Ta)	0.2 mg	0.0000003%	• Has no known biological use.
Vanadium (V)	0.11 mg	0.0000002%	• Is important for bone and teeth development. • Helps the body convert some foods into energy. • Stabilizes blood sugar levels.
Thorium (Th)	0.1 mg	0.0000001%	• Has no known biological use.

Uranium (U)	0.1 mg	0.0000001%	• Has no known biological use.
Samarium (Sm)	50 µg	0.00000007%	• Has no known biological use.
Beryllium (Be)	36 µg	0.00000005%	• Has no known biological use.
Tungsten (W)	20 µg	0.00000003%	• Is used by a small number of enzymes in a fashion similar to that of molybdenum.

Note: The raw data on which this table is based on is from John Emsley, The Elements, 3rd ed., Clarendon Press, Oxford, 1998. Percentage of each element is calculated based on the raw data. Biological function is summarized from various sources.

2. Human Body Chemical Compositions

The major component of the human body is water. The fat and protein compositions are relatively small, with the remainders being minerals and carbohydrate. The fat composition will vary considerably between individuals in terms of absolute amounts. Fat mass consists of 20% water and 80% adipose tissue, and can, in obese people be twice as much as in lean people. Table 1-2 summarizes the chemical compositions of a lean man and an obese man.

Table 1-2 Comparison of chemical compositions of lean man and obese man

Composition	70-kg lean man	100-kg obese man
Water	62%	48%
Protein	17%	13%
Fat	17%	35%
Carbohydrate	1%	1%
Minerals	3%	3%

Water, protein, fat, minerals, and carbohydrate contents in various organs/tissues in the human body are different. I searched all the published results, finding only three research papers that have determined the composition of an adult human body by chemical analysis. By comparing the data, I managed to organize the range of various compositions into a table, which is presented in Table 1-3.

**Table 1-3 Chemical compositions of various organs/tissues
in normal adult human body**

Ogans/tissues	Water(%)	Protein (%)	Fat(%)	Minerals (%)*	Carbohydrate (%)**
Brain	70–76	10–14	10–14	0.3–0.5	0
Lungs	75–85	13–20	1–2	0.1–0.2	0
Liver	70–73	16–23	3–10	0.1–0.2	1–2
Heart	60–75	15–18	9–18	0.1–0.2	0
Spleen	76–80	17–19	1–2	0.2–0.3	0
Kidneys	70–80	14–20	4–8	0.2–0.3	0
Skeleton (bones)	25–35	18–20	ND	35–38	0
Teeth	5***	23***	ND	35–38	0
Skin	56–65	21–28	12–15	0.05–0.1	0
Muscle	70–80	16–22	3–7	0.1–0.2	0.5–1
Pancreas	70–75	10–15	9–14	0.1–0.2	0
Adipose tissues	20–30	5–8	65–75	0.1–0.2	0
Alimentary tract	75–80	10–15	5–10	0.1–0.2	0

Minerals estimated based on the analytical data of calcium and phosphorus
**Carbohydrate determined by 100–water–protein–fat–ash*
***Assumed*
ND: not determined

From Table 1-3, it can be observed that the water content in all organs/tissues except skeleton, teeth, and adipose tissues is more than 50%, with a maximum of up to 85% in the lungs. In all the organs/tissues except adipose tissues, the protein content of each organ/tissue is more than its fat content. Mineral content of skeleton and teeth is in the range of 14%–16% and 35%–38%, while the rest is only in the range of 0.05%–0.5%. The carbohydrate stored in the liver and muscle is in the range of 0.5%–2%.

The carbohydrate is stored in the body typically as glycogen in liver and muscle, and can vary between individuals ranging from approximately 500 grams in normal individuals to over 1 kg in trained athletes and obese individuals. Values also vary depending on body size and previous carbohydrate ingestion.

Water has various functions in the human body. Water is an essential component of all body organs/tissues. As a solvent, it makes many nutrients available for cell function and is the medium needed for millions of chemical and biological reactions. Water is essential for the physiological processes of digestion, absorption, and excretion. It plays a key role in the structure and function of the circulatory system and acts as a transport medium for nutrients and all body substances. Water maintains the physical and chemical constancy of intracellular and extracellular fluids and has a direct role in maintaining body temperature. Evaporation of perspiration cools the body during warm weather; 600 kcal of body heat dissipates during the evaporation of 1 liter of perspired water.

In moderate weather, adults can live up to 10 days without water, and children can live up to 5 days. In contrast, it is quite possible to survive for several weeks without food.

From the chemical compositions in various organs/tissues in the human body, it is observed that all organs/tissues are composed of water, fat, proteins, and minerals. Due to metabolism, our bodies lose all of these compositions in different amounts every day. Thus, we must supplement these compositions daily to meet the needs of our metabolisms. Chapters Two, Three, and Four will discuss human nutrition in detail.

Chapter Two
Human Nutrition—Macronutrients

Based on its amounts required daily by the human body, human nutrition can be divided into macronutrients and micronutrients. Macronutrients include oxygen, water, protein, fat, carbohydrate, and fiber, each being required daily in amounts of grams. Micronutrients are all the vitamins and minerals required daily in amounts of milligrams or micromilligrams.

Macronutrients and micronutrients are essential to life. Without oxygen, life cannot sustain for more than five minutes. Without water, life cannot live for more than ten days. Without food life cannot maintain for more than thirty days. Without important vitamins and minerals, life cannot live for more than two years.

1. Oxygen

Due to its importance to life, oxygen should be considered the most important nutrient because life can sustain for only a few minutes without it.

From the time a baby enters the world, his/her first need is oxygen. When a baby breathes his/her first breath, oxygen fills the lungs. Of course, oxygen continues to be the most important need throughout our entire lives.

A normal human would utilize about 3.5 ml oxygen/kg/min. By calculation, a 70 kg human breathes 352.8 liters (504 g) of oxygen each day (24 hours) from air that is equivalent to 1680 liters of air based on the 21% of oxygen in the air.

Oxygen is by far the most important necessity of human life. It performs hundreds of tasks in the body, but **its first and most important function is energy production**. The production of energy in the body is accomplished by the reaction of carbohydrates, fats, and proteins in our diets with oxygen, producing adenosine triphosphate (ATP). Low oxygen levels mean low energy levels, which means low vitality. Energy is life, and the production of energy in the body depends on oxygen.

The second most important function of oxygen is detoxification. It is to combine with metabolic waste products to allow their elimination from the body. This process is called the oxidation reduction cycle. When insufficient oxygen is available, the detoxification process slows down, wastes pile up, circulation becomes sluggish, and oxygen is prevented from reaching the cells and the result is disease. Dr. Otto Warburg, who was awarded the Nobel Prize for research on the cause of cancer, was convinced that cancer cells can only begin to proliferate in the human body when cells become oxygen deficient. More important, his research showed that cancer cells cannot proliferate at all when exposed to an oxygen-rich environment. Renowned molecular biologist and geneticist Dr. Stephen Levin concluded that the lack of oxygen in human cells and tissues is the underlying root cause of not just cancer, but, quite possibly, of all chronic degenerative diseases. Continued research appears to conclusively back-up Warburg's and Levin's conclusions.

All functions of our bodies are regulated by oxygen. Our brain processes billions of bits of information each second, largely because of oxygen. Other important benefits of oxygen are: oxygen appears to dramatically aid nervous system response, promote brain function, relieve mental fatigue, and restore mental clarity to optimal levels. This is due to the electrical conductivity of oxygen. All of our organs need a great deal of oxygen to function efficiently. The ability to think, feel, move, eat, talk, and even sleep all depends on energy generated from oxygen. Oxygen energizes cells so they can regenerate. Oxygen must be replaced every moment because 90% of our lives depend on it.

Oxygen is the only element capable of combining with almost every other element to form the essential components necessary to build and maintain our bodies. For example: oxygen + nitrogen + hydrogen = protein; oxygen + carbon + hydrogen = carbohydrates; oxygen + hydrogen = water.

Oxygen is absorbed by hemoglobin in the blood and is transferred to every cell in the body. Cellular homeostasis is dependent on an adequate supply of oxygen in the blood. A lack of oxygen results in sickness, poor vitality, poor stamina, fatigue, and a general weak disposition. Authorities stress that most diseases, especially yeast or fungal infections like candida albicans occur most frequently in an oxygen poor environment in the body. Dr. Stephen Levin, a molecular biologist and geneticist has also stated, "We can look at oxygen deficiency as the single greatest cause of disease." Thus, the development of a shortage of oxygen in the blood could very well be the starting point for the loss of the immune system and the beginning of feared health problems such as cancer, leukemia, seizures, nerve deterioration, and candida. Low oxygen levels are undesirable because they affect the body's cell metabolism and may even cause it to manufacture improper chemicals and/ or give rise to various health problems. Oxygen provides life and energy to every living cell. If the cells are deprived of vital oxygen, the immune system may weaken. Many experts conclude that a lack of oxygen in human cells and tissues is linked to a vast variety of quite possibly all health problems and diseases. It plays a very important role in the body, acting as a guardian and a protector against unfriendly bacteria and disease organisms. **Most scientists and doctors reiterate that metabolic disorders are the result of blood deficiency in oxygen.**

The air we breathe is generally composed of 78% nitrogen and 21% oxygen by volume. The other gases together, called trace gases, comprise the remaining 1%. These are argon, carbon dioxide, neon, helium, methane, krypton, hydrogen, and xenon. Therefore, the length of human life depends on the quality of air that is breathed in. The quality of the air can determine the level of health that is attained throughout life.

2. Water

Water should be considered the second most important nutrient because life can sustain for only a few days without it. Water is one of the most essential nutrients to our survival.

Depending on our activity and environmental temperature, the average adult in the United States loses one half (1/2) gallon of water/fluids per day through perspiration, respiration, urination, and defecation. If we don't replace this amount of water on a daily basis, we slowly dehydrate. Rapid dehydration causes heart and kidney failure and even death. Gradual dehydration leads to a litany of signs, signals, and symptoms often mistaken as disease. The most obvious sign of dehydration is dry, flaky, and wrinkled skin. An estimated seventy-five percent of Americans have mild, chronic dehydration. Signs and consequences of dehydration are summarized in Tabe 2-1.

**Table 2-1 Signs and consequences of the percentage
of body weight lost due to dehydration**

Body weight lost	Sign and consequence
1%	Thirst
2%	Strong thirst, vague discomfort, loss of appetite
3%	Decreased blood volume, impaired physical performance
4%	Increased effort for physical work, nausea
5%	Difficulty in concentrating
6%	Failure to regulate excess temperature
8%	Dizziness, labored breathing during exercise, increased weakness

10%	Muscle spasms, delirium, and wakefulness
11%	Inability of deceased blood volume to circulate normally; Failure to renal and heart function
20%	Can cause death

Water is important to the mechanics of the human body. Our bodies cannot work without it, just as a car cannot run without gas and oil. In fact, all the cells and organs made up in our entire anatomy and physiology depend on water for their functioning.

Water is an important structural component of all body organs/tissues. The brain in an average man is composed of 70%–76% of water, the lungs: 75%–85%, the liver: 70%–73%, the heart: 60%–75%, the spleen: 76%–80%, the kidneys: 70%–80%, the skeleton (bones): 25%–35%, the teeth: 5%, the skin: 56%–65%, the muscle: 70%–80%, the pancreas: 70%–75%, the adipose tissues (fat): 20%–30%, and the alimentary tract: 75%–80%. Except for the teeth, the fat, and the bones, the water contents of all other organs/tissues are more than 50%, with a maximum of up to 85% in the lungs.

Water is a perfect conductor of electricity and this becomes important for the day to day operation of our bodies. For example, the electrical potential is shared between the brain neurons through electrochemical transmitters. This electrical potential of brain chemistry must be present for any of our "thoughts" to take place.

Water is a universal solvent. Digestion, absorption, and excretion of food we eat cannot happen without water. The digestion of food is the combination of the mechanical and chemical process by which food is absorbed into our bodies. Chunks of meat, potatoes, and vegetables don't just float around in our bodies after we eat a meal. Food cannot be used until they are digested and converted into simple substances, such as fatty acids, amino acids, and glucose that can pass through the cells of the small intestine and then into the blood or lymph. Enzymes, coenzymes, hormones, vitamins, and minerals from the foods or supplements are all dissolved into watery body fluids. Water also serves as a solvent for waste products such as urea, carbon dioxide, and various electrolytes that the body excretes. As a solvent containing these substances, water is necessary for transporting them to and from over 70 trillion cells in our bodies.

Water is a medium needed for millions of chemical and biological reactions in our bodies.

Water serves as a lubricant in digestion and almost all other body processes. The water in saliva facilitates chewing and swallowing, ensuring that food will slide easily down the esophagus. Water in other digestive fluids sustains movement throughout the gastrointestinal system. The watery fluid surrounding body parts, such as joints and eyeballs, helps them move smoothly and is in fact, their only lubricant.

Water maintains the physical and chemical constancy of intracellular and extracellular fluids. Approximately 60% of the total water content in the human body is contained inside the cells and makes up the intracellular compartment. The balance of the extracellular compartment has two major divisions. The intravascular fluid represents 20% of the extracellular fluid in the body, is the liquid component of the blood, and is present in our heart, arteries, veins, and capillaries. The interstitial and transcellular fluid accounts for 80% of the extracellular fluid in the body. These fluids include the fluids that bathe all the cells, spinal fluids, ocular fluid for lubricating the eyes, the synovial fluid that lubricates joints, various secretions (such as saliva, bile, gastric juice, mucus), and lymph.

Water regulates the body temperature, as cooling and heating is distributed through perspiration. Evaporation of perspiration cools the body during warm weather; 600 kcal of body heat dissipates during the evaporation of 1 liter of perspired water.

Water helps alleviate constipation by moving food through the intestinal tract, thereby eliminating waste – the best detoxified agent.

In addition to the daily maintenance of our bodies, **water also plays a key role in the prevention of disease**. Drinking enough water daily can decrease the risk of colon cancer by 45%, bladder cancer by 50% and it can potentially even reduce the risk of breast cancer. And those are just a few examples!

3. Protein

Both animal and plant proteins are made up of 20 common amino acids, in which amino nitrogen accounts for approximately 16% of the weight of the proteins. Amino acids are required for the synthesis of body protein and other important nitrogen-containing compounds, such as creatine, peptide hormones, and some neurotransmitters. Some amino acids are lost in the human body by oxidative catabolism. Metabolic products (urea, creatinine, uric acid, and other nitrogenous products) are excreted in the urine. Nitrogen is also lost in feces, sweat, and other body secretions and in sloughed skin, hair, and nails. So, a continuous supply of dietary amino acids is required to replace these losses, even after growth has ceased.

The proteins we eat must first be digested in our stomach into the form of various amino acids that are then absorbed by the small intestine into the blood. Amino acids consumed in excess of the amounts needed for the synthesis of nitrogenous tissue constituents are not stored but are degraded.

Eleven of the 20 common amino acids in both animal and plant proteins can be synthesized by mammals, but nine of them: histidine, isoleucine, leucine, lysine, methionine, phenylalanine, threonine, tryptophan, and valine, cannot be synthesized by our human bodies. Therefore, these are dietary essential or indispensable nutrients and commonly called the essential amino acids. Histidine is an essential amino acid for infants, but was not demonstrated to be required by adults until recently.

Products of dietary protein digestion and protein secreted into the gut lumen are available for absorption and transportation into the portal vein leading to the liver. Homeostatic regulations control the concentrations of specific acids in the amino acid pool and the rate at which muscle and plasma proteins are synthesized and broken down. Body protein synthesis and breakdown, or turn over, is regulated. In healthy individuals, the amount of protein taken in is balanced by protein used for body maintenance, and excreted in feces, urine, and from skin.

Protein is an important structural component of all body organs/ tissues. The brain of an average man is composed of 10%–14% of protein, the lungs: 13%–20%, the liver: 16%–23%, the heart: 15%–18%, the spleen: 17%–19%, the kidneys: 14%–20%, the skeleton (bones): 18%–20%, the teeth: 23%, the skin: 21%–28%, the muscle: 16%–22%, the pancreas: 10%–15%, the adipose tissues (fat): 5%–8%, and the alimentary tract: 10%–15%.

Dietary protein is essential for growing children. Children should ingest more protein in order to maintain a positive nitrogen balance.

Dietary protein is essential for the body maintenance of adults. In a series of 11 studies involving more than 200 adults ranging in the ages of 20 to 77 years old, daily obligatory nitrogen losses averaged 53 mg (in the range of 41–69 mg) per kilogram daily. Every day, your body loses protein constantly. Your muscles, your immune system, and every enzyme, et al. in your body are composed of protein, as stated above. Your body requires incoming protein on continual basis to repair and maintain its critical systems. Without adequate incoming dietary protein, these critical body functions begin to run down.

Another important function of dietary protein is to stimulate the hormone glucagon. Glucagon has the opposite physiological action to insulin. Glucagon's primary job is to release stored carbohydrates in the form of glucose from the liver. Once released by glucagon, the glucose enters the bloodstream, and helps maintain the tight balance of blood sugar required for the brain to function adequately. In fact, glucagon acts as the major governor of excessive insulin production. It is excess insulin that makes you fat, hungry, mentally foggy, decreases your physical performance, and increases the likelihood of chronic diseases.

Deficiency of protein is very rare in the United States, and is most commonly seen in deprived children in poor countries. Where protein intake is exceptionally low, there are physical signs: stunting, poor musculature, edema, thin and fragile hair, skin lesions, and biochemical changes that include low serum albumin and hormonal imbalances. Edema and the loss of muscle mass and hair are the prominent signs in adults.

4. Fat

Dietary fat is triglycerides (also called triacylglvcerols) that are composed of three fatty acids esterified to glycerol. Glycerol ($C_3H_8O_3$), having three hydroxyl groups (a trihydric alcohol), is the invariable component of all glycerides (esters). Such esters may contain one fatty acid (monoglycerides), two fatty acids (diglycerides) or three fatty acids (triglycerides). More than 95% of lipids in the food supply are in the triglyceride storage form.

Food fats are hydrolyzed after ingestion in the stomach into free fatty acids, which are then absorbed. The efficiency of fatty acid absorption in healthy adults is high, ranging from 95% to 99%, whereas that of cholesterol ranges from 30% to 70%.

Fatty acids are classified according to the extent of saturation as saturated fatty acids (SFAs), monounsaturated fatty acids (MFAs), and polyunsaturated fatty acids (PUFAs). In SFAs, all binding sites not linked to carbon are saturated with hydrogen. MFAs contain only one double bond and PUFAs contain two or more double bonds. Fatty acids are also characterized by the location of their double bonds. With usually convention, lowercase Greek letters are used to refer to the placement of the carbons within the fatty acid. Alpha (α) refers to the first carbon adjacent to carboxyl group, beta (β) to the second carbon, and omega (ω) to the last carbon which is referred to as the fatty acid's omega number. Double bonds labeled with ω are counted from the terminal methyl carbon. For example, the arachidonic acid (20: 4 ω-6) is an omega-6 fatty acid that has four double bonds and the first of which is six carbons from the terminal methyl group. Eicosapentaenoic acid (EPA) (20: 5 ω-3) is an omega-3 fatty acid that has five double bonds, the first of which is three carbons from the terminal methyl group. Docosahexaenoic acid (DHA) (22: 6 ω-3) is an omega-3 fatty acid that has six double bonds, the first of which is three carbons from the terminal methyl group.

Essential fatty acids (EFAs) are fatty acids that can be defined as those which either cannot be synthesized at all or cannot be synthesized in sufficient quantities by humans, who require them for growth, maintenance, and the proper function of a variety of physiological processes. Therefore, these EFAs must be obtained from the diet. There are a total of eight essential fatty acids, which fall into two classes: omega-3 and omega-6 fatty acids. Omega-3 mainly includes α-linolenic acid or ALA (18: 3 ω-3), EPA (20: 5 ω-3) and DHA (22: 6 ω-3), while omega-6 includes gamma-linolenic acid or GLA (18:3 ω-6), dihomo-gamma-linolenic acid or DGLA (20:3 ω-6), and arachidonic acid or AA (20:4 ω-6).

Fat is an important structural component of most body organs/tissues. The brain of an average man is composed of 10%–14% of fat, the lungs: 1%–2%, the liver: 3%–10%, the heart: 9%–18%, the spleen: 1%–2%, the kidneys: 4%–8%, the skeleton (bones): 16%–26%, the teeth: not available, the skin: 12%–15%, the muscle: 3%–7%, the pancreas: 9%–14%, the adipose tissues (fat): 65%–75%, and the alimentary tract: 5%–10%. The structural fat pads hold the body organs and nerves in position and protect them against traumatic injury and shock. Fat pads on the palms and buttocks protect the bones from mechanical pressure. Humans also have a subcutaneous layer of fat that insulates the body, preserving body heat and maintaining body temperature. In addition, humans use a large amount of fat in the adipose tissues in order to survive without food for weeks and sometimes, for even months.

Fat provides the most concentrated energy in an average mixed diet 9 kilocalories per gram, being more than twice the number per gram supplied by protein and carbohydrate, both of which only provide 4 kilocalories per gram.

Fat is renown for its ability to increase the palatability of food. In part, this may be due to its lubricating effect. In large measure, however, the increased palatability stems from the taste impaired to the food by fats. Fat increases the satiety of a diet by decreasing the sense of hunger between meals, since its peak absorption is delayed until about 3.5 hours after its ingestion.

Fat in a meal causes the release of a hormone called cholecystokinin (CCK) from the stomach. This hormone tells the brain that you are satisfied, and to stop eating.

Dietary fat is also essential for the digestion, absorption, and transport of the fat-soluble vitamins such as vitamins A, D, E, and K, and fat-soluble phytochemicals such as carotenoids and lycopenes. Dietary fat depresses gastric secretions, slows gastric emptying, and stimulates biliary and pancreatic flow, thereby facilitating the digestive process. Eating fat together with carbohydrate will slow the entry rate of glucose into the bloodstream.

Dietary fat provides essential fatty acids that control the production of eicosanoids – the body's superhormones which controls all of the body's hormonal systems. In the human body, there are hundreds of hormones that play various roles, for examples insulin and glucagon control blood sugar, while eicosanoids manage all of these hormones. Omega-3 and omega-6 fatty acids from dietary fat can be made into eicosanoids, with omega-6 being the most important for them.

Trans fat is the common name for a type of unsaturated fat with *trans*-isomer fatty acid(s). Trans fats may be monounsaturated or polyunsaturated but never saturated. *Cis* and *trans* are terms that refer to the arrangement of the chains of carbon atoms across the double bond. In the *cis* arrangement, the two carbons participate in a double bond with two hydrogens on the same side of the bond. In the *trans* arrangement, the two carbons participate in a double bond with one hydrogen on opposite sides of the bond.

The process of hydrogenation is intended to add hydrogen atoms to *cis*-unsaturated fats, eliminating a double bond and making them more saturated. These saturated fats have a higher melting point, which makes them attractive for baking and extends their shelf-life. However, the process frequently has a side effect that turns some *cis*-isomers into *trans*-unsaturated fats instead of hydrogenating them completely.

There is another class of trans fats, vaccenic acid, which occurs naturally in trace amounts in meat and dairy products from ruminants.

Unlike other dietary fats, **trans fats are not essential**, and they do not promote good health. The consumption of trans fats increases one's risk of coronary heart disease by raising levels of "bad" low-density lipoprotein (LDL) cholesterol and lowering levels of "good" high-density lipoprotein (HDL) cholesterol. Health authorities worldwide recommend that consumption of trans fats be reduced to trace amounts. Trans fats from partially hydrogenated oils are more harmful than naturally occurring oils.

Major sources of trans fats in our diets are partially hydrogenated margarine, shortening, commercial frying fats, high-fat baked goods, and salty snacks containing these fats. Butter and animal fat can also contain trans fats from bacterial fermentation.

Cholesterol is a peculiar molecule. It is often called a lipid or a fat. Because cholesterol is insoluble in water and thus also in blood, it is transported in our blood inside spheric particles composed of fats (lipids) and proteins, the so-called lipoproteins. Lipoproteins are easily dissolved in water because their outside is composed mainly of water-soluble proteins. The inside of the lipoproteins is composed of lipids, and there is room for water-insoluble molecules such as cholesterol. Like submarines, lipoproteins carry cholesterol from one place in the body to another. The highest concentration of cholesterol in the body is found in the brain and other parts of the nervous system.

Cholesterol has many biological functions in our bodies:

- Cholesterol contributes to cell membrane rigidity and strength, just like saturated fats do.

- Cholesterol acts as an antioxidant, actually protecting us against cellular damage that leads to heart disease and cancer.

- Cholesterol helps maintain a healthy intestinal lining, which offers protection against autoimmune illnesses.

- Cholesterol is used to make bile that is needed for digesting fat in our foods.

- Cholesterol is converted to vitamin D.

- Cholesterol is used to make hormones that help us deal with stress.

Our bodies produce three to four times more cholesterol than we can eat. The production of cholesterol increases when you eat little cholesterol and decreases when you eat more. The association between high serum cholesterol concentration and risk for heart disease has led to dietary restrictions of cholesterol-rich foods such as eggs, each of which has 250 mg of cholesterol. However, serum cholesterol levels are homeostatically controlled, and individual responses to dietary cholesterol are highly variable. Recent research found that there is no direct relationship between serum cholesterol level and dietary cholesterol intake. Therefore, the most recent recommendation for cholesterol dietary reference intake from the Institute of Medicine, National Academies is that cholesterol intake should be as low as possible while consuming a nutritionally adequate diet, rather than not more than 300 mg per day that have been set up by them previously.

EPA (Eicosapentaenoic Acid) and DHA (Docosahexaenoic Acid). EPA and DHA are two of the most important essential fatty acids. DHA and EPA are present in fatty fish and in a mother's milk, and are present at low levels in meat and eggs. More than 8,000 studies published over the past 35 years have consistently shown that Omega-3 EPA and DHA are important to your health throughout every stage of your life. Omega-3 EPA and DHA have complementary roles in human health: DHA plays a structural role as a component of cell membranes, while EPA plays a physiological role by helping reduce inflammation. Together, Omega-3 EPA and DHA have a wide variety of health benefits, which can be grouped into four general categories: heart health, brain health, normal growth and development, and overall health and well-being. Some of their health benefits are summarized as follows:

- Reduces the risk of heart attacks and strokes

- Reduces blood thickness (viscosity)

- Lowers blood pressure

- Reduces triglycerides (blood fat levels)

- Protects against the hardening of the arteries (atherosclerosis)

- Protects against plaque rupture

- Reduces the risk of developing memory problems, including Alzheimer's disease and other types of dementia

- Improves cognition and IQ in babies and children

- Improves learning, reading, and writing ability

- Helps reduce the risk of inflammatory conditions, including asthma, colorectal and prostate cancer, and diabetes

5. Carbohydrate

Carbohydrate is the main energy source for the human body. Chemically, carbohydrates are organic molecules in which carbon, hydrogen, and oxygen bond together in the ratio: $C_x(H_2O)_y$, where x and y are whole numbers that differ depending on the specific carbohydrate to which we are referring. Animals (including humans) break down carbohydrates during the process of metabolism to release energy. For example, the chemical metabolism of the sugar glucose is shown below:

$$C_6H_{12}O_6 + 6O_2 \rightarrow 6CO_2 + 6H_2O + energy$$

Animals obtain carbohydrates by eating foods that contain them, for example potatoes, rice, breads, and so on. These carbohydrates are manufactured by plants during the process of photosynthesis. Plants harvest energy from sunlight to run the reaction just described in reverse:

$$6CO_2 + 6H_2O + energy \text{ (from sunlight)} \rightarrow C_6H_{12}O_6 + 6O_2$$

A potato, for example, is primarily a chemical storage system containing glucose molecules manufactured during photosynthesis. In a potato, however, those glucose molecules are bound together in a long chain. As it turns out, there are two types of carbohydrates, the simple sugars and those carbohydrates that are made of long chains of sugars—the complex carbohydrates.

From the above description, carbohydrate can be classified into simple carbohydrate and complex carbohydrate. Simple carbohydrate includes monosaccharides, such as glucose and fructose, and disaccharides, such as sucrose (table sugar), maltose, and lactose (milk sugar). Complex carbohydrate (polysaccharides) comprises starches and dietary fibers. Starches are polymers of glucose. Fibers include: cellulose, hemicellulose and pectin that are in plant cell walls, a variety of gums, mucilages, and algal polysaccharides.

Starch is the principal polysaccharide used by plants to store glucose for later use as energy. Plants often store starch in seeds or other specialized organs. For example, common sources of starch include rice, beans, wheat, corn, potatoes, and so on. When humans eat starch, an enzyme, called amylase, which occurs in saliva and in the intestines, breaks the bonds between the repeating glucose units, thus allowing the sugar to be absorbed into the bloodstream. Once absorbed into the bloodstream, the human body distributes glucose to the areas where it is needed for energy or stores it as its own special polymer—glycogen. Glycogen, another polymer of glucose, is the polysaccharide used by animals to store energy. Excess glucose is bonded together to form glycogen molecules, which the animal stores in the liver and muscle tissue as an "instant" source of energy. Both starch and glycogen are polymers of glucose; however, starch is a long, straight chain of glucose units whereas glycogen is a branched chain of glucose units.

Another important polysaccharide is cellulose. Cellulose is yet a third polymer of the monosaccharide glucose. Cellulose differs from starch and glycogen because the glucose units form a two-dimensional structure, with hydrogen bonds holding together nearby polymers, thus giving the molecule added stability. Cellulose, also known as plant fiber, cannot be digested by humans, therefore it passes through the digestive tract without being absorbed into the body. Some animals, such as cows and termites, contain bacteria in their digestive tract that helps them digest cellulose. Cellulose is a relatively stiff material, and in plants cellulose is used as a structural molecule to add support to the leaves, stem, and other plant parts. Despite the fact that it cannot be used as an energy source in most animals, cellulose fiber is essential in the diet because it helps exercise the digestive track and keep it clean and healthy.

The principle function of carbohydrates in human nutrition is the maintenance of the blood glucose concentration within the range of 70 to 110 mg/dl. Ingested carbohydrate is hydrolyzed to glucose and then absorbed into the bloodstream. The blood glucose, in an acceptable range, is the fuel of choice for most organs but is absolutely essential for the proper function of the brain. When excess carbohydrate enters the body by the ingestion of sugars or starches, insulin—a storage hormone is to take excess glucose and store it as glycogen (glycogensis) in the liver, muscle, brain, and other tissues or as fat. When the blood glucose concentration is lower than 70 mg/dl, glucagon—a mobilization hormone (glucagon) is to release glycogen stored in the liver. So, insulin and glucagon control the blood glucose level.

Carbohydrates are the major source of energy for the human body. The human body needs energy to power muscles and to fuel the millions of chemical and biological reactions that take place throughout our system every day. Carbohydrates are not essential nutrients in humans: the body can obtain all its energy from protein and fats. However, the brain and neurons generally cannot burn fat by themselves and need glucose for energy; the body can make some glucose from a few of the amino acids in protein and also from the glycerol backbone in triglycerides (fat). Carbohydrates and proteins contain 4 kilocalories per gram, respectively, while fats contain 9 kilocalories per gram. In the case of protein, this is somewhat misleading as only some amino acids are usable for fuel. Likewise, in humans, only some carbohydrates are usable for fuel, such as many monosaccharides and some disaccharides. Other carbohydrate types can be used, but only with the assistance of gut bacteria. Some animals, such as ruminants and termites, can even process cellulose, while most animals cannot. Once our immediate energy needs are satisfied, the remaining glucose is handled in one of two ways. Either it is converted to liquid glycogen (a temporary source of readily available energy) and stored in the liver or muscles, or it is converted into fatty acids by the liver and stored in adipose cells (fat-cells) around the body. So, excessive consumption of carbohydrates can lead to obesity.

Carbohydrate is the principal vehicle of sweetness in human food. An acquired taste for sweets developed during childhood is usually carried over into the mature and older years of life. Carbohydrates and particularly sucrose rank with fats and salt as major components imparting desired flavors to many food products.

Carbohydrate is the components of major dietary fibers. Technically, fiber is a complex carbohydrate. Dietary fibers include insoluble fibers and soluble fibers. Both fibers have different functions and health benefits, which will be discussed in the following section on fiber.

6. Fiber

Based on their solubility, dietary fibers are divided into **insoluble fiber** and **soluble fiber**. Both types of fiber are present in all plant foods, with varying degrees of each according to a plant's characteristics. For example, plums (or prunes) have a thick skin covering a juicy pulp. The plum's skin is an example of an insoluble fiber source, whereas soluble fiber sources are inside the pulp. Other sources of insoluble fiber include whole wheat, wheat, corn bran, flax seed lignans, and vegetables such as celery, nopal, green beans, and potatoes.

Insoluble fiber is a type of fiber found in certain complex carbohydrate foods and some common supplements used as bulking agents. Insoluble fiber is not digested in the intestinal tract or absorbed into the bloodstream. Sources of **insoluble fiber** include: whole grain foods, bran, nuts and seeds, and vegetables such as green beans, cauliflower, zucchini (courgette), and celery.

Insoluble fiber possesses water-attracting properties. In water one gram of insoluble fiber swells to about twenty times its original size. The unique properties of insoluble fiber can create a feeling of fullness in the stomach, which can help obese people lose weight and healthy people maintain their weight. In addition, it helps to increase bulk, soften stool, and shorten transit time through the intestinal tract, therefore eliminating constipation problems. Furthermore, this also plays an important role in the prevention of colon cancer—the second leading cause of cancer deaths in North America.

Soluble fiber is found in varying quantities in all plant foods, including: legumes (peas, soybeans, and other beans), oats, rye, chia, barley, some fruits and juices (particularly prune juice, plums and berries), certain vegetables such as broccoli, carrots and Jerusalem artichokes, root vegetables such as potatoes, sweet potatoes, and onions (skins of these vegetables are sources of insoluble fiber), and psyllium seed husk (a mucilage soluble fiber).

Soluble fiber undergoes metabolic processing via fermentation, yielding short chain fatty acids (SCFA) with broad, significant health effects. SCFA are used by the intestinal mucosa or absorbed through the colonic wall into the portal circulation (supplying the liver) that transports them into the general circulatory system. The major SCFA in humans are butyrate, propionate, and acetate. Butyrate is the major energy source for colonocytes. Propionate is destined for uptake by the liver. And acetate enters the peripheral circulation to be metabolized by peripheral tissues. Collectively, SCFA have extensive physiological actions promoting health effects, among which major functions are:

- stabilizes blood glucose levels by acting on pancreatic insulin release and liver control of glycogen breakdown

- stimulates gene expression of glucose transporters in the intestinal mucosa, regulating glucose absorption

- provides nourishment of colonocytes, particularly by butyrate

- suppresses cholesterol synthesis by the liver and reduce blood levels of low-density lipoprotein (LDL) cholesterol and triglycerides is responsible for atherosclerosis

- lowers colonic pH (i.e., raises the acidity level in the colon) which protects the lining from formation of colonic polyps and increases absorption of dietary minerals

- stimulates production of T helper cells, antibodies, leukocytes, cytokines, and lymph mechanisms, having crucial roles in immune protection

- improves barrier properties of the colonic mucosal layer, inhibiting inflammatory and adhesion irritants, contributing to immune functions

Summarizing these effects: upon fermentation, prebiotic fibers yield SCFA that affect major regulatory systems, such as blood glucose and lipid levels, the colonic environment and intestinal immune functions.

Chapter Three
Human Nutrition—Micronutrients: Vitamins

Based on their solubility, vitamins are usually classified into two groups: fat-soluble vitamins and water-soluble vitamins. Fat-soluble vitamins include vitamin A, vitamin D, vitamin E, and vitamin K, and water-soluble vitamins are vitamin B_1 (thiamine), vitamin B_2 (riboflavin), vitamin B_3 (niacin), vitamin B_5 (pantothenic acid), vitamin B_6 (pyridoxine), vitamin B_7 (biotin), vitamin B_9 (folic acid or folate), vitamin B_{12} (cobalamin), vitamin C (ascorbic acid or calcium ascorbate), and choline.

Vitamins are a group of organic compounds distinct from protein, fat, and carbohydrate, which neither provide energy nor serve as structural components of tissue, but are essential for life in minute amount for normal physiological function, such as maintenance, growth, development and reproduction. Vitamins are not synthesized by the body in amounts adequate to meet normal physiological needs that can be supplemented from natural components of food or supplements containing various vitamins. Deficiency of vitamins or their insufficient use can cause a specific deficiency syndrome.

Fat-soluble vitamins are usually absorbed passively and must be transported with dietary fat. They tend to be found in the lipid portions of the cell such as membranes and lipid droplets. Water-soluble vitamins are absorbed by passive and active mechanisms, transported by carriers, and not stored in appreciable amounts in the body. Fat-soluble vitamins are generally excreted with feces via enterohepatic circulation, whereas water-soluble vitamins or their metabolites are excreted in the urine.

Fat-Soluble Vitamins

1. Vitamin A

Vitamin A, as its name implies, was the first name of all vitamins, which was identified in 1913. Vitamin A includes three preformed compounds: retinol, retinal, and retinoic acid, and one provitamin: β-carotene. The three preformed vitamin A exist only in animal products in the form of complexes with proteins in foods, whereas β-carotene exists in plants that contain a group of compounds known collectively as carotenoids that can yield retinoids when metabolized in the body. Although several hundred carotenoids exist in foods naturally, only a few have significant vitamin A activity. The most important of these are β-carotene, lutein, and zeaxanthin. Lutein and zeaxanthin help protect against photodamage of the retina by filtering out blue light, help protect against peroxidation of fatty acids in the photoreceptor membrane, and help protect the blood vessels that supply the macular region.

Absorption of retinol and carotenoids, especially β-carotene, differs in several ways. For example, in physiological amounts, retinol is more efficient than most carotenoids, e.g. 70%–90% compared to 20%–50%. However, carotenoids present in oils are well absorbed. As the amount ingested increases, the efficiency of retinol absorption usually remains high (60%–80%), whereas carotenoids absorption falls markedly to levels as low as 10% or less.

Functions

Vitamin A has various functions in vision, normal cell differentiation, cell recognition, growth and development, immunity, and reproduction, et al.

- Retinal is a structural component of the visual pigments of the rod and cone cells of the retina in our eyes. As such, it is essential to photoreception.

- Vitamin A (specifically retinoic acid) acts as hormones to affect gene expression.

- Vitamin A involves glycoprotein synthesis. Glycoprotein is important for normal cell surface functions, such as cell aggregation and cell recognition. Also, it plays an important role in cell growth.

- Vitamin A is essential for normal reproduction (retinol).

- Vitamin A is essential for bone development and function.

- Vitamin A is essential for immune system function.

- β-carotene acts as an antioxidant.

- β-carotene regulates cell growth.

- β-carotene induces some enzymes.

- β-carotene promotes gap junction communications.

- β-carotene is used as retinoid-dependent signaling.

Health Benefits

Many health benefits of vitamin A have been found from clinical studies and doctors' practices.

- Prevents both infectious and noninfectious diseases of the respiratory system.

- Protects against lung cancer due to air pollution.

- Reduces the incidence of gastrointestinal cancer.

- Lowers the incidence of breast cancer in women and prostate cancer in men.

- Maintains eye and skin health.

Deficiency Symptoms

Deficiencies of vitamin A result from inadequate intakes of preformed vitamin A or provitamin A, carotenoids. In addition, they may result from malabsorption caused by insufficient dietary fat. Deficiencies of vitamin A can cause the following symptoms.

- Night blindness. Low-level night blindness is becoming more common in the United States and may eventually become recognized as a subclinical deficiency.

- Other eye problems.

- Skin disorders

- Suboptimal growth

- Reproductive failure

2. Vitamin D

Vitamin D is known as the sunshine vitamin because modest exposure to sunlight is usually sufficient for most people to produce their own vitamin D using the ultraviolet light and cholesterol in the skin. Vitamin D (calciferol) includes vitamin D_3 (cholecalciferol) and vitamin D_2 (ergocalciferol). Ergocalciferol is the product of ultraviolet light-induced conversion of ergosterol in plants, whereas cholecalciferol is synthesized from 7-dehydrocholestrol under the catalysis of ultraviolet light. Vitamins D_2 and D_3 require further metabolism to yield the metabolically active forms of 1, 25-dihydroxyvitamin

D_2 and D_3 (calcitriol). Calcitriol increases calcium and phosphate absorption in the intestine, increases calcium and phosphate absorption in bone, and acts on the kidney to decrease calcium loss in urine. The efficiency of dietary vitamin D absorption is about 50%.

Functions

Vitamin D has various functions in the metabolism of calcium and phosphorus in the body and mineral homeostasis, etc.

- Calcitriol (1, 25-dihydroxyvitamin D_3) acts like a steroid hormone, involving interaction with cell membrane receptors and nuclear vitamin D receptor (VDR) proteins to affect gene transcription in a wide variety of tissues.

- Vitamin D increases the absorption of calcium and phosphorus in the intestine.

- Vitamin D increases the uptake of minerals by the bones.

- Vitamin D maintains a homeostasis of calcium and phosphorus.

- Calcitriol stimulates differentiation of intestinal epithelial cells and osteoblasts.

- Calcitriol seems to inhibit cell proliferation and growth.

Health Benefits

Vitamin D has the following health benefits.

- Vitamin D, combined with calcium, has been found to possess anti-cancer properties.

- Active vitamin D plays a role in the treatment of some immunological disorder.

- Improves psoriasis.

- Affects biological rhythms, mood, and behavior.

- Improves muscle strength.

Deficiency Symptoms

Vitamin D deficiencies are associated with the following symptoms.

- Rickets in children. The symptoms are stunted growth, delayed tooth development, weakness, softened skulls (in infants), and irreversible bone deformities.

- Osteomalacia in adults. The disease involves generalized reductions in bone density and the presence of pseudofractures, especially in the spine, femur, and humerus.

- Osteoporosis in postmenopausal women and the elderly. It is a very different bone disease from osteomalacia, involving the reduction in total bone mass but the retention of a normal historic appearance.

- Women's difficulties in giving birth because of irregularities in the pelvic bones.

3. Vitamin E

Since its discovery in 1922, vitamin E has been widely investigated on its biological activity, function, and health benefits. Vitamin E has two groups: tocopherols and tocotrienols. There are four members of the tocopherols group: α-, β-, γ-, and δ-tocopherols. The most active form of vitamin E, α-tocopherols, is also the most widely distributed in nature.

Vitamin E is absorbed in the upper small intestine by micelle-dependent diffusion, and like the other fat-soluble vitamins, its use depends on the presence of dietary fat and adequate biliary and pancreatic function. The absorption of vitamin E is highly variable, and efficiency ranges from 20% to 80%.

Functions

Vitamin E has the important biological functions in trapping free radicals.

- Vitamin E is the most important lipid-soluble antioxidant in the cell.

- Vitamin E prevents oxidation of unsaturated fatty acids in phospholipids of the membrane by reducing free radicals into harmless metabolites by donating a hydrogen to them. This process is called free radical scavenging.

- Vitamin E is an important component of cellular antioxidant defense system, which involves other enzymes.

- Vitamin E protects the body against a variety of carcinogens and toxins, including mercury, lead, carbon tetrachloride, benzene, ozone, and nitrous oxide.

Health Benefits

Many health benefits of vitamin E combined with other related nutrients such as selenium, copper, zinc, magnesium, and vitamin C have been found from clinical studies and doctors' practices.

- Anti-aging

- Treats arthritis

- Prevents cancers

- Prevents cardiovascular diseases

- Prevents diabetes

- Prevents cataracts

- Anti-infection

- Prevents Alzheimer's disease

- Helps alleviate the symptoms associated with premenstrual syndrome (PMS)

- Is important for normal functioning of the nervous system

Deficiency Symptoms

Vitamin E deficiencies are associated with the following symptoms. These symptoms appear only when there is a severe fat malabsorption that occurs in people with disorders of the pancreas, tropical sprue, celiac, and cystic fibrosis, and in premature infants.

- Neuromuscular disease such as difficulty in walking, frequent falling, and abnormal reflexes

- Premature aging

- Anemia resulting from the death of red blood cells

- Fragile capillaries

4. Vitamin K

Vitamin K was discovered by a Danish Scientist in 1929. The new vitamin received the letter K because the initial discoveries were reported in a German journal, in which it was designated as Koagulationsvitamin. Vitamin K includes vitamin K_1 (from plants), vitamin K_2 (made by our intestinal bacteria), and vitamin K_3 (synthetic). Vitamin K_3 is a synthetic compound: menadione. Menadione is twice as potent biologically as the naturally occurring forms vitamins K_1 and K_2.

Vitamin K_1 is absorbed by an energy dependent process in the small intestine, whereas vitamins K_2 and K_3 are absorbed in the small intestine and colon by passive diffusion. Like the other fat-soluble vitamins, absorption depends on a minimum amount of dietary fat, bile salts, and pancreatic juices.

Functions

Vitamin K has some key biological functions in the body.

• Vitamin K plays an essential role in blood clotting.

• Vitamin K plays a role in bone formation.

• Vitamin K plays an essential role in the posttranslational carboxylation of glutamic acid residues in proteins to form carboxyglutamate (Gla) and in the residues binding calcium.

Health Benefits

Vitamin K nutrition has many health benefits, especially for newborn infants and elderly people.

• Prevents hemorrhagic disease of the newborn infants.

• Corrects hypoprothrombinemia induced iatrogenically by excessive doses of vitamin K antagonists among the elderly.

• Decreases incidence of advanced prostate cancer.

• Protects against bone fractures.

Deficiency Symptoms

Vitamin K deficiencies are associated with the following symptoms.

• Hemorrhage.

• Hypoprothrombinemia

• Hip fracture in older adults

- Stomach pains

- Cartilage calcification and severe malformation of developing bone, or deposition of insoluble calcium salts in the walls of arteries

Water-Soluble Vitamins

5. Vitamin B₁ (Thiamin)

Thiamin was first discovered in 1910 by Umetaro Suzuki in Japan when researching how rice bran cured patients of beriberi. Vitamin B_1 is the term for a family of molecules sharing a common structural feature responsible for its activity as a vitamin. It is one of the B vitamins. Its most common form is a colorless chemical compound with a chemical formula $C_{12}H_{17}N_4OS$. This form of thiamin is soluble in water, methanol, and glycerol and practically insoluble in acetone, ether, chloroform, and benzene.

Vitamin B_1 is activated by phosphorylation into thiamin triphosphate (TTP), or cocarboxylase, which serves as a coenzyme in energy metabolism and the synthesis of pentoses. Thiamin is absorbed from the proximal small intestine by active transport in low doses and passive diffusion in high doses (i.e., > 5 mg/day). Approximately 90% of circulating thiamin is carried as TPP by erthrocytes.

Functions

Vitamin B_1 has various biological functions in the body.

- Vitamin B_1 plays an essential role in the metabolism of carbohydrates in the body, in which it acts as a catalyst in burning carbohydrates.

- Vitamin B_1 plays an essential role in the neural function.

- Vitamin B_1 is involved with converting fatty acids into steroids in the body.

- Vitamin B_1 is necessary for proper growth and for the maintenance of healthy skin.

- Vitamin B_1 acts as an antioxidant to decrease oxidation of lipids (fats) in the body.

Health Benefits

Vitamin B_1 nutrition has some health benefits.

- Prevents beriberi disease

- Promotes metabolism of carbohydrates and fats

- Maintains the function of the brain and the nerves

Deficiency Symptoms

The classic deficiency disease of vitamin B_1 is beriberi, which is associated with the following symptoms.

- Fast pulse

- High blood pressure

- Urine volume reduction

- loss of immediate memory

- Difficulty in walking

- Confusion

- Delusion

- Jerky movements of eyes

- Tense calf muscles

6. Vitamin B_2 (Riboflavin)

Vitamin B_2 is a water-soluble vitamin that functions primarily as a component of two flavin coenzymes: flavin mononucleotide (FMN) and flavin adenine dinucleotide (FAD) that catalyze many oxidation-reduction reactions. Vitamin B_2 is readily absorbed, largely in the proximal small intestine, and excreted with its metabolites in the urine. In men, urinary excretion of less than 10% of vitamin B_2 intake may reflect potential vitamin B_2 deficiency.

Functions

Vitamin B_2 has different biological functions in the body.

- Vitamin B_2 plays an essential role in the metabolism of carbohydrates, proteins and fats. In the protein metabolism, it forms enzymes necessary to transform oxygen to the cells.

- Vitamin B_2 is needed for tissue repair.

- Vitamin B_2 is required in the blood for red blood cell production.

- Vitamin B_2 is required in the pigment of the retina in the eyes for adaptation to light.

- Vitamin B_2 is required for the conversion of pyridoxine (vitamin B_6) to its functional form, pyridoxal phosphate.

- Vitamin B_2 is required for the biosynthesis of the vitamin niacin from amino acid tryptophan.

Health Benefits

Vitamin B_2 nutrition has the following health benefits.

- Promotes metabolism of carbohydrates, proteins and fats

- Reduces physical stress

- Avoids anemia

- Maintains eye health

Deficiency Symptoms

The deficiency of vitamin B_2 is associated with the following symptoms.

- Poor appetite

- Photophobia

- Tearing

- Burning and itching of eyes

- Loss of visual acuity

- Soreness

- Burning of lips, mouth, and tongue

- Cheilosis (fissuring of the lips)

- Angular stomatisis (cracks in the skin at the corners of the mouth)

- Swollen tongue

- Capillary overgrowth around the cornea of the eyes

- Neuropathy

- Anemia

7. Vitamin B₃ (Niacin)

Niacin, including nicotinic acid and nicotinamide, is referred to as vitamin B_3 because it was the third of the B vitamins to be discovered. Vitamin B_3 is converted to nicotinamide and then to nicotinamide adenine dinucleotide (NAD) and nicotinamide adenine dinucleotide phosphate (NADP) *in vivo*. Although the two are identical in their vitamin activity, nicotinamide does not have the same pharmacological effects of niacin, which occur as side-effects of niacin's conversion. Thus, nicotinamide does not reduce cholesterol or cause flushing, although nicotinamide may be toxic to the liver at doses exceeding 3 g/day for adults.

Vitamin B_3 is absorbed in the stomach and small intestine by carrier-mediated facilitated diffusion. It is transported in the plasma in free form and taken up by most tissues from passive diffusion, although some tissues (for example the erythrocytes, kidneys, and the brain) also have a transport system for vitamin B_3.

Functions

Vitamin B_3 has some key biological functions in the body.

- Vitamin B_3 plays essential roles as cosubstrates of more than 200 enzymes involved in the metabolism of carbohydrates, fatty acids, and amino acids.

- Vitamin B_3 is a coenzyme in several important biochemical functions, particularly those needed to maintain healthy skin, gastrointestinal tract, and the nervous system.

- Vitamin B_3 is used to treat high levels of cholesterol.

Health Benefits

Vitamin B_3 nutrition has the following health benefits.

- Reduces both cholesterol and triglyceride levels in the blood.

- Keeps a healthy skin.

- Maintains a normal nervous system.

- Keeps a good gastrointestinal tract function.

Deficiency Symptoms

The deficiency of vitamin B$_3$ is associated with the following symptoms.

* Muscular weakness

* Anorexia

* Indigestion

* Skin eruptions

* Dermantitis

* Dementia

* Diarrhea

* Tremors

* Sore tongue

* Confusion

* Depression

* Loss of memory

* Disorientation

* Neuritis

8. Vitamin B$_5$ (Pantothenic Acid)

Pantothenic acid, also called vitamin B$_5$ (a B vitamin), is a water-soluble vitamin required to sustain life (essential nutrient). Within most foods, pantothenic acid is in the form of coenzyme A (CoA) or acyl-carrier protein (ACP). In order for the intestinal cells to absorb this vitamin it must be converted into free pantothenic acid. Free pantothenic acid is absorbed into intestinal cells via a saturable, sodium-dependent active transport system. At high levels of intake, when this mechanism is saturated, some pantothenic acid may also be absorbed via passive diffusion. It is then transported in the free acid form in solution in the plasma and taken up by diffusion into erythrocytes, which carries most of the vitamin in the blood. Within the cell, the vitamin is converted to coenzyme A (CoA), which is its predominant form in most tissues, particularly in the liver, adrenals, kidneys, the brain, and the heart.

Functions

Vitamin B_5 has some key biological functions in the body.

- Vitamin B_5 plays an essential role in the metabolism of carbohydrates, proteins, and fats by coenzyme A.

- Vitamin B_5 is vital for the healthy functioning of the adrenal gland.

- Vitamin B_5 plays an essential role in the synthesis of steroids, cholesterol, bile, and hemoglobin.

- Vitamin B_5 is needed for the production of two very important substances involved in nerve transmission: sphingosine and acetylcholine.

Health Benefits

Vitamin B_5 nutrition has the following health benefits.

- Maintains a healthy functioning of the adrenal gland, from which it has long been considered an "anti-stress: vitamin".

- Keeps a normal nervous system.

- Promotes metabolism of carbohydrates, proteins, and fats.

- Keeps a healthy immune system.

Deficiency Symptoms

The deficiency of vitamin B_5 is associated with the following symptoms.

- Paresthesia in the toes

- Soles of the feet

- Burning sensations in the feet

- Depression

- Fatigue

- Insomnia

- Weakness

- Headache

- Rheumatoid arthritis

9. Vitamin B$_6$ (Pyridoxine)

Vitamin B$_6$ is a water-soluble compound that was discovered in the 1930s during nutrition studies on rats. The vitamin was named pyridoxine to indicate its structural homology to pyridine. Later it was determined that vitamin B$_6$ could exist in two other, slightly different, chemical forms, termed pyridoxal and pyridoxamine. All three forms of vitamin B$_6$ are converted in the liver, erythrocytes, and other tissues to pyridoxal 5'-phosphate (PLP), which plays a vital role as the cofactor of a large number of essential enzymes in the human body.

Vitamin B$_6$ is absorbed in the jejunum and ileum via passive diffusion. The absorption of pyridoxal phosphate and pyridoxamine phosphate involves their phosphorylation catalyzed by a membrane-bound alkaline phosphatase. Those products and non-phosphorylated vitamers in the digestive tract are absorbed by diffusion, which is driven by the trapping of the vitamin as 5'-phosphates through the action of phosphorylation (by a pyridoxal kinase) in the jejunal mucosa. The trapped pyridoxine and pyridoxamine are oxidized to pyridoxal phosphate in the tissue.

Functions

Vitamin B$_6$ has many biological functions in the body.

- Vitamin B$_6$ plays an essential role in the processes of amino acid, glucose, and lipid metabolisms.

- Vitamin B$_6$ plays an essential role in the synthesis of neurotransmitter.

- Vitamin B$_6$ plays an essential role in the synthesis of histamine.

- Vitamin B$_6$ plays an essential role in the synthesis and function of hemoglobin.

- Vitamin B$_6$ plays an essential role in the expression of genes.

- Vitamin B$_6$ plays a role in the metabolism of glucogen.

- Vitamin B$_6$ plays a role in the metabolism of heme.

- Vitamin B$_6$ is required for the conversion of tryptophan to niacin.

Health Benefits

Vitamin B$_6$ nutrition has the following health benefits.

- Keeps a normal nervous system.

- Promotes metabolism of carbohydrates, proteins, and fats.

- Maintains healthy blood and blood vessels.

- Keeps kidneys healthy.

- Prevents melanoma cancer.

- Keeps skin healthy.

- Prevents women from having premenstrual syndrome (PMS).

- Alleviates some of the many symptoms of an alcoholic hangover and morning sickness from pregnancy

Deficiency Symptoms

The deficiency of vitamin B_6 is associated with the following symptoms.

- Weakness

- Sleeplessness

- Peripheral neuropathies

- Cheilosis

- Glossitis

- Stomotitis

- Impaired cell-mediated immunity

- Impaired glucose tolerance

10. Vitamin B_7 (Biotin)

Biotin, also known as vitamin H or vitamin B_7, with the chemical formula $C_{10}H_{16}N_2O_3S$ (Biotin; Coenzyme R, Biopeiderm), is a water-soluble B-complex vitamin that is composed of an ureido (tetrahydroimidizalone) ring fused with a tetrahydrothiophene ring. A valeric acid substituent is attached to one of the carbon atoms of the tetrahydrothiophene ring. Biotin is a cofactor in the metabolism of fatty acids and leucine, and in gluconeogenesis.

Vitamin B_7 is a component of various foods and is synthesized in the lower gastrointestinal tract by microorganisms and some fungi. It is absorbed in the proximal small intestine primarily by carrier-mediated diffusion. Smaller amounts of biotin can be also absorbed from the colon, which facilitates the use of the vitamin produced hind gut microflora. Biotin is transported in the plasma primarily as free biotin, but approximately 12% is also bound to protein and biotinidase.

Functions

Vitamin B_7 has some important biological functions in the body.

- Vitamin B_7 is a coenzyme, which plays an essential role in the metabolism of carbohydrates, proteins, and fats.

- Vitamin B_7 plays a role in the citric acid cycle, which is the process by which biochemical energy is generated during aerobic respiration.

- Vitamin B_7 helps transfer carbon dioxide in the body.

Health Benefits

Vitamin B_7 nutrition has the following health benefits.

- Helps maintain a steady blood glucose level.

- Strengthens hair and nails.

- Counteracts the problem of hair loss in both children and adults.

- Improves seborrheic dermatitis.

Deficiency Symptoms

The deficiency of vitamin B_7 is associated with the following symptoms.

- Dermatitis

- Hair loss

- Glossitis

- Anorexia

- Nausea

- Loss of appetite

- Depression

- Hepatic steatosis

- Hypercholesterolemia

11. Vitamin B₉ (Folic Acid or Folate)

Folic acid (also known as Vitamin M and Folacin) and Folate (the anionic form) are both forms of the water-soluble Vitamin B_9. These occur naturally in food and can also be taken as supplements. Folate gets its name from the Latin word *folium* ("leaf").

A key observation by researcher Lucy Wills in 1931 led to the identification of folate as the nutrient needed to prevent anemia during pregnancy. Dr. Wills demonstrated that anemia could be reversed with brewer's yeast. Folate was identified as the corrective substance in brewer's yeast in the late 1930s and was extracted from spinach leaves in 1941. It was first synthesized in 1946 by Yellapragada Subbarao.

Dietary vitamin B_9 is absorbed only as the monoglutamate forms of folic acid, 5-methyltetrahydrofolic acid, and 5-formyltetrahydrofolic acid. Absorption of vitamin B_9 occurs mainly in the jejunum by active transport, but the vitamin can also be absorbed by passive diffusion when ingested in large amounts.

Functions

Vitamin B_9 has various biological functions in the body.

- Vitamin B_9 plays an essential role in the metabolism of carbohydrates, proteins, and fats.

- Vitamin B_9 is required for the production of RNA and DNA.

- Vitamin B_9 is necessary for the production and maintenance of new cells.

- Vitamin B_9 derivatives are coenzymes for neurotransmitters.

- Vitamin B_9 is essential for the formation of red and white blood cells in the bone marrow and for their maturation.

- Vitamin B_9 is a single-carbon carrier in the formation of heme.

- Vitamin B_9 is necessary for fertility in both men and women.

Health Benefits

Vitamin B_9 nutrition has the following health benefits.

- Helps protect against a number of congenital malformations including neural tube defects at the time just before and just after a woman becomes pregnant.

- Enhances memory and mental agility.

- Prevents colorectal, postmenopausal breast, and pancreatic cancers.

- Reduces the risk of stroke.

- Improves the condition of a certain congenital form of mental redardation.

- Corrects the anemia associated with vitamin B_{12} deficiency

Deficiency Symptoms

The deficiency of vitamin B_9 is associated with the following symptoms.

- Megaloblastic anemia

- General weakness

- Depression

- Polyneuropathy

- Poor growth

- Dermatologic lesions

- Neural tube defects

- Low IQ

12. Vitamin B_{12} (Cobalamin)

The term vitamin B_{12} refers to a family of cobalamin compounds containing the porphyrin-like, cobalt-centered corrin nucleus. Of the several cobalamin compounds that exhibit vitamin B_{12} activity, cyanocobalamin and hydroxy-cobalamin are the most active. The majority of vitamin B_{12} is absorbed by active transport, and intrinsic factor, a specific binding protein for vitamin B_{12} produced in the stomach, is essential for the process. Only about 1% can be absorbed by simple diffusion even in high amounts.

Individuals who lack intrinsic factor have a decreased ability to absorb vitamin B_{12}. This results in 80%–100% excretion of oral doses in the feces versus 30%–60% excretion as seen in individuals with adequate intrinsic factor. The total amount of vitamin B_{12} stored in the body is about 2–5 mg in adults. Around 80% of this is stored in the liver.

Functions

Vitamin B_{12} has many biological functions in the body in two coenzyme forms: adenosylcobalamin and methylcobalamin.

- Vitamin B_{12} is normally involved in the metabolism of every cell in the body.

- Vitamin B_{12} plays an important role in the synthesis and regulation of DNA.

- Vitamin B_{12} plays an essential role in the metabolism of carbohydrates, proteins and fats.

- Vitamin B_{12} plays an essential role in the metabolism of propionate.

- Vitamin B_{12} is involved in the production of myelin, which is the sheath that covers our nerves.

Health Benefits

Vitamin B_{12} nutrition has the following health benefits.

- Maintains healthy nerve cells.

- Keeps healthy red blood cells to help iron function better in the body.

- Helps make DNA, the genetic material in all cells.

- Helps support the higher energy levels.

- Prevents the formation of cancer combined with ascorbic acid.

- Helps lessen the risk of heart disease.

Deficiency Symptoms

The deficiency of vitamin B_{12} is a common disorder in older adults associated with the following symptoms.

- Pernicious anemia

- A lemon yellow-colored tint on the skin

- Eyes resulting from concurrent anemia and jaundice from ineffective erythropoiesis

- A smooth, beefy, red tongue

- Neurologic disorders

13. Vitamin C (Ascorbic Acid or L-Ascorbate)

Vitamin C is a water-soluble antioxidant that can be synthesized by many mammals, but not by humans. Vitamin C is purely the L-enantiomer of ascorbate; the opposite D-enantiomer has no physiological significance. Both forms are mirror images of the same molecular structure. When L-ascorbate, which is a strong reducing agent, carries out its reducing function, it is converted to its oxidized form, L-dehydroascorbate. L-dehydroascorbate can then be reduced back to the active L-ascorbate form in the body by enzymes and glutathione.

L-ascorbate is a weak sugar acid structurally related to glucose which naturally occurs either attached to a hydrogen ion, forming ascorbic acid, or to a metal ion, forming a mineral ascorbate. So, vitamin C includes ascorbic acid (the mostly used form in supplements) and sodium ascorbate, calcium ascorbate et al.

Vitamin C is absorbed in the intestine by a sodium-dependent transport process. The efficiency of enteric absorption of the vitamin is high (80%–90%) at low intakes, but declines markedly at intakes greater than about 1 g/day. Vitamin C is transported in the plasma in the reduced form (dehydroascorbate).

Functions

Vitamin C has many important biological functions in the body.

- Vitamin C is a highly effective antioxidant, acting to lessen oxidative stress.

- Vitamin C blocks the formation of nitrosamines, potentially cancer-causing compounds.

- Vitamin C helps the inactive form of folic acid turn into the active form.

- Vitamin C increases the absorption of iron, while it decreases the absorption of copper.

- Vitamin C stimulates the excretion of lead, thereby reducing the concentration of lead in the body tissues.

- Vitamin C is a substrate for ascorbate peroxidase that detoxifies peroxides such as hydrogen peroxide.

- Vitamin C is an enzyme cofactor for the biosynthesis of many important biochemicals.

- Vitamin C acts as an electron donor for eight different enzymes. Three are very important in the synthesis of collagen that is essential for the development and maintenance of scar tissue, blood vessels, and cartilage. Two is necessary for the synthesis of carnitine that is essential for the transport of fatty acids into mitochondria for adenosine triphosphate (ATP) generation. In the remaining three, one participates in the biosynthesis of norepinephrine, and one adds amide groups to peptide hormones to increase their stability, and another one modulates tyrosine metabolism.

- Vitamin C promotes resistance to infection through its involvement with the immunologic activity of leukocytes, the production of interferon, the process of inflammatory reaction, and the integrity of the mucous membranes.

Health Benefits

Vitamin C nutrition has the following health benefits.

- Enhances the immune system, thereby helping increase resistance to diseases including infections and cancers.

- Lessens all types of physical and mental stress.

- Repairs tissues in all parts of the body.

- Promotes growth of tissues in all parts of the body.

- Reduces neurological deficits and mortality following stroke.

- Reduces the risk of cancer of the stomach, colon, bladder, lung, esophagus, and cervix.

- Helps prevent high blood pressure and atherosclerosis.

Deficiency Symptoms

The deficiency of vitamin C leads to scurvy in adults and children associated with the following symptoms.

- Liver spots on the skin

- Swollen, bleeding gums

- Tooth loss

- Lethargy

- Fatigue

- Rheumatic pains in the legs

- Depression

14. Choline

Choline is an organic compound, classified as a water-soluble essential nutrient, and usually grouped within the Vitamin B complex. Choline was discovered by Andreas Strecker in 1864 and chemically synthesized in 1866. In 1998, choline was classified as an essential nutrient by the Food and Nutrition Board of the Institute of Medicine of the National Academy of Sciences (U.S.A.). Adequate intakes (AI) of this micronutrient are between 425 to 550 milligrams daily for adults, having been established by scientists.

Choline can be biosynthesized from ethanolamine by sequential methylations using S-adenosylmethionine, but most humans obtain choline from dietary phosphatides. Choline is widely distributed in fat, existing predominantly in the form of lecithin in eggs, animal livers, soybeans, beef, milk, and peanuts. Free choline is present in animal livers, oatmeal, soybeans, iceberg lettuce, cauliflower, kale, and cabbage. When choline is metabolized by the body, it may form trimethylamine, a compound with a fishy odor. Hence, when large amounts of choline are taken, the person may suffer from a fishy body odor.

Choline is released by the hydrolysis of lecithin by pancreatic and intestinal lipases and is absorbed by a carrier-mediated process and passive diffusion. Absorbed choline is transported via chylomicrons in lymphatic circulation primarily in the form of lecithin. Then, it is transferred to lipoproteins in this form for distribution to peripheral tissues.

Functions

Choline has some key biological functions in the body.

- As phosphatidylcholine (lecithin), choline is a structural component of membranes, a precursor to the sphingolipids, and a promoter of lipid transport that keeps your cell membranes, the gates through which nutrients enter and through which wastes leave your cells, functioning properly

- As acetylcholine, choline is a neurotransmitter and an element of platelet-activating factor, which allows your nerves to communicate with your muscles.

- Choline prevents the build-up of homocysteine in your blood. Homocysteine is a harmful compound that is associated with cardio-vascular disease and osteoporosis.

Health Benefits

Choline nutrition has the following health benefits.

- Enhances memory in brain development.

- Prevents cardiovascular disease

- Prevents cancer

- Boosts energy levels

- Delays fatigue

- Reduces chronic inflammation

- Diminishes the short-term memory loss associated with Alzheimer's disease

- Alleviates symptoms of tardive dyskinesia and Huntington's disease in very high doses (up to 20 g per day)

Deficiency Symptoms

The deficiency of choline is associated with the following symptoms.

- Heart disease

- High blood pressure

- Fatigue

- Insomnia

- Poor ability of the kidneys to concentrate urine

- Accumulation of fats in the blood

- Nerve-muscle problems

Chapter Four
Human Nutrition—Micronutrients: Minerals

Minerals can be divided into macrominerals (bulk elements), microminerals (trace elements), and ultratrace minerals. Macrominerals are required in amounts of 100 mg/day or more. They include: calcium, phosphorus, magnesium, sulfur, sodium, potassium, and chloride. Microminerals (trace elements) are required in smaller amounts of less than 15 mg/day. They include: iron, zinc, copper, and fluoride. Ultratrace minerals are consumed only in microgram (μg) quantities each day. They include: iodine, selenium, manganese, chromium, cobalt, and molybdenum.

Macrominerals

1. Calcium

Calcium is the most abundant mineral in the human body, which makes up of about 1.5%–2% of the body weight. Approximately 99% of the calcium exists in the bones and teeth and the remaining 1% of calcium is in the blood and extracellular fluids and within the cells of all tissues.

A hormone called calcitonin manufactured from the thyroid takes up excess calcium from the blood and deposits it in the bones when the calcium level begins to go up too high. Also, urine and feces take extra calcium out of the body. Conversely, when calcium levels in the blood go down too low, a hormone produced from the parathyroid pulls stored calcium from the bones and sends it into the blood. Thus, the two hormones keep the levels of calcium in your blood dynamically balanced at a normal concentration of about 10 mg per 100 ml of blood serum. However, if the bones are depleted of calcium for a long time, they will become thin and weak.

Calcium is mostly absorbed by active transport and passive transfer in all parts of the small intestine. Vitamin D increases calcium uptake at the brush border of the intestinal mucosal cell. Usually only 30% of ingested calcium is absorbed by adults.

Functions

- Calcium plays a key role in building and maintaining strong and healthy bones and teeth.

- Calcium activates the enzymes involved in fat and protein digestion and in the production of energy.

- Calcium initiates the formation of a blood clot by stimulating the release of thromboplastin from blood platelets.

- Calcium controls the release of neurotransmitters that pass impulses from one nerve to the next, carrying messages throughout the body.

- Calcium regulates the contraction and relaxation of muscles, including heartbeats.

- Calcium influences the transport functions of cell membranes and the transmission of ions across membranes of cell organelles.

- Calcium affects the function of hormones and the release or activation of intracellular and extracellular enzymes.

- Calcium may help regulate blood pressure.

- Calcium aids in the absorption of many nutrients, particularly vitamin B_{12}.

Health Benefits

- Calcium intake prevents the development of osteoporosis.

- Calcium intake reduces high blood pressure.

- There is some evidence that calcium intake may help prevent colon cancer.

- Calcium intake lowers the risk of developing premenopausal breast cancer

- Calcium acts as a weight-limiting aid.

Deficiency Symptoms

- Osteoporosis

- Colon cancer

• Hypertension

2. Phosphorus

Phosphorus is the second most abundant mineral in the body. Approximately 700 g of phosphorus exist in adult tissues, in which about 85% is present in the bones and teeth, while the rest is distributed throughout the body in cells, blood, and other fluids. The serum inorganic phosphorus level is closely maintained by parathyroid hormone (PTH) at 3–4 mg per100 ml in adults. Almost 50% of the inorganic phosphate is present in serum as free ions. Smaller percentages are bound to protein (~10%) or complexed (~40%). The ratio of calcium to phosphorus in the bones is about 2:1; however, we have a much higher proportion of phosphorus in soft tissues.

Regardless of the form, most phosphates are absorbed in the inorganic state in the intestine. The efficiency of phosphate absorption is 60%–70% in adults, almost twice as high as calcium's. In addition, phosphate absorption is much more rapid than that of calcium's. For example, the peak of absorption of phosphates occurs approximately 1 hour after ingestion of a meal, whereas the peak of calcium's entry into the blood appears 3–4 hours after a meal.

Functions

• Phosphorus as phosphates is a key structural component of deoxyribonucleic acid (DNA) and ribonucleic acid (RNA), which controls heredity and the replication of cells.

• Living cells use phosphate to transport cellular energy via adenosine triphosphate (ATP). Nearly every cellular process that uses energy obtains it in the form of ATP. ATP is also important for phosphorylation, a key regulatory event in cells.

• Phospholipids are the main structural components of all cellular membranes.

• Cyclic adenosine monophosphate (CAMP) acts as a secondary signal within cells following peptide hormone activation of many membrane receptors.

• Numerous phospholipid molecules act as secondary messengers within the cytosol.

• Phosphorus is involved in the transport of fats in the circulatory system.

- Phosphorus is involved in protein synthesis, hormone secretion, and muscle contraction.

- Phosphate ions combine with calcium to form hydroxyapatite, the major inorganic molecule in teeth and bones, which assists in stiffening them.

- Phosphate buffer system is important in keeping the body pH in balance.

- Many of the B-vitamins are effective only when combined with phosphate in the body.

Health Benefits

- Phosphorus intake strengthens the bones and teeth.

- Phosphorus intake prevents the development of osteoporosis.

- Phosphorus intake facilitates the effective digestion of vitamin B_2 and vitamin B_3 in a proficient manner.

- Phosphorus intake keeps the kidneys at a normal condition by ensuring the proper release of wastes from the kidneys by the process of excretion.

- Phosphorous intake has the ability to remove minor health problems such as weakness, numbness, fatigue, and other similar ailments. Sexual weakness can also be cured with an adequate presence of phosphorous in the body.

- The proper level of phosphorous helps maintain proper brain functions.

- Phosphorus intake helps the process of reproduction. It also facilitates the maximum utilization of protein in the human body to ensure the proper growth of cells, along with their repair from time to time.

- Phosphorus intake helps to utilize carbohydrates as well as fats.

- Phosphorus intake regulates the balance of hormones in the human body. It ensures that hormones, especially those required for good reproductive health, are always present in balanced form.

- Phosphorus intake ensures that body cells are developed properly and remain active for admirable health conditions.

- Phosphorus intake helps utilize various nutrients entering the body.

Deficiency Symptoms

- Weak bones

- Tooth decay

- Discomfort in various body joints

- Loss of appetite

- Numbness

- Loss of weight

- Tremor

- Restricted growth

- Anxiety

3. Magnesium

Magnesium is the second most abundant intracellular cation after potassium in the human body. The adult human body contains approximately 20–28 g of magnesium, of which 60% is found in the bones, 26% in the muscles, and the remainder, in the soft tissues and body fluids. Normal serum levels are in the range of 1.5–2.1 mEq/L (0.75–1.1 mmol/L). About half of the magnesium in the plasma is free, approximately one third is bound to albumin, and the remainder is complexed with citrate, phosphate, or their anions. Magnesium homeostasis is governed by intestinal absorption and renal excretion. No hormone is known to have a major role in the control of serum magnesium.

The efficiency of absorption of magnesium varies from 35% to 45%. Magnesium may be absorbed along the length of the small intestine, but most absorption occurs in the jejunum by two mechanisms: a carrier-facilitated process and simple diffusion. Vitamin D has little or no effect on magnesium absorption.

Functions

- Along with calcium and phosphorus, magnesium is required for strong, healthy bones and teeth.

- Magnesium is a cofactor for more than 300 enzymes involved in the metabolism of food components, and the synthesis of fatty acids and proteins, and phosphorylation of glucose.

- Magnesium plays a role in neuromuscular transmission and activity, working in concert with and against the effects of calcium. After calcium flows into muscles to help them contract, magnesium replaces the calcium and allows them to relax.

- Magnesium maintains the function of the nerves.

- Magnesium works with the enzymes in the body to break down sugar stored in the liver to create energy. These reactions are essential whenever energy is needed.

- Magnesium interacts with other minerals such as sodium, potassium, and calcium to affect the muscle tone of the blood vessels.

- Magnesium plays a key role in the homeostasis of calcium and potassium.

- Magnesium helps stabilize the rhythm of the heart and helps prevent abnormal blood clotting in the heart.

Health Benefits

- Magnesium intake may help reduce high blood pressure.

- Magnesium intake may prevent the development and progression of diseases of the blood vessels.

- Magnesium intake aids in the recovery from a heart attack or stroke.

- Magnesium intake reduces the risk of cardiovascular disease.

- Magnesium may prove useful in preventing certain pregnancy complications such as prematurity and intrauterine growth retardation.

- Magnesium intake helps prevent severe vision problem and even blindness.

- Magnesium intake assists in preventing osteoporosis.

- Magnesium intake helps prevent asthma.

- Magnesium intake helps prevent diabetes.

Deficiency Symptoms

- Tremor

- Muscle spasm

- Anorexia

- Nausea

- Vomiting

- Mental derangement

- Personality change

- Hypocalcemia

- Hypokalemia

4. Sodium

Sodium is the major cation of extracellular fluid: the water and dissolved substances in the spaces outside cells. The normal serum concentration of sodium is 136–145 mEq/L. Various intestinal secretions, such as bile and pancreatic juice contain substantial amounts of sodium. About 35%–40% of the total body's sodium is in the skeleton; however, most of it is unexchangeable or slowly exchangeable with that in body fluids. Contrary to common belief, sweat is hypotonic and contains a relatively small amount of sodium.

Sodium is readily absorbed from the intestine and is carried to the kidneys, where it is filtered and returned to the blood to maintain appropriate levels. The amount absorbed is proportional to the intake. Approximately 90%–95% of a normal body's sodium loss is through the urine; the rest is lost in feces and sweat.

Sodium balance is regulated by aldosterone, a mineralocorticoid secreted by the adrenal cortex. When blood sodium levels rise, the thirst receptors in the hypothalamus stimulate the thirst sensation. Ingestion of fluids returns sodium levels to normal. When blood sodium levels are low, sodium excretion through the urine decreases.

Functions

- Sodium regulates the plasma volume.

- Sodium regulates the volume of extracellular fluid in the body.

- Sodium plays a pivotal role in enzyme operation and muscle contraction.

- Sodium aids in the nerve impulse conduction in the body.

- Sodium helps in the absorption of glucose by cells for the smooth transportations of nutrients in body cell membranes.

- Sodium balances the osmotic pressure in the body due to regulation of fluid in body cells.

- Sodium shares an association with chlorides and bicarbonates in maintaining a sound balance between the two types of ions, positively charged ions as well as negatively charged ions.

- Sodium plays an important role in the removal of excess amounts of carbon dioxide accumulated in the body.

- Sodium helps restore youthful and healthy skin.

- Sodium assists in metabolic process of various nutrients like fats, proteins, and carbohydrates.

Health Benefits

- Sodium intake prevents dehydration.

- Sodium intake keeps the mind sharp.

- Sodium intake prevents sunstroke, or heat prostration by replacing the loss of essential electrolytes. Sunstroke is caused by continuous exposure to very high temperatures, in which the body loses its capacity to maintain its normal temperature

- Sodium intake prevents muscle cramps.

- Sodium intake maintains youthful healthy skin.

- Sodium intake maintains a healthy condition of the heart.

Deficiency Symptoms:

- Diarrhea

- Vomiting

- Headache

- Weakness

- Low blood pressure

- Lethargy

- Weight loss

- Confusion

- Dizziness

5. Potassium

Potassium is the major cation of intracellular fluid, and only small amounts of it is present in extracellular fluid. The normal serum potassium concentration is 3.5–5 mEq/L.

Potassium is readily absorbed from the small intestine. Approximately 80%–90% of ingested potassium is excreted in urine; the remainder is lost in the feces. The kidneys maintain normal serum levels through their ability to filter, reabsorb, and excrete potassium under the influence of aldosterone. Ionized potassium is excreted in place of ionized sodium through the renal tubule exchange mechanism.

Functions

- With sodium, potassium is involved in maintaining a normal water balance, osmotic equilibrium and the acid-base balance in the body.

- In addition to calcium, potassium is important in the regulation of neuromuscular activity.

- Potassium promotes cellular growth.

- Potassium in muscle plays an important role in maintaining muscle mass and in storing glycogen.

- Potassium helps boost the spirit of nerve reflexes to transmit messages from one body part to another. This, in turn, helps muscle contractions to perform various activities everyday.

- Potassium helps regulate the level of fluids in the human body and thus, performs a number of critical body functions.

- Potassium assists the kidneys in removing waste by the process of excretion.

- Potassium assists in the metabolic processes of various nutrients like fats, proteins, and carbohydrates.

- Potassium plays an important role in regular muscle contraction.

- Potassium acts as a vital component, which maintains the normality of blood pressure in the human body.

- Potassium plays an irreplaceable role in regulating the functions of the heart.

Health Benefits

- Potassium intake prevents the occurrence of stroke in the human brain.

- Potassium intake prevents loss of memory.

- Potassium intake prevents muscle cramps.

- Potassium intake abolishes the possibilities of heart diseases and hypertension.

- Potassium intake ensures efficient mental performance of the human body.

- Potassium intake maintains muscular strength.

- Potassium intake prevents dehydration.

- Potassium intake prevents sweating, headache, weakness, trembling, and nervousness resulting from low blood sugar.

Deficiency Symptoms

- Fatigue and weakness in muscles.

- Inactive reflexes

- Abnormal heartbeat

- Heart palpitations

- Anemia

- Severe headaches.

- High blood pressure

- Pain in the intestines

- Swelling in the glands

- Diabetes is a serious effect of this deficiency

6. Chloride

Chloride is a type of electrolyte that works in conjunction with sodium and potassium. As the principle anion of extracellular fluids, chloride is widely distributed throughout the body. The normal serum chloride concentration is 96–106 mEq/L. The amount of chloride in the blood is carefully controlled by the kidneys. The highest concentrations of chloride are found in cerebrospinal fluid, bile, and gastric and pancreatic juices. In the stomach, chloride is secreted by gastric mucosa as hydrochloric acid, providing an acid medium for digestion and enzyme activation.

Chloride is almost completely absorbed in the intestines and excreted in urine and sweat. Chloride loss parallels sodium loss. Excessive loss through sweat is minimized by aldosterone, which acts directly on sweat glands. Extra chloride may be needed to correct the metabolic alkalosis resulting from disease, the use of diuretics, or gastric losses from gastric suctioning or vomiting.

Functions

- Working with sodium and potassium, chloride helps to maintain water balance and osmotic pressure.

- Chloride is crucial for maintaining the acid-base balance in the human body.

- Within the stomach, you'll find that chloride appears in the form of hydrochloric acid. In order for your body to effectively digest food, hydrochloric acid helps break the food down so that it can be absorbed by the small intestine.

- In the liver, chloride may help in the process of removing waste.

- Chloride may regulate the rennin-angiotensin-aldosterone system.

- In the central nervous system, the inhibitory action of glycine and some of the action of gamma-aminobutyric acid (GABA) relies on the entry of Cl⁻ into specific neurons.

- The chloride-bicarbonate exchanger biological transport protein relies on the chloride ion to increase the blood's capacity of carbon dioxide, in the form of the bicarbonate ion.

Health Benefits

- Chloride intake prevents dehydration.

- Chloride intake raises the efficiency of food absorption.

- Chloride intake maintains the functioning of the central nervous system.

- Chloride intake prevents low blood pressure.

- Chloride intake prevents alkalosis.

- Chloride intake, along with potassium, prevents hypokalemia.

Deficiency Symptoms

- Low blood pressure

- A general feeling of weakness

- Diarrhea

- Vomiting

- Weight loss

Microminerals

7. Iron

The adult human body contains iron in two major pools: (1) functional iron in hemoglobin, myoglobin, and enzymes, and (2) storage iron in ferritin, hemosiderin, and transferrin (a transport protein in blood). Healthy adult men have about 3.6 g of total body iron, whereas women have about 2.4 g. Approximately 76% of iron is found in functional iron in adult men, compared with about 87% in adult women. Adult women have much lower amounts of iron in storage with about 13%, while men have about 24%. Iron is highly conserved by the body; approximately 90% is recovered and reused everyday. The rest is excreted, primarily in the bile. Dietary iron must be available to maintain iron balance in order to meet this 10% gap. Otherwise, iron deficiency occurs.

Dietary iron exists in two chemical forms: (1) heme iron, which is found in hemoglobin, myoglobin, and some enzymes, and (2) nonheme iron, which is found predominantly in plant food but also in some animal foods. Absorption of heme iron may be as high as 25%, compared with only 5% or so for nonheme iron. Iron absorption is enhanced by the coingestion of vitamin C because ascorbic acid reduces ferric to ferrous iron. Other food molecules such as sugars and sulfur-containing amino acids may also enhance iron entry by forming chelates with ionic iron.

Functions

- Iron is an important part of hemoglobin that combines with oxygen in the lungs and then transports oxygen to the body cells, where it picks up carbon dioxide and then releases it in the lungs after it returns from the tissues.

- Iron is an important part of myoglobin that is present in the muscle tissues and helps supply oxygen required for contraction of muscles.

- Iron is a facilitator for regulating body temperature.

- Iron acts as a carrier of oxygen and thus participates in transferring oxygen from one body cell to another. This is an important function of iron, as oxygen is required by each and every body part in order to perform routine functions.

- Iron actively takes part in the synthesis of a number of essential neurotransmitters like dopamine, norepinephrine, along with serotonin. These chemicals play major roles in different activities involving neurons and the human brain.

- Iron plays a key role in providing strength for the immune system.

- Iron is an important spectator of energy metabolism in the human body, by which the energy is extracted from the food consumed and distributed to different body parts.

- Iron is the most important constituent of different enzyme systems and other important constituents such as myoglobin, the cytochromes, and catalase.

Health Benefits

- Iron intake prevents iron deficiency anemia.

- Iron intake ensures optimal brain functions. Oxygen supply in blood is aided by iron and the brain uses approximately 20% of that oxygen.

- Iron intake prevents restless leg syndrome.

- Iron intake helps treat chronic disorders like renal failure anemia.

- Iron intake may exhibit its health benefits in curing anemia resulting in women during pregnancy or menstruation.

- Iron intake eradicates different causes of fatigue, which may occur in men as well as women. Iron deficiency is a natural cause of fatigue since it is an important component of hemoglobin.

- Iron intake treats insomnia in the human body and also improves the sleeping benefits of an individual.

- Iron, when consumed in sufficient amounts in the diet, builds concentration amongst students and professional people, so they can carry out their work efficiently.

- Iron intake fights against a number of diseases and infections.

Deficiency Symptoms

- Feeling tired and weak

- Decreased work and school performance

- Slow cognitive and social development during childhood

- Difficulty in maintaining body temperature

- Decreased immune function, which increases susceptibility to infection

- Glossitis (an inflamed tongue)

- Hypochromic and microcytic anemia

8. Zinc

Except for iron, no other micromineral is as prevalent in the body as zinc. The human body has about 2–3 g of zinc, with the highest concentrations in the liver, pancreas, kidneys, bones, and muscles. Other tissues with high concentrations include various parts of the eye, prostate gland, spermatozoa, skin, hair, fingernails, and toenails. Relatively, large amounts of zinc are deposited in the bones and muscles, but these stores of zinc are not in rapid equilibrium with the rest of the organism. Zinc is primarily an intracellular ion, functioning in association with more than 300 different enzymes of various classes. Even though zinc is abundant in the cytosol, virtually, all of it is bound to proteins, but it is in equilibrium with a small ionic fraction.

Zinc absorption and excretion is controlled by poorly understood homeostatic mechanisms. The mechanism of absorption involves two pathways similar to those of calcium: (1) a saturable carrier mechanism operating most efficiently at low zinc intakes when luminal zinc concentrations are low, and (2) a passive mechanism involving paracellular movement when zinc intakes and luminal concentrations are high.

Zinc absorption is affected not only by the level of zinc in the diet but also by the presence of interfering substances, especially phytate. Phytate decreases zinc absorption, but other complexing agents (e.g., tannins) do not. Copper and cadmium compete for the same carrier protein, so they reduce zinc absorption. High intakes of iron and calcium can also reduce the amount of zinc absorbed. Folic acid may reduce zinc absorption if zinc intake is low. Zinc absorption may be enhanced by glucose or lactose and by soy protein consumed alone or mixed with beef. Like iron, zinc is better absorbed from human's milk than from cow's milk.

Functions

- Zinc participates in reactions involving either synthesis or degradation of major metabolites: carbohydrates, lipids, proteins and nuclei acids.

- Zinc plays important structural roles as components of several proteins.

- Zinc functions as an intracellular signal in brain cells.

- Zinc is involved in the stabilization of protein and nuclei acid structure and the integrity of subcellular organelles.

- Zinc helps promote the healing of wounds.

- Zinc is required for the immune system to function properly.

- Zinc is involved in the expression of genetic information. It stabilizes RNA and DNA structures and is required for the activity of RNA polymerases, important in cell division.

- Zinc functions in chromatin proteins, involved in transcription and replication.

- Zinc appears in the crystalline structure of bone, in the bone enzymes, and at the zone of demarcation.

- Zinc is required for activating many enzymes.

- Zinc is necessary for taste buds to function normally.

- Zinc is an essential mineral for the normal functioning of the reproductive organs.

Health Benefits

- Zinc intake prevents prostate disorder.

- Zinc intake helps cure acne and pimples.

- Zinc intake helps decrease the severity and duration of cold illnesses.

- Zinc intake controls the appetite, thereby, it helps people lose weight.

- Zinc intake accelerates the healing of wounds.

- In males, zinc intake assists in spermatogenesis and the development of sex organs. In females, it aids in all the reproductive phases, including parturition and lactation stages.

- Zinc intake helps a person's taste and smell senses.

- Zinc intake helps promote fetus growth.

- Zinc intake helps protect against infectious disorders and fungal infections, which includes pneumonia and conjunctivitis.

- Zinc intake improves vision.

- Zinc intake helps prevent the loss of hair in both children and adults.

- Zinc intake makes the bone matrix strong and hard.

Deficiency Symptoms

- Growth retardation

- Low blood pressure

- Retarded bones

- Loss of appetite

- Loss of sense of smell and taste

- Depression

- Rough skin

- Weight loss

- Pale skin

- Diarrhea

- Hair loss

- Fatigue

- White spots under finger nails.

- Eye lesions, including photophobia and night blindness

- Impaired taste (hypogeusia)

9. Copper

The average adult has about 100–150 milligrams of copper in the body. Concentrations of copper are highest in the liver, brain, heart, and kidneys. The muscles contain a low level of copper, but due to its large mass, skeletal muscle contains almost 40% of all the copper in the body.

Copper absorption occurs in the small intestine by facilitated diffusion and active transport. Net absorption of copper varies from 25% to 60%. Approximately 90% of the copper in the serum is incorporated into ceruloplasmin; the rest is bound loosely to albumin, transcuprein, other proteins, and free amino acids, possibly histidine. Copper is transported in the blood to other tissues, primarily bound to albumin.

Fiber and phytate may slightly inhibit copper absorption. In amounts of 150 mg/day, zinc has been shown to induce copper deficiency. High ascorbic acid intake (1500 mg/day) also reduces blood concentrations of copper, which may decrease the role of ceruloplasmin in red cell formation.

Functions

- Copper is a constituent of a number of enzymes of energy production, the oxidation of fatty acids, and the formation of melanin, a skin pigment.

- Copper in ceruloplasmin has a well-documented role in oxidizing iron before it is transported in the plasma.

- Lysyl oxidase, a copper-containing enzyme is essential in the lysine-derived cross-linking of collagen and elastin, connective tissue proteins with great tensile strength.

- As a part of copper-containing enzymes such as superoxide dismutase (SOD), copper protects against oxidants and free radicals and promotes the synthesis of melanin and catecholamines.

- Copper is involved in the metabolism of ascorbic acid.

- Copper plays a role in maintaining the integrity of myelin (the outer covering of the nerves).

- Copper is needed for taste sensitivity and bone development.

- Copper is essential for the synthesis of adenosine triphosphate (ATP), which is an energy storehouse in the human body.

- Copper can destroy or inhibit the growth of bacterial strains such as E. Coli.

- Copper has an important role in ensuring the proper functioning of thyroid glands.

Health Benefits

- Copper intake assists in reducing the symptoms of arthritis by its anti-inflammatory ability.

- Copper intake helps protect skeletal, nervous, and cardiovascular systems.

- Copper intake helps protect against graying hair.

- Copper intake helps in the absorption of iron from the intestinal tract and releasing it from its primary storage sites like the liver.

- Copper intake helps utilize the sugar in the body.

- Copper intake ensures better wound healing.

- Copper intake helps cure anemic problems.

- Copper intake enhances the flexibility of connective tissues.

- Copper intake lowers total cholesterol and raises high-density lipoprotein (HDL) cholesterol.

Deficiency symptoms

- Anemia

- Low body temperature

- Osteoporosis

- Osteoarthritis and rheumatoid arthritis

- Uneven heartbeat

- Elevated cholesterol levels

- Low resistance to infections

- Birth defects

- Low skin pigmentation

- Neutropenia and leucopenia in children

- Hair loss

- Anorexia

- Diarrhea

- Reproductive problems

- Impaired brain function

- Colon cancer

10. Fluoride

Fluorine occurs naturally in the Earth's crust, water, and food as the negatively charged ion, fluoride (F^-). Fluoride is considered a trace element because only small amounts are present in the body (about 2.5 grams in adults), and because the daily requirement for maintaining dental health is only a few milligrams a day. About 95% of the total body fluoride is found in the bones and teeth.

Fluoride is absorbed in the stomach and the small intestine. Once in the blood stream it rapidly enters mineralized tissue (bones and developing teeth). At usual intake levels, fluoride does not accumulate in soft tissue. The predominant mineral elements in bone are crystals of calcium and phosphate, known as hydroxyapatite crystals. Fluoride's high chemical reactivity and small radius allow it to either displace the larger hydroxyl (-OH) ion in the hydroxyapatite crystal, forming fluoroapatite, or it increases crystal density by entering spaces within the hydroxyapatite crystal. Fluoroapatite hardens tooth enamel and stabilizes bone mineral.

Both calcium and magnesium form insoluble complexes with fluoride and are capable of significantly decreasing fluoride absorption when present in the same meal. However, the absorption of fluoride in the form of monofluorophosphate (unlike sodium fluoride) is unaffected by calcium. A diet low in chloride (salt) has been found to increase fluoride retention by reducing urinary excretion of fluoride. The primary route of fluoride excretion is the kidneys, and urine generally accounts for approximately 90% of the total fluoride excreted.

Functions

- Fluoride strengthens the teeth's enamel by strengthening the mineral composition of the teeth themselves.

- Fluoride aids in strengthening the bone structure by either displacing the larger hydroxyl (-OH) ion in the hydroxyapatite crystal, forming fluoroapatite, or increasing crystal density by entering spaces within the hydroxyapatite crystal.

- Fluoride acts as an antibacterial agent in the oral cavity, serving as an enzyme inhibitor.

Health Benefits

- Fluoride intake prevents tooth decay (dental caries)

Deficiency Symptoms

- Dental caries

- Loss of teeth

Ultratrace minerals

11. Iodine

Our bodies contain 20–30 mg of iodine. More than 75% of it is stored in our thyroid glands, and the rest is distributed throughout the body, mostly in the fluid that bathes our cells.

Iodine is absorbed as easily as iodide. Iodide is rapidly and almost completely absorbed in the thyroid gland for synthesis of the thyroid hormones, and in salivary and gastric glands and in the kidneys for excretion into gastrointestinal tract and urine. In the circulation, iodine exists freely and protein bound, but the bound iodide predominates. Excretion is primarily via urine, but small amounts are found in the feces as a result of biliary secretion. So, urinary excretion is a reliable indicator of iodine status under normal circumstances.

Functions

- Iodine plays a very important role in the normal functioning of the thyroid glands, which secretes thyroid hormones: triiodothyronine (T_3) and thyroxine (T_4) that control the basic metabolic rate of the body, and influence heart rate, blood pressure, body weight, and temperature.

- Iodine helps synthesize proteins.

- Iodine plays an important role in maintaining optimum energy levels of the body by ensuring optimum utilization of calories, without allowing them to be deposited as excess fats.

- Iodine helps in the normal growth and maturity of reproductive organs.

- Iodine can flush out chemical toxins such as fluoride, lead, mercury etc., apart from biological toxins.

- Iodine can strengthen the immune system by increasing the antioxidant status of human serum similar to that of vitamin C.

- Iodine aids hair growth.

Health Benefits

- Iodine intake keeps a good heart rate, blood pressure, body weight, and temperature.

- Iodine intake maintains healthy and shiny skin, teeth, and hair.

- Iodine intake prevents goiter.

- Iodine intake prevents still births or neurocognitive conditions like cretinism in babies.

- Iodine intake prevents breast cancer.

- Iodine intake prevents surgical wound infections.

- Iodine intake prevents hearing loss.

- Iodine intake prevents the absorption of radioactive iodine in the event of a nuclear accident by thyroid to protect against thyroid damage, and possibly thyroid cancer.

Deficiency Symptoms

- Poor cognition in schoolchildren

- Mental retardation

- Endemic or simple goiter

- Cretinism in infants

12. Selenium

Not until 1979 was selenium considered a nutrient essential to human health. Selenium is present in all the tissues of the body, but is concentrated most highly in the kidneys, liver, spleen, pancreas, and testes.

Absorption of selenium occurs in the upper segment of the small intestine, being more efficient under conditions of deficiency. Increased intake frequently results in increased excretion of selenium in the urine. Erythrocyte selenium measurement is an indicator of long-term intake. Selenium is transported bound to albumin initially and subsequently to α_2-globulin.

Functions

- Selenium is a key component of glutathione peroxidase (GPX), a selenium-dependent enzyme, which can promote activities of other antioxidants and free radical scavengers in the body.

- Selenium is a key component of delenoprotein P, a selenium-containing molecule, which may act as a free radical scavenger or a transporter of selenium.

- Selenium, as selenomethionine or selenocystein, exists in a family of enzymes such as cellular glutathione peroxidase that is widely distributed in the body, which may help provide reserve of selenium in proteins that can be drawn on when needed.

- Selenium, as selenomethionine or selenocystein, exists in phospholipid hydroperoxide glutathione peroxidase that has a distribution in lipid-soluble fractions of the cell, which may have other roles in lipid and eicosanoid metabolism.

- Selenium plays a role in iodine metabolism because selenium in one enzyme is responsible for forming active T_3 from thyroglobulin stored in the thyroid gland.

- Selenium keeps the pancreas, heart, and liver, functioning properly.

- Selenium decreases MAO-B (monoamine oxidase B) enzyme activity in the brain that is increased during aging.

Health Benefits

- Selenium intake helps prevent cancers including lung, colorectal, prostate, and mammary cancer.

- Selenium intake helps prevent heart disorders.

- Selenium intake prevents Keshan's disease (a heart disease).

- Selenium intake helps improve asthma symptoms.

- Selenium intake combined with copper and zinc may increase the rate of burn wound healing.

- Selenium intake may affect the development of cataracts.

- Selenium-containing shampoos help get rid of dandruff.

- Selenium intake helps prevent osteoarthritis.

- Selenium intake helps prevent Alzheimer's disease.

- Selenium intake helps prolong longevity by delaying the progression of aging.

Deficiency Symptoms

- Muscular weakness and discomfort

- Heart attack

- Keshan's disease

- Osteoarthritis

- Cataracts

- Alzheimer's disease

- Cancers

13. Manganese

Our bodies contain 10–20 mg of manganese that is concentrated in our kidneys, pancreas, liver, and is mostly in our bones. Manganese deficiency in humans was first reported in 1972. The essentiality of manganese in humans is well established.

Manganese is absorbed throughout the small intestine. Iron and cobalt compete for common sites of absorption. Manganese is transported bound to a macroglobin, transferrin, and transmanganin. Excretion of manganese occurs mainly in the feces after secretion into the intestine via bile.

Functions

- Manganese is very important for the normal functioning of the brain and nerve areas of our body.

- Manganese is very essential for the proper and normal growth of the human bone structures.

- Manganese has antioxidant properties with a special function of controlling the flow of free radicals in the human body. These radicals are capable of damaging human cells.

- Manganese exhibits its efficiency in controlling the level of sugar in human blood.

- Manganese activates many enzymes to help in the metabolisms of cholesterol, amino acids, carbohydrates, as well as some vitamins such as vitamin E and the B vitamins and some minerals like magnesium.

- Manganese is helpful in maintaining the functioning of the digestive track. This further improves the absorption of fat in the process of digestion.

- Manganese is a component in some enzymes, including glutamine synthetase, pyruvate carboxylase, and mitochondrial superoxide dismutase.

Health Benefits

- Manganese intake aids in increasing the mineral density of spinal bone, especially in case of post menopausal women.

- Manganese intake may prevent the occurrence of certain diseases like diabetes.

- Manganese intake helps alleviate sprains and inflammation.

- Manganese intake prevents osteoporosis and osteoarthritis syndrome.

- Manganese intake prevents premenstrual syndrome for women. In such situations, manganese helps to alleviate the mood swings, headaches, depression, and irritability to a considerable extent.

- Manganese intake helps treat specific nervous disorders.

- Manganese intake aids in glucose metabolism in the human body.

- Manganese intake helps absorb fat and some vital vitamins like the B vitamins and vitamin E and some minerals like magnesium.

Deficiency Symptoms

- High blood pressure

- High cholesterol levels

- Poor eyesight

- Hearing trouble

- Severe memory loss

- Heart disorders

- Infertility in women

- Osteoporosis

- Muscular contraction

- Shivering

14. Chromium

As adults, our bodies contain approximately 14 mg of chromium that is most highly concentrated in the spleen, kidneys, testes, and hair. The heart, pancreas, lungs, and brain also contain this trace element, but in lower concentrations.

As with other minerals, organic and inorganic forms of chromium are absorbed differently. Organic chromium is readily absorbed but quickly passes out of the body. Less than 2% of the trivalent chromium consumed is absorbed. The type of dietary carbohydrate consumed modifies absorption from chromium chloride: starch rather than sugar increases absorption. The absorption of chromium ions from chromium picolinate is greater than that from chromium chloride, whose absorption efficiency is 2% or less.

The kidneys primarily excrete inorganic chromium, with small amounts being excreted through hair, sweat, and bile. Organic chromium is excreted through bile. Strenuous exercise, physical trauma, or an increased intake of simple sugar results in increased chromium being excreted.

Functions

- Chromium balances blood sugar levels by regulating insulin production.

- Chromium controls fat and cholesterol levels in the blood.

- Chromium, similar to that of zinc, helps regulate gene expression.

- Chromium assists with the functioning of neurotransmitters.

- Chromium helps balance hormones in the body by the brain.

Health Benefits

- Chromium intake helps regulate hunger by reducing food cravings.

- Chromium intake helps prevent diabetes and hypoglycemia.

- Chromium intake helps prevent hypertension.

- Chromium intake lowers high blood pressure.

- Chromium intake aids in protecting DNA and RNA

Deficiency Symptoms

- Impaired growth

- Possible advancement of arteriosclerosis and diabetes

- Hypoglycemia

- Cold sweats, dizziness or irritability after six hours without any food

- Frequent hunger

- Cold hands

- Addiction to sweet foods

- Frequent urination

- Excessive thirst

- Elevated serum cholesterol and triglyceride concentrations

- Increased incidence of aortic plaques and corneal lesions

- Decreased fertility and sperm count

15. Molybdenum

Our bodies contain approximately 5 mg of molybdenum that is most highly concentrated in the liver, kidneys, adrenal gland, and bone, with the lowest quantities found in the tissues.

Molybdenum is readily absorbed from the stomach and the small intestine, with the rate of absorption being higher in the proximal small intestine than in the distal small intestine. As with other minerals, molybdenum is absorbed by two mechanisms: carrier mediated and passive diffusion. Molybdenum is excreted primarily in the urine. Excretion rather than absorption is the homeostatic mechanism. Some molybdenum is also excreted in the bile.

Functions

- Molybdenum is a key component of the prosthetic group in xanthine oxidase, sulfite oxidase, and aldehyde oxidase, which catalyze oxidation-reduction reactions in the human body.

- Xanthine oxidase (XO) plays an important role in the normal functioning of the liver. During severe liver damage, xanthine oxidase is released into the blood, so a blood assay for XO is a way to determine if liver damage has happened.

- Sulfite oxidase plays a particular role in the normal functioning of the brain because of its importance in the sulfation of various compounds, especially in the brain.

- Aldehyde oxidase is involved not only in the oxidation of aldehydes to carboxylic acids but also in the oxidation of nitrogen-containing heterocyclic compounds and the reduction of nitro-aromatic compounds, isoxazole, and isothiazole ring systems.

- Molybdenum is a facilitator of liver detoxification.

- Molybdenum is involved in breaking down certain amino acids (the building blocks of protein) and the production of waste products for excretion in the urine.

- Molybdenum is involved in the chemical reactions that form bone, cartilage, and blood.

Health Benefits

- Molybdenum intake improves all-around health, keeping your body and mind in good shape.

- Molybdenum intake prevents liver disease.

- Molybdenum promotes normal growth of the brain.

- Molybdenum intake reduces allergy symptoms.

- Molybdenum can help prevent anemia by enabling your body to use iron.

- Molybdenum intake is useful in cases of impotence in older men.

- Molybdenum intake helps protect against dental caries and tooth decay.

- Molybdenum intake may protect against certain cancers.

Deficiency Symptoms

- Anemia

- Tooth decay

- Impotence

- Irritability

- Poor general health

- Irregular heartbeat

- Premature death in early childhood

Chapter Five
ORAC of Foods and Human Health

1. ORAC

ORAC is an abbreviation for Oxygen Radical Absorbance Capacity. ORAC is a method of measuring antioxidant capacities of different foods or dietary supplements. The research behind ORAC has been around for more than a century, but it wasn't until 1990 that the ORAC assay was first used to test food against an extract at the National Institute on Aging. It was developed by the scientists at the National Institute on Aging in the National Institutes of Health (NIH) in Maryland. The U.S. Department of Agriculture (USDA) listed a database of the ORAC values on its home page (www.usda.gov). A wide variety of foods have been tested using this methodology, with certain spices, berries, and legumes rated very highly. Correlation between the high antioxidant capacity of fruits and vegetables, and the positive impact of diets high in fruits and vegetables, is believed to play an important role in the free-radical theory of aging.

2. Free-Radical Theory of Aging and Disease

In 1956, Dr. Denham Harman proposed the free-radical theory of aging, which suggests that aging is caused by highly reactive molecules called free radicals. The theory received less than enthusiastic acceptance from the scientific community. Since that time, however, many scientists throughout the world have studied the complex relationship between free radicals and aging. Their findings have supported Dr. Harman's original hypothesis. Today, the free-radical theory of aging is widely accepted as one of the foremost explanations for the aging process and recognized as a practical guide to a longer, healthier life span.

A free radical is an atom, molecule or molecular fragment that contains at least one unpaired electron, in contrast to normal molecules, which contain only paired electrons. Free radicals, together with non-radicals that contribute to free radical production, are often referred to as reactive oxygen species.

Free radicals are a byproduct of aerobic, or oxygen-using, metabolism that generates ATP, the cell's energy source, from the foods we eat. During this process, which occurs in specialized cell parts called mitochondria, electrons are passed from molecule to molecule. Most of the electrons (97%–99%) are taken up by oxygen at the end of the transport chain. The remaining electrons combine incorrectly with oxygen to form superoxide, a free radical that is the major source of other free radicals in the cell.

Having an unpaired electron makes a free radical unstable, so it tries to stabilize itself by either gaining an additional electron or losing its unpaired electron. It can only accomplish this by reacting with other cell molecules, such as proteins, lipids, and DNA. When the free radical gains or loses an electron, it converts the donor/recipient molecule into a free radical, thus initiating a destructive cascade of free radical reactions.

Free radical reactions cause widespread damage to the cell molecules and, subsequently, the cells themselves. Many of the detrimental effects of free radical reactions occur within the mitochondria, particularly the mitochondrial DNA, which contains the genetic information needed for the production of proteins and other molecules used during energy production. Unlike damage to the DNA of the cell nucleus, damage to mitochondrial DNA is not often repaired. Instead, it accumulates, leading to ever-increasing functional impairment. Other molecules also cease to function normally when damaged by free radical reactions. This, in turn, disrupts the vital cellular systems that require those molecules for proper functioning. When the damage inflicted by free radical reactions becomes so severe that the cell cannot repair it or compensate for it, the cell dies. If this process occurs in many cells throughout an organ or tissue, the result can be irreversible organ failure.

Research has shown that the damaging effects of free radicals on molecular and cellular functions are involved not only in aging, but also in diseases, such as atherosclerosis, cancer, and Alzheimer's disease. If the attack of free radicals is in the arteries, a do-it-yourself bandage that uses cholesterol and calcium heals the wound, and then you get "hardening of the arteries" and high blood pressure. If it happens in the capillaries, they may begin to leak, thereby causing easy bruising and loss of blood internally. If it happens in the joints, it's called arthritis. In the pancreas it's called diabetes. On neurons, it's called Parkinson's or Multiple Sclerosis. Free radical damage has been associated with many types of cancer. Most chronic degenerative diseases have been linked to free radicals.

3. Daily Free-Radical Amounts in the Human Body

Free radicals in the human body can be caused by (1) metabolic processes, (2) cigarette-smoking, (3) exposure to electromagnetic radiation such as copy machines, computer monitors, cell phones, and television sets, (4) exposure to free radicals in the air we breathe and in the water we drink, (5) processed foods that have many added chemicals, (6) smog, (7) pesticides, (8) drugs, and/or (9) emotional stress. Emotional stress, including anxiety, tension, frustration, and anger require more oxygen to meet your accelerated and intensified heart and breathing rates, thus more free radicals could be generated. So, in order to reduce the free radical amounts, we should pay much more attention to causes (2) to (9).

In the human body, the following types of free radicals can be produced:

- Superoxide radical (O_2^-). This is the most "famous" one that accounts for 97%–99% of the total free radical amounts. It is produced by phagocytic cells and can be beneficial because it inactivates viruses and bacteria.

- Hydroxyl radical ($\cdot OH$). It is always harmful.

- Nitric oxide ($NO\cdot$). It has beneficial effects in that it is a vasodilator agent, can function as a neurotransmitter and can be produced by macrophages and act to kill parasites. Nitric oxide may also be harmful when it reacts with superoxide to form the peroxynitrite anion.

- Peroxyl radical ($ROO\cdot$). This is the most common radical in biological systems.

Free radicals are produced as products of normal cellular oxidative metabolism through the following metabolic processes:

$$O_2 \text{ (Oxygen)} \rightarrow O_2^- \rightarrow H_2O_2 \rightarrow \cdot OH \rightarrow H_2O \text{ (water)}$$

A normal adult would utilize about 3.5 mL oxygen/kg/min. By calculation, a 70-kg human breathes 352.8 liters (504 g) of oxygen each day (24 hours) from air. The literature suggests that anywhere from 2% to 5% of the total oxygen intake during both rest and exercise have the ability to form the highly damaging superoxide radical via electron escape. A 70 kg human produces about 10–25 g of free radicals. The calculated results of the free radical amounts produced by different body weights are presented in Table 5-1.

Table 5-1 Daily free radical amounts produced in our bodies

Body weight(kg[lb])	Daily free radical amount (g)		
	Minimum	Maximum	Average
44 [97]	6.3	15.8	11.1
46 [101]	6.6	16.6	11.6
48 [106]	6.9	17.6	12.3
50 [110]	7.2	18.0	12.6
52 [115]	7.5	18.7	13.1
54 [119]	7.8	19.4	13.6
56 [124]	8.1	20.2	14.1
58 [128]	8.4	20.9	14.6
60 [132]	8.6	21.6	15.1
62 [137]	8.9	22.3	15.6
64 [141]	9.2	23.0	16.1
66 [146]	9.5	23.8	16.6
68 [150]	9.8	24.5	17.1
70 [154]	10.1	25.2	17.6
72 [159]	10.4	25.9	18.1
74 [163]	10.7	26.6	18.6
76 [168]	10.9	27.4	19.2
78 [172]	11.2	28.1	19.7
80 [176]	11.5	28.8	20.2
82 [181]	11.8	29.5	20.7
84 [185]	12.1	30.2	21.2
86 [189]	12.4	31.0	21.7
88 [194]	12.7	31.7	22.2
90 [198]	13.0	32.4	22.7

During exercise, oxygen consumption increases 10–20 folds to 35–70 ml/kg/min. Thus, during exercise, a person will increase 10–20 times the free radical amounts in his/her body. In addition, cigarette-smoking, exposure to electromagnetic radiation, air and water pollution, pesticides, drugs, emotional stress, et al. also will increase the total amount of free radicals in your body.

4. ORAC Scores of Selected Foods

In 2007, scientists in the United States Department of Agriculture (USDA) published an updated list of ORAC values for 277 foods commonly consumed by the U.S. population (fruits, vegetables, nuts, seeds, spices, grains, etc.). Values were reported as micromoles of Trolox equivalents (TE, vitamin E derivative) per 100 grams both for lipid-soluble ("lipophilic" as for carotenoids) and water-soluble ("hydrophilic" as for phenolics) antioxidant chemicals in foods, thus it is a sum of lipophilic and hydrophilic values or total ORAC. These values are considered to be more accurate than previously published ORAC numbers because lipophilic values were being included for the first time. The data showed that all plants have variable amounts of both lipophilic and hydrophilic phytochemicals that contribute to the total ORAC. Table 5-2 summarizes total ORAC values (scores) of 147 foods in the following order: vegetables, fruits, legumes, cereal and grain, dairy, bread, nuts and seeds, oil, beverage, and spice. According to the scores per 100g, I calculated the scores per normal portion (NP) for the selected foods, which are also listed in Table 5-2.

Table 5-2 ORAC scores per 100g and per normal portion (NP) of selected foods

Food name	ORAC/100g	Normal portion	Amount (g)	ORAC /NP
Vegetables				
Artichoke, raw	6552	base & ends-leaves	100	6552
Asparagus, raw	2150	4 large spears	100	2150
Beets, green, raw	1945	1 cup	150	2918
Broccoli, raw	1362	1 med. stalk	180	2452
Cabbage, raw	508	1 cup finely	90	457
Cabbage, red, raw	2252	1 cup shredded	100	2252
Carrots, raw	666	1 carrot 7.5 × 1.125 in.	80	533
Cauliflower, raw	829	1 cup whole floweretes	100	829
Celery, raw	497	1 cup chopped	120	596
Corn, raw	728	1 cob 5×1.75 in. (kernels)	140	1019

Cucumber, raw	214	1 small 6.5 × 1.5 in.	180	385
Eggplant, raw	14500	1 cup diced	200	29000
Garlic, raw	5346	1 clove (1.3×0.5×0.3 in.)	3	160
Leeks, raw	490	3–4 (5 inches)	100	490
Lettuce, iceberg, raw	438	wedge 0.125 in. of head	90	394
Lettuce, green leaf, raw	1447	1 cup chopped	55	796
Lettuce, red leaf, raw	2380	1 cup chopped	55	1309
Onions, white, raw	863	1 cup chopped	160	1381
Onions, red, raw	1521	1 cup chopped	160	2434
Parsley, raw	1301	1T. chopped	4	52
Peppers, sweet, green, raw	923	1 cup strips	100	923
Peppers, sweet, green, salted	615	1 cup strips	100	615
Peppers, sweet, yellow, raw	965	1 cup strips	100	965
Peppers, sweet, red, raw	791	1 cup strips	100	791
Potatoes, white, flesh and skin, raw	1058	2.75 × 4.25 in.	250	2645
Potatoes, white, flesh and skin, baked	1138	2.75 × 4.25 in.	250	2845
Potatoes, red, flesh and skin, raw	1098	2.75 × 4.25 in.	250	2745
Potatoes, red, flesh and skin, baked	1326	2.75 × 4.25 in.	250	3315
Radishes, red, raw	1736	10 small (1 in. diam.)	100	1736
Spinach, raw	1515	1 cup chopped	55	833
Squash, summer, skin, raw	180	1 cup cubed	130	234
Squash, winter, butternut, raw	396	1 cup cubed	130	515

Tomatoes, red, ripe, raw, yr. round ave.	367	2.5 inch diam.	100	367
Fruits				
Apples, Fuji, raw, with skin	2589	1 med. 2.75 in. diam.	150	3884
Apples, Gala, raw, with skin	2882	1 med. 2.75 in. diam.	150	4323
Apples, Golden, raw, with skin	2670	1 med. 2.75 in. diam.	150	4005
Apples, Golden, raw, without skin	2210	1 med. 2.75 in. diam.	150	3315
Apples, Red, raw, with skin	4234	1 med. 2.75 in. diam.	150	6351
Apples, Red, raw, without skin	2936	1 med. 2.75 in. diam.	150	4404
Apples, raw, with skin	3082	1 med. 2.75 in. diam.	150	4623
Apples, raw, without skin	2573	1 med. 2.75 in. diam.	150	3860
Apricots, raw	1115	1 med.	40	446
Avocados, Hass, raw	1933	1 cup	150	2900
Bananas, raw	879	1 med.	150	1319
Blackberries, raw	5347	1 cup	140	7486
Blueberries, raw	6552	1 cup	140	9173
Chokeberries, raw	16062	1 cup	140	22487
Cranberries, raw	9584	1 cup	140	13418
Elderberries, raw	14697	1 cup	140	20576
Figs, raw	3383	2 large/3 small	100	3383
Grapefruit, pink&red, raw, all areas	1548	sections 1 cup	190	2941
Grape, white or green, raw	1118	1 cup	150	1677
Grape, red, raw	1126	1 cup	150	1689
Honeydew melons, raw	241	1 med. Slice	20	48
Limes, raw	82	1 med.	100	82

Kiwi fruit (Chinese gooseberries), raw	882	1 med.	50	441
Kiwi, gold, raw	1210	1 med.	50	605
Mangos, raw	1002	1cup diced	140	1403
Nectarine, raw	750	2 med.	100	750
Oranges, raw, navels	1819	1 med.	180	3274
Oranges, mandarin, tangerines, raw	1620	1 med.	100	1620
Peaches, raw	1814	1 med.	100	1814
Pears, raw	2941	1 med.	100	2941
Pears, green cultivars, raw	1911	1 med.	100	1911
Pears, red anjou, raw	1746	1 med.	100	1746
Pineapples, raw, all varieties	385	1 cup diced	140	539
Plums, raw	6259	2 med.	100	6259
Raisins, seedless	3037	2 table spoon	18	547
Raspberries, raw	4482	¾ cup	100	4482
Strawberries, raw	3577	1 cup whole	150	5366
Watermelon, raw	142	1 med. Slice	300	426
Legumes				
Beans, black, mature seeds, raw	8040	½ cup	100	8040
Beans, kidney, red mature seeds, raw	8459	½ cup	100	8459
Beans, navy, mature seeds, raw	1530	½ cup	100	1530
Beans, pink, mature seeds, raw	8320	½ cup	100	8320
Beans, pinto, mature seeds, raw	7779	½ cup	100	7779
Beans, pinto, mature seeds, cooked	904	½ cup	100	904
Beans, snap, green, raw	759	½ cup	100	759

Chickpeas (garbanzo beans), raw	847	¼ cup	50	424
Cowpeas, common, mature seeds, raw	4343	½ cup	70	2128
Lentils, raw	7282	½ cup	100	7282
Peas, yellow, mature seeds, raw	741	1 cup	140	1037
Peas, split, mature seeds, raw	524	1 cup	140	734
Soybeans, mature seeds, raw	5764	¼ cup	50	2882
Cereal and Grain				
Cereals, oats, old fashioned, uncooked	1708	1 cup	80	1366
Cereals, oats, quick, uncooked	2169	1 cup	80	1735
Cereal, oats, instant, fortified, dry	2380	1 cup	80	1904
Cereal, ready-to-eat, corn flakes	2359	1 cup	60	1415
Chocolate, dutched powder	40200	¼ cup	50	20100
Cocoa, dry powder, unsweetened	80933	¼ cup	50	40467
Corn, sweet, yellow, raw	728	½ cup	100	728
Popcorn, air-popped	1743	3 cups	42	732
Sorghum, grain, black	21900	¼ cup	50	10950
Sorghum, grain, hi-tannin	45400	¼ cup	50	22700
Sorghum, grain, red	14000	¼ cup	50	7000
Sorghum, grain, white	2200	¼ cup	50	1100
Sumac, grain, raw	86800	¼ cup	50	43400
Sumac, bran, raw	312400	1 cup	80	249920
Rice bran, crude	24287	1cup	80	19430

Dairy				
Milk, chocolate, fluid, reduced fat	1263	1 cup	244	3082
Bread				
Bread, butternut whole grain	2104	1 slice	25	526
Bread, mixed-grain	1421	1 slice	25	355
Bread, oatnut	1318	1 slice	25	330
Bread, pumpernickel	1963	1 slice	32	628
Nuts and Seeds				
Almonds	4454	1 table spoon	8	356
Cashew, raw	1948	14 large	28	545
Peanuts, all types, raw	3166	15 whole	9	289
Pecans	17940	10 large	9	1615
Walnuts, English	13541	7 in shell	28	3792
Oil				
Olive oil, extra-virgin	1150	1 table spoon	14	161
Peanut oil	106	1 table spoon	14	15
Beverage				
Apple juice, canned or bottled	408	1 cup	244	996
Blueberry juice	2906	1 cup	244	7086
Concord grape juice	2377	1 cup	244	5800
Cranberry juice, white	232	1 cup	244	566
Grape juice, red	1788	1 cup	244	4363
Strawberry juice	1002	1 cup	244	2445
Grape juice, white	793	1 cup	244	1935
Grapefruit juice, white, raw	1238	1 cup	244	3009
Lemon juice, raw	1225	1 cup	244	2989
Lime juice, raw	823	1 cup	244	2008
Orange juice, raw	726	1 cup	244	1771
Pear juice, all varieties	704	1 cup	244	1718

Pineapple juice, canned	568	1 cup	244	1386
Prune juice, canned	2036	1 cup	244	4968
Tomato juice, canned	486	1 cup	244	1186
Vegetable juice cocktail, canned	548	1 cup	244	1337
Wine, table, red	3873	¼ cup	61	2363
Wine, table, red, Cabernet Suavignon .	5034	¼ cup	61	3071
Wine, table, rose,	1005	¼ cup	61	613
Wine, table, white	392	¼ cup	61	239
Spice				
Basil, dried	67553	1 table spoon	8	5404
Cardamom	2764	1 table spoon	8	221
Chili powder	23636	1 table spoon	8	1891
Cinnamon, ground	267536	1 table spoon	8	21403
Cloves, ground	314446	1 table spoon	8	25156
Cumin seed	76800	1 table spoon	8	6144
Curry powder	48504	1 table spoon	8	3880
Garlic powder	6665	1 table spoon	8	533
Ginger, ground	28811	1 table spoon	8	2305
Mustard seed, yellow	29257	1 table spoon	8	2341
Onion powder	5735	1 table spoon	8	459
Oregano, dried	200129	1 table spoon	8	16010
Paprika	17919	1 table spoon	8	1434
Parsley, dried	74349	1 table spoon	8	5948
Pepper, black	27618	1 table spoon	8	2209
Poppy seed	481	1 table spoon	8	38
Turmeric, ground	159277	1 table spoon	8	12742

5. ORAC and Human Health

An antioxidant is any substance that, when present at low concentrations compared to those of an oxidizable substrate, significantly delays or prevents the oxidation of substrates. The normal antioxidant defense system in biological systems consists of both enzymatic and nonenzymatic systems. Although both are important in biological systems, when we consider the role of food antioxidants, we will be considering the nonenzymatic antioxidant systems which include substances such as: alpha-tocopherol (vitamin E), ascorbic acid (vitamin C), glutathione, flavonoids, β-carotene (vitamin A precursor), uric acid, and plasma proteins such as albumin, ceruloplasmin, transferrin, metalothionein, etc.

According to the studies on antioxidant for aging conducted by some researchers, foods with high ORAC scores generally have the following benefits:

• Raises the antioxidant for aging power of human blood by 10 to 25 percent

• Prevents some loss of long-term memory and learning ability

• Maintains the ability of brain cells to respond to a chemical stimulus—a function that normally decreases with age

• Protects tiny blood vessels and capillaries against oxygen damage

Based on these apparent results, it is the contention of antioxidant for aging nutritionist Ronald L. Prior that, if it is shown that there is a relationship between ORAC scores and health outcome in peoples, then there will come a point when ORAC scores may become a new standard for good antioxidant for aging power.

The higher the score, the more powerful the food is as an antioxidant. High ORAC foods are critical for your health, as they help eliminate free radicals that contribute to or cause cancer, aging, heart disease, and other diseases and conditions.

Free radicals, or oxygen radicals, are chemicals formed by natural cellular energy processing, and most are carried away as waste by your body and are either excreted or recycled. Exercise creates free radicals; sunlight, pollution, and even digestion also create free radicals. These chemicals are highly reactive, and recent studies indicate that they can damage DNA or cellular structures, causing disease as well as the sort of damage that results in cancer. Normally, these free radicals are eliminated by normal processes in the body. But if you've had a lot of free radical activity, your body may not be able to eliminate all of them. In cases like this, it is a good idea to ramp up your consumption of high ORAC foods.

For most people, eating a diet that adheres to the USDA food pyramid will give you an adequate supply of high ORAC foods, especially if you focus on eating a rainbow of fruits and vegetables, especially the dark-colored ones.

By eating a diet with a minimum of 5000 ORAC units per day, you can increase your blood plasma level of antioxidants by more than 25%.

If you work out a lot, such as heavy labor and physical activity, or if you've had a lot of sun or have been sick, boosting your ORAC is probably a good idea.

The average life expectancy of many species has been increased by more than 20 percent by adding antioxidants to the diet. This increase is equivalent to raising the average human life span from the present 74.8 years to 97.8 years.

Chapter Six
pH of Blood and Human Health

1. Composition of Blood

Normally, 7%–8% of human body weight is blood. Blood is a red liquid connective tissue that measures about 4–6 liters in an adult, depending on the body size. Its normal pH range is from 7.35 to 7.45. This essential fluid carries out the critical functions of transporting oxygen and nutrients to our cells and getting rid of carbon dioxide, ammonia, and other waste products. In addition, it plays a vital role in our immune system and in maintaining a relatively constant body temperature. Blood is a highly specialized tissue composed of many different kinds of components. Four of the most important ones are red blood cells, white blood cells, platelets, and plasma. Of the total blood volume in the human body, 50%–60% is plasma or the liquid portion of the blood. The rest of the blood volume, including "formed elements" (red blood cells, white blood cells, and platelets), antibodies, and inorganic butters, accounts for 40%–50%. All humans produce these blood components—there are no populational or regional differences.

Red blood cells, or erythrocytes, are relatively large microscopic cells that don't have any nuclei. In this latter trait, they are similar to the primitive prokaryotic cells of bacteria. Red blood cells normally make up 40%–50% of the total blood volume. They transport oxygen from the lungs to all of the living tissues of the body and carry away carbon dioxide. The red cells are produced continuously in our bone marrow from stem cells at a rate of about 2–3 million cells per second. Hemoglobin is the gas transporting protein molecule that makes up 95% of a red blood cell. Each red blood cell has about 270,000,000 iron-rich hemoglobin molecules. People who are anemic generally have a deficiency in red blood cells. The red color of blood is primarily due to oxygenated red blood cells.

White blood cells, or leukocytes, exist in variable numbers and types but make up a very small part of the blood's volume—normally only about 1% in healthy people. Leukocytes are not limited to blood. They occur elsewhere in the body as well, most notably in the spleen, liver, and lymph glands. Most are produced in our bone marrow from the same kind of stem cells that produce red blood cells. Others are produced in the thymus gland, which is at the base of the neck. Some white blood cells (called lymphocytes) are the first responders for our immune system. They seek out, identify, and bind to alien protein on bacteria, viruses, and fungi so that they can be removed. Other white blood cells (called granulocytes and macrophages) then arrive to surround and destroy the alien cells. They also get rid of dead or dying blood cells as well as foreign matter such as dust and asbestos. Red blood cells remain viable for only about 4 months before they are removed from the blood and their components recycled in the spleen. White blood cells usually only last 18–36 hours before they also are removed, even though some types live for as much as a year. The description of white blood cells presented here is a simplification. There are actually many specialized sub-types of them that participate in different ways in our immune responses.

Platelets, or thrombocytes, are cell fragments without nuclei that work with blood clotting chemicals at the site of wounds. They do this by adhering to the walls of blood vessels, thereby plugging the rupture in the vascular wall. They can also release coagulating chemicals which cause clots to form in the blood that can plug up narrowed blood vessels. There are more than a dozen types of blood clotting factors and platelets that need to interact in the blood clotting process. Recent research has shown that platelets help fight infections by releasing proteins that kill invading bacteria and some other microorganisms. In addition, platelets stimulate the immune system. Individual platelets are about 1/3 the size of red blood cells. They have a lifespan of 9–10 days. Like the red and white blood cells, platelets are produced in the bone marrow from stem cells.

Plasma is the relatively clear liquid water, sugar, fat, protein, and salt solution that carries red blood cells, white blood cells, platelets, and some other chemicals. Normally, 55% of our blood's volume is made up of plasma. About 95% of plasma consists of water. As the heart pumps blood to cells throughout the body, plasma brings nourishment to them and removes the waste products of metabolism. Plasma also contains blood clotting factors, sugars, lipids, vitamins, minerals, hormones, enzymes, antibodies, and other proteins. It is likely that plasma contains some of every protein produced by the body—approximately 500 have been identified in human plasma so far.

2. Functions of Blood

Blood functions as a transport medium. The general functions of blood include transportation, regulation, and protection. These categories overlap and interact as the blood carries out its role in providing suitable conditions for cellular functions. The detailed functions of blood are summarized as follows:

- Carries oxygen and nutrients to cells.

- Transports carbon dioxide and wastes from tissues to the lungs and the kidneys, where wastes can be removed from the body.

- Carries hormones to the endocrine glands to the target tissues.

- Helps regulate body temperature by removing heat from active areas, such as skeletal muscles, and transporting it to other areas of the skin so that the heat can be dissipated.

- Plays a significant role in fluid and electrolyte balance because salt and plasma proteins contribute to osmotic pressure by providing weight and bulk to our blood.

- Functions in pH regulation through the action of buffer systems in the blood.

- Clotting mechanisms prevent fluid loss when blood vessels are damaged.

- Certain cells in the blood, phagocytic white blood cells, help protect the body against diseases by engulfing and destroying the agents.

- Antibodies in the plasma help protect against diseases by their reaction with offending agents.

3. Amount of Blood in the Human Body

Normally, blood accounts for 7%–8% of human body weight. Thus, different body weights have different blood weights, thereby, different blood volumes. By using 7.5% of the human body weight, I calculated the average blood weights of different body weights. The results are shown in Table 6-1. The density of blood is in the range of 1.0475 to 1.0537 g/ml. I computed the blood volumes of different body weights by taking the medium value of the density: 1.0506 g/ml. The computed results are also listed in Table 6-1.

Table 6-1 Blood weights and volumes of different body weights

Body weight (kg [lb])	Blood weight (kg [lb])	Blood volume (L)
44 [97]	3.30 [7.3]	3.14

46 [101]	3.45 [7.6]	3.28
48 [106]	3.60 [7.9]	3.43
50 [110]	3.75 [8.3]	3.57
52 [115]	3.90 [8.6]	3.71
54 [119]	4.05 [8.9]	3.85
56 [124]	4.20 [9.3]	4.00
58 [128]	4.35 [9.6]	4.14
60 [132]	4.50 [9.9]	4.28
62 [137]	4.65 [10.3]	4.43
64 [141]	4.80 [10.6]	4.57
66 [146]	4.95 [10.9]	4.71
68 [150]	5.10 [11.2]	4.85
70 [154]	5.25 [11.6]	5.00
72 [159]	5.40 [11.9]	5.14
74 [163]	5.55 [12.2]	5.28
76 [168]	5.70 [12.6]	5.43
78 [172]	5.85 [12.9]	5.57
80 [176]	6.00 [13.2]	5.71
82 [181]	6.15 [13.6]	5.85
84 [185]	6.30 [13.9]	6.00
86 [189]	6.45 [14.2]	6.14
88 [194]	6.60 [14.6]	6.28
90 [198]	6.75 [14.9]	6.42

Everyone with weights in the range of 44 kg (97 lb)–90 kg (198 lb) can find his or her blood weight and blood volume. Blood volume and its quality are very important to the functions of all the cells and organs in our body, and ultimately, to our health.

4. Blood pH Theory of Disease and Aging

Blood is the river of life, as the Bible states: "*For the Life of the flesh is in the blood ...*" (Leviticus 17:11). In Table 6-1, humans with the weights of 44 to 90 kg have blood volumes between 3.14 to 6.42 liters, which flows into 60,000 miles of veins and arteries. As stated before, blood has many vital functions, particularly in our immune system because of its prevention of diseases. The pH in blood controls various functions of blood and must be kept in a very narrow range of 7.35–7.45 in order to ensure its normal functions. Below or above this range means symptoms and diseases.

If the pH of your blood falls below 7.35, the result is a condition called acidosis, a state that leads to central nervous system depression. Severe acidosis, where the blood pH falls below 7.00, can lead to a coma and even death. If the pH of your blood rises above 7.45, the result is alkalosis. Severe alkalosis can also lead to death, but through a different mechanism. Alkalosis causes all of the nerves in your body to become hypersensitive and overexcited, often resulting in muscle spasms, nervousness, and convulsions. The convulsions usually cause death in severe cases.

Mild acidosis can cause problems such as:

- Cardiovascular damage, including the constriction of blood vessels and the reduction of oxygen.

- Weight gain, obesity, and diabetes.

- Bladder and kidney conditions, including kidney stones.

- Immune deficiency.

- Acceleration of free radical damage, possibly contributing to cancerous mutations.

- Hormone concerns.

- Premature aging.

- Osteoporosis; weak, brittle bones, hip fractures, and bone spurs.

- Joint pain, aching muscles, and lactic acid buildup.

- Low energy and chronic fatigue.

- Slow digestion and elimination.

- Yeast/fungal overgrowth.

pH is a measure of how acidic or alkaline a liquid is. The pH scale ranges from 0 (the highest acidic) to 14 (the highest alkaline). A liquid with a pH of 7 is neutral. At pH 7, water or a liquid contains equal amounts of H^+ and OH^- ions. Liquid with a pH of less than 7 is acidic because it contains a higher concentration of H^+ ions. Liquid with a pH of more than 7 is alkaline because it contains a higher concentration of OH^- ions. The pH scale is from

0 to 14 and is logarithmic, which means that each step is ten times the previous one. In other words, a pH of 5 is 10 times more acidic than 6, 100 times more acidic than 7, and 1000 times more acidic than 8. In this light, you can see how a slight change in your blood pH value can have a great impact on your internal environment and your health.

A very important function of blood is to carry oxygen that comes into cells by breathing. About 90% of the body's life energy is created by oxygen. In fact, all functions of the body are regulated by oxygen. At pH 7.0 of blood, the oxygen content of blood is less than 15% compared to that at pH 7.2, and is less than 25% compared to that at pH 7.4. So, a lower pH of blood can greatly affect all functions of the body because pH controls the speed of the body's millions of biochemical reactions. It does this by controlling the speed of enzyme activity as well as the speed that electricity moves through the body.

More and more research is showing that low oxygen delivery to cells under a low pH of blood is a major factor in most, if not all, degenerative conditions. Fully breath of each cell in your body depends on having an optimum pH balance.

In general, degenerative diseases are the result of acid waste build-up within weak cells and organs. When we are born, we have the highest alkaline mineral concentration, establishing the highest pH. That is why most degenerative diseases do not occur when you are young. They usually occur after 40 years of age.

Cancer cell growth is caused by acid. All healthy cells carry an electromagnetic negative charge, but all fermented cells and their acids carry an electromagnetic positive charge. These rotting cells and their acids act like glue to attract healthy cells. This leads to oxygen deprivation where healthy cells begin to rot. This is cancer. It is Dr. Gary Tunsky's conclusion based on years of research and study that cancer are nothing more or less than a cellular disturbance of the electromagnetic balance due to acid pH disorganization of the cellular microzymas, their morbid evolution to bacteria, yeast fungus and molds, and their production of exotoxins and mycotoxins. Cancer, therefore, is a four-letter word: ACID, especially lactic acid as a waste product due to the low oxygen level and waste products of yeast and fungus.

Nobel laureate, Dr. Otto Warburg of Germany, won his Nobel Prize for his discovery of oxygen deficiency in the cancer growth process. As stated above, when our pH is off and our bodies are running more acidic, our cells are getting less oxygen. Cancer thrives under an acid tissue pH/oxygen deficient environment. If you cover your mouth and nose, oxygen is cut off and carbon dioxide is built up as an acid waste and you will eventually pass out through asphyxiation. And **if your body's blood pH goes below seven, oxy-**

gen is cut off and you will be put into a coma or death will occur. Blood performs a balancing act in order to maintain the blood pH within a safe range of 7.35–7.45. Some cells don't die as normal cells do in an acid environment, instead they may adapt and survive by becoming abnormal cells like primitive yeast cells. These abnormal primitive yeast cells are called malignant cells. Malignant renegade cells do not communicate with brain function, or with their own DNA memory code. Therefore, malignant cells grow indefinitely and without order. This biological disorder is what science calls cancer.

Diabetes is caused by acid. The pancreas produces one of the highest pH body fluids—pancreatic juice with a pH of 8.8. A shortage of calcium ions in the body impairs the production and the release of the insulin hormone. This eventually leads to an acidic blood condition. With the accumulated acidic waste products coating the receptor sites of the insulin producing beta cells, insulin is prevented from being synthesized or utilized, so that the glucose concentration could not be decreased to normal level. Diabetes is the result.

Allergies are acid related. Allergies are an irritation/inflammation reaction appearing as allergy symptoms as a means of dealing with acid toxins. If a beneficial cleansing substance is taken, such as wheat grass or fresh vegetable juice, symptoms like sinus swelling, runny nose, skin reactions, tearing eyes, etc., are all ways of eliminating acid toxins. Thus, yeast and fungus, whose poisons are acid, may contribute significantly to your hay fever and sneezing. If you have no symptogenic yeast or fungus, it would be impossible for you to have allergies.

Obesity is linked to acid pH. Over ingestion of carbohydrates, proteins, and fats and not enough exercise to burn them as fuel causes our bodies to store fatty acids. Acetic acid, lactic acid and LDL (low-density lipoprotein) cholesterol are the derivatives of fatty acid. Lactic acids and acetic acids lower the pH of body fluids drastically. This prevents the cellular engines from burning on all cylinders reducing metabolic rate. So, a combination with a lack of exercise, toxic acidic residues around the cell, infiltration of morbid microforms in and around the cell, and a reduction of peak performance energy burning from the mitochondria engines, causes obesity to set in.

Arthritis is caused by acidity. Many different forms of arthritis are the result of acid accumulation from the blood into the joints and wrists. It is this accumulated acid that damages cartilage and coats the cells that produce synovial and bursa fluids causing a dryness which irritates the joints, manifesting swelling.

Most diseases are acid related. The underlying causes of cancer, heart disease, arteriosclerosis, high blood pressure, diabetes, arthritis, gout, kidney disease, asthma, allergies, psoriasis and other skin disorders, indigestion, diarrhea, nausea, obesity, tooth and gum diseases, osteoporosis, eye diseases, etc., are the accumulation of acids in tissues and cells. Poor blood and lymph circulation, and poor cell activity are due to toxic acidic residues accumulating around the cell membrane which prevent nutritional elements from entering the cells. The accumulation of toxic acids is caused by the low pH of blood that leads to a lack of oxygen in cells and tissues. All these diseases accelerate the aging process.

5. Blood pH Balance in the Human Body

As stated above, the pH of blood must be kept in the narrow range of 7.35–7.45 in order to achieve good health. If the pH is out of range, symptoms, diseases, and even death will occur. Therefore, everyone is concerned with if his/her blood pH is within the range of 7.35–7.45. The following paragraphs will discuss the causes of the pH of blood being out of range, and will then explain how to make the blood pH balance in the range.

Diet, metabolism, and a stressful lifestyle can directly affect the pH levels of all body fluids, which determines how well your immune system functions. A weakened immune system, of course, means low resistance to infections. High acid also allows LDL-cholesterol (the bad cholesterol) to build up faster in your arteries, damaging artery walls, and creating plaque buildup.

When you ingest foods and liquid drinks, the end products of digestion and assimilation of nutrients often results in an acid or alkaline-forming effect. The end products are sometimes called acid ash or alkaline ash. High acidity enters your body when you eat processed foods, pre-packaged foods, sugary foods, pastas, dairy products (milk, cheese, ice cream, etc.), alcoholic beverages, coffee, cola, or drugs. Meat also promotes acidity.

In addition, as your cells produce energy on a continual basis, a number of different acids are formed and released into your body fluids. These acids, generated by your daily metabolic activities, are unavoidable; as long as your body generates energy to survive, it will produce a continuous supply of acids.

Also, stress plays a significant role in creating excess acid. This is why people with type A personalities, who tend to live in a perpetual state of tension and rigidity, are prone to developing acidic conditions. If you don't get enough sleep or exercise, or face life-changing events (loss of a job, divorce, moving to a new city, etc), your body probably has more acid than it can handle.

So, there are three main forces at work on a daily basis that can disrupt the pH of your body fluids (these forces are the acid or alkaline): (1) forming effects of foods and liquids that you ingest, (2) the acids that you generate through regular metabolic activities, and (3) stress.

Fortunately, your body has five major mechanisms at work at all times to prevent these forces from shifting the pH of your blood to outside the 7.35 to 7.45 range, much like our internal thermostat that tries to maintain a 98.6-degree Fahrenheit (37-degree Celsius) body temperature. These mechanisms are (1) buffer systems including a carbonic acid-bicarbonate buffer system, a protein buffer system, and a phosphate buffer system, (2) exhalation of carbon dioxide, (3) elimination of hydrogen ions via kidneys, (4) elimination of acidic residues through the skin, and (5) pushing blood acid residues and accumulated toxins into outer extremities as a storage bin away from vital organs. The wrist, joints, fingers, toes, and skin are the major target areas to keep the toxins away from saturating internal vital organs like the heart and the lungs.

When dietary, metabolic, and stressful factors pushes the pH of your blood outside the 7.35–7.45 range, they work together to make your blood pH in balance. For example, your phosphate buffer system uses different phosphate ions in your body to neutralize strong acids and bases. About 85% of the phosphate ions that are used in your phosphate buffer system come from calcium phosphate salts, which are structural components of your bones and teeth. If your body fluids are regularly exposed to large quantities of acid-forming foods and liquids, your body will draw upon its calcium phosphate reserves to supply your phosphate buffer system to neutralize the acid-forming effects of your diet. Over time, this may lead to structural weakness in your bones and teeth.

Drawing on your calcium phosphate reserves at a high rate can also increase the amount of calcium that is eliminated via your genito-urinary system, which is why a predominantly acid-forming diet can increase your risk of developing calcium-rich kidney stones.

This is just one example of how your buffering systems can be overtaxed to a point where you experience negative health consequences. Since your buffering systems have to work all the time anyway to neutralize the acids that are formed from daily metabolic activities, it is in your best interest to optimize your diets to make sure it doesn't create unnecessary work for your buffering systems.

6. Effects of Common Foods on Blood pH Balance

Generally speaking, most vegetables and fruits have an alkaline-forming effect on your body fluids. Most grains, meat, and highly processed foods have an acid-forming effect on your body fluids. Your health is best served by a good mix of nutrient-dense alkaline and acid-forming foods; ideally, you want to eat more alkaline-forming foods than acid-forming foods to have the net acid and alkaline-forming effects of your diet match the slightly alkaline pH of your blood.

The following lists indicate which common foods have an alkaline-forming effect on your body fluids, and which ones result in acid ash formation when they are digested and assimilated into your system.

- Foods that have a moderate to strong alkaline-forming effect are: watermelon, cantaloupe, celery, limes, kale, mango, honeydew, papaya, parsley, seaweed, sweet seedless grapes, watercress, asparagus, kiwi, pears, pineapple, raisins, vegetable juices, apples, apricots, alfalfa sprouts, avocados, bananas, garlic, ginger, peaches, nectarines, grapefruit, oranges, peas, lettuce, broccoli, cauliflower, carrots, lettuce, mushrooms, spinach, onions, peppers, tomatoes, blackberries, blueberries, strawberries, and most herbs.

- Foods that have a moderate to strong acid-forming effect are: soft drinks, coffee, white sugar, refined salt, artificial sweeteners, antibiotics, white flour products (including pasta), rice, rice flour, rice, noodles, seafood, white vinegar, most boxed cereals, cheese, most beans, flesh meats, chicken, beef, fish, and most types of bread.

Different drinks have different pH values:

pH of a popular brand of cola: 2.5

pH of soft drinks: 3.2

pH of popular brand beers: 4.7

pH of coffe: 5.2–6.9

pH of tap water: 8.3

pH of distilled water: 7.0

pH of green fresh vegetable juice: 8.9

pH of alkaline water: 10.0

Please note that it will take 32 glasses of a 10.0 pH alkaline water to neutralize one can of cola.

These lists of acid and alkaline-forming foods and drinks are not comprehensive. If you're eating mainly grains, flour products, meat, and washing these foods down with coffee, soda, and cola, you can almost certainly improve your health by replacing some of your food and beverage choices with fresh vegetables and fruits.

Although our body is already designed to keep the pH of our blood in a tight, slightly alkaline range, what we eat and drink has a big influence on the pH of our blood. How to choose foods and drinks to meet the requirements of blood pH and other nutrients will be discussed in the following chapters.

So far, we can say: life is in the blood, but our health is in the pH of the blood, and the pH of the blood is in what we drink and eat.

Chapter Seven
Human Body Daily Energy and Nutrition Requirements

1. Human Body Daily Energy Requirements

Life requires energy to grow and sustain. That energy comes from the foods we eat. The Energy in foods is released in the body by oxidation, yielding the chemical energy needed to sustain metabolism, nerve transmission, respiration, circulation, and physical work. The heat produced during these processes is used to maintain body temperature.

The Food and Agriculture Organization/World Health Organization/United Nations University (FAO/WHO/UNU) Expert Consultation on Energy and Protein requirements defines energy requirements as follows:

The energy requirement of an individual is the level of energy intake from food that will balance energy expenditure when the individual has a body size and composition, and level of physical activity, consistent with long-term good health; and that will allow for the maintenance of economically necessary and socially desirable physical activity. In children and pregnant or lactating women the energy requirement includes the energy needs associated with the deposition of tissues or the secretion of milk at rates consistent with good health.

Unlike other nutrient requirements, body weight is an indicator of energy adequacy or inadequacy. The body has the unique ability to convert the fuel mixture of carbohydrates, proteins, and fats into energy needs. However, consuming too much or too little over time results in body weight changes. Therefore, body weight reflects adequacy of energy intake but it is not a reliable indicator of macronutrient or micronutrient adequacy, i.e., energy balance doesn't indicate macronutrient or micronutrient balance.

Body mass index (BMI). Even though body weight is an indicator of energy balance, how do we know if our body weights are in the normal range? Body mass index is used as an indirect indicator of body composition, and is used to classify underweight and overweight individuals. BMI is defined as weight in kilograms divided by the square of height in meters.

The National Institutes of Health (NIH) clinical guidelines on the identification, evaluation, and treatment of normal, overweight, and obese adults and the World Health Organization have defined BMI cutoffs for adults over 19 years of age, regardless of age or gender. Underweight is defined as a BMI of less than 18.5 kg/m², overweight as a BMI from 25 up to 30 kg/m², and obese as a BMI of 30 kg/m² or higher. A healthy or desirable BMI is considered to be from 18.5 to 25 kg/m². Body weight classification by BMI and body fat content are summarized in Table 7-1.

We must keep our BMIs in the normal range because research has shown that being out of the range, especially beyond 25 kg/m², gives you an increasing risk of getting diabetes, hypertension, and coronary heart disease.

Table 7-1 Body weight classification by body mass index (BMI) and body fat content

BMI Range (kg/m²)	Classification	Body Fat (%)	
		Men	Women
From 18.5 up to 25	Normal	13–21	23–31
From 25 up to 30	Overweight	21–25	31–37
From 30 up to 35	Obese	25–31	37–42
35 or higher	Clinically obese	> 31	> 42

Reference Weights. Weights corresponding to BMIs from 18.5 up to 25 kg/m² are tabulated for adult men and women with heights ranging from 1.47 to 1.98 m in Table 7-2 (men) and Table 7-3 (women). Reference weights used here correspond to a BMI of 22.5 kg/m² for men and a BMI of 21.5 kg/m² for women, which match the 50th percentile among 19-year-old individuals.

Table 7-2 Reference heights and weights for men based on a body mass index (BMI) range from 18.5 up to 25 kg/m²

Height (m[in])	Weight at BMI of 18.5 kg/m2 (kg [lb])	Weight at BMI of 22.5 kg/m2 (kg [lb])	Weight at BMI of 25 kg/m2 (kg [lb])
1.47 (58)	40 (88)	49 (108)	54 (119)
1.50 (59)	42 (93)	51 (112)	56 (123)
1.52 (60)	43 (95)	52 (115)	58 (128)
1.55 (61)	44 (97)	54 (119)	60 (132)
1.57 (62)	46 (101)	55 (121)	62 (137)
1.60 (63)	47 (104)	58 (128)	64 (141)

1.63 (64)	49 (108)	60 (132)	66 (146)
1.65 (65)	50 (110)	61 (134)	68 (150)
1.68 (66)	52 (115)	64 (141)	70 (154)
1.70 (67)	53 (117)	65 (143)	72 (159)
1.73 (68)	55 (121)	67 (148)	75 (165)
1.75 (69)	57 (126)	69 (152)	76 (168)
1.77 (70)	58 (128)	70 (154)	78 (172)
1.78 (70)	59 (130)	71 (156)	79 (174)
1.80 (71)	60 (132)	73 (161)	81 (178)
1.83 (72)	62 (137)	75 (165)	84 (185)
1.85 (73)	63 (139)	77 (170)	86 (190)
1.88 (74)	65 (143)	80 (176)	88 (194)
1.91 (75)	67 (148)	82 (181)	91 (201)
1.93 (76)	69 (152)	84 (185)	93 (205)
1.96 (77)	71 (156)	86 (190)	96 (212)
1.98 (78)	72 (159)	88 (194)	98 (216)

Table 7-3 Reference heights and weights for women based on a body mass index (BMI) range from 18.5 up to 25 kg/m²

Height (m[in])	Weight at BMI of 18.5 kg/m2 (kg [lb])	Weight at BMI of 21.5 kg/m2 (kg [lb])	Weight at BMI of 25 kg/m2 (kg [lb])
1.47 (58)	40 (88)	46 (101)	54 (119)
1.50 (59)	42 (93)	48 (106)	56 (123)
1.52 (60)	43 (95)	50 (110)	58 (128)
1.55 (61)	44 (97)	52 (115)	60 (132)
1.57 (62)	46 (101)	53 (117)	62 (137)
1.60 (63)	47 (104)	55 (121)	64 (141)
1.63 (64)	49 (108)	57 (126)	66 (146)
1.65 (65)	50 (110)	59 (130)	68 (150)
1.68 (66)	52 (115)	61 (134)	70 (154)
1.70 (67)	53 (117)	62 (137)	72 (159)
1.73 (68)	55 (121)	64 (141)	75 (165)

1.75 (69)	57 (126)	66 (146)	76 (168)
1.77 (70)	58 (128)	67 (148)	78 (172)
1.78 (70)	59 (130)	68 (150)	79 (174)
1.80 (71)	60 (132)	70 (154)	81 (178)
1.83 (72)	62 (137)	72 (159)	84 (185)
1.85 (73)	63 (139)	74 (163)	86 (190)
1.88 (74)	65 (143)	76 (168)	88 (194)
1.91 (75)	67 (148)	78 (172)	91 (201)
1.93 (76)	69 (152)	80 (176)	93 (205)
1.96 (77)	71 (156)	82 (181)	96 (212)
1.98 (78)	72 (159)	84 (185)	98 (216)

Basal Energy Expenditure (BEE). BEE can be simply defined as the minimal amount of energy expected that is compatible with life. A person's BEE reflects the amount of energy over 24 hours while physical resting (i.e., lying down) and mental resting in a thermoneutral environment that prevents the activation of heat-generating processes such as shivering. Basal energy rate (BMR) describes the rate of energy expenditure that occurs in the postabsorptive state, defined as the particular condition that prevails after an overnight fast, the subject having not consumed food for 12 to 14 hours and resting comfortably, supine, awake, and motionless in a thermoneutral environment. This standardized metabolic state corresponds to the situation in which food and physical activity have minimal influence on metabolism. The BMR thus reflects the energy needed to sustain the metabolic activities of cells and tissues, plus the energy needed to maintain blood circulation, respiration, and gastrointestinal and renal processing (i.e., the basal cost of living). BMR is commonly extrapolated to 24 hours to be more meaningful, and it is then referred to as basal energy expenditure (BEE), expressed as kcal/24 hours.

Resting Energy Expenditure (REE). REE is the energy expended in the activities necessary to sustain normal body functions and homeostasis. These activities include respiration and circulation, the synthesis of organic compounds, the pumping of ions across membranes, the energy required by the central nervous system, and the maintenance of body temperature. Resting metabolic rate (RMR), energy expenditure under resting conditions, tends to be somewhat higher (10%–20%) than under basal conditions due to increases in energy expenditure caused by recent food intake (i.e., by the "thermic effect of food") or by the delayed effect of recently completed physical activity. REE is the energy by extrapolating RMR to 24 hours, expressed as kcal/24 hours. Thus, it is important to distinguish between BMR and RMR and between BEE and REE.

Factors Affecting Resting Energy Expenditure. Body size, body composition, age, sex, hormonal status, fever, extremes in environmental temperature, and food digestion, et al. all have a large impact on the resting energy expenditure. Basal, resting, and sleeping energy expenditures are related to body size, being most closely correlated with the size of the fat-free mass (FFM), which is the weight of the body minus the weight of its fat mass. The size of the FFM generally explains about 70%–80% of the variance in RMR. However, RMR is also affected by age, gender, nutritional state, inherited variations, and by differences in the endocrine state, notably (but rarely) by hypo- or hyperthyroidism. Larger people generally have higher metabolic rates than smaller people, yet tall, thin people have higher metabolic rates than short, wide people. The loss of FFM with aging is associated with a decline in RMR, amounting to about 2%–3% decline per decade after early adulthood. Women, who generally have more fat in proportion to muscle than men, have metabolic rates that are approximately 5%–10% lower than men of the same weight and height. The metabolic rate of women fluctuates with the menstrual cycle. An average of 359 kcal/day difference in the BMR has been measured between the low point and the high point. The average increase in energy expenditure is about 150 kcal/day during the second half of the menstrual cycle. Fevers increase the metabolic rate by about 7% for each degree increase in body temperature above 98.6° Fahrenheit (i.e., 13% for each degree above 37° Celsius). People living in tropical climates usually have RMRs that are 5%–20% higher than those living in temperate areas. The thermic effect of food (TEF) accounts for approximately 10% of total energy expenditure.

Energy Expenditure of Physical Activity (EEPA). EEPA varies greatly among individuals as well as from day to day. In sedentary individuals, about two thirds of total energy expenditure goes to sustain basal metabolism over 24 hours (the BEE), while one-third is used for physical activity. In very active individuals, the 24-hour total energy expenditure can rise to twice as much as basal energy expenditure, while even higher total expenditures can occur among heavy laborers and some athletes.

Total Energy Expenditure (TEE). Total Energy Expenditure (TEE) is the sum of BEE (which includes a small component associated with arousal, as compared to sleeping), TEF, physical activity, thermoregulation, and the energy expended in depositing new tissues and in producing milk. With the emergence of information on TEE by the doubly labeled water (DLW) method, it has become possible to determine the energy expenditure of infants, children, and adults under free-living conditions. TEE from doubly labeled water does not include the energy content of the tissue constituents laid down during normal growth and pregnancy or the milk produced during lactation, as it refers to energy expended during oxidation of energy-yielding nutrients to water and carbon dioxide. It should be noted that direct measurements of TEE represent a distinct advantage over previous TEE evaluations, which had to rely on the factorial approach and on food intake data, which have limited accuracy due to the inability to reliably determine the average physical activity cost and nutrient intakes.

Physical Activity Level (PAL). The level of physical activity is commonly described as the ratio of the total energy expenditure to the basal energy expenditure (TEE/BEE). This ratio is known as the Physical Activity Level (PAL), or the Physical Activity Index. Describing physical activity habits in terms of PAL is not entirely satisfactory because the increments above basal needs in energy expenditure, brought about by most physical activities where body weight is supported against gravity (e.g., walking, but not cycling on a stationary cycle ergometer), are directly proportional to body weight, whereas BEE is more nearly proportional to body weight 0.75. However, PAL is a convenient comparison and is used to describe and account for physical activity habits. Physical activity level (PAL) categories associated with walking equivalence are summarized in Table 7-4.

Table 7-4 Physical activity level categories and walking equivalence

PAL category	PAL range	PAL	Walking equivalence (miles/day at 3-4 mph)		
			Light-weight individual (44 kg)	Middle-weight Individual (70 kg)	Heavy-weight individual (120 kg)
Sedentary	1.0-1.39	1.25	~ 0	~ 0	~ 0

Low active Mean	1.4-1.59	1.5	2.9	2.2	1.5
Active Minimum Mean	1.6-1.89	1.6 1.75	5.8 9.9	4.4 7.3	3.0 5.3
Very active Minimum Mean Maximum	1.9-2.49	1.9 2.2 2.5	14.0 22.5 31.0	10.3 16.7 23.0	17.5 12.3 17.0

From the Institute of Medicine, Food and Nutrition Board: Dietary reference intakes for energy, carbohydrate, fiber, fat, fatty acids, protein, amino acids, Washington DC, 2002/2005, The National Academies Press.

How to Determine PAL. The impact of various physical activities is often described and compared in terms of metabolic equivalents (METs) (i.e., multiples of an individual's resting oxygen uptake), and one MET is defined as a rate of oxygen (O_2) consumption of 3.5 ml/kg/min in adults. Taking the oxygen energy equivalent of 5 kcal/L consumed, this corresponds to 0.0175 kcal/minute/kg (3.5 ml/min/kg × 0.005 kcal/ml). A rate of energy expenditure of 1.0 MET thus corresponds to 1.2 kcal/min in a man weighing 70 kg (0.0175 kcal/kg/minute × 70 kg) and to 1.0 kcal/minute in a woman weighing 57 kg (0.0175 kcal/kg/min × 57 kg) based on the reference body weights for adults in Tables 7-2 and 7-3. Knowing the intensity of a type of physical activity in terms of METs (see Table 7-5 for the METs of various activities) allows a simple assessment of its impact on the energy expended while the activity is performed (number of METs × minutes × 0.0175 kcal/kg/minute). However, the increase in daily energy expenditure is somewhat greater because exercise induces an additional small increase in expenditure for some time after the exertion itself has been completed. This "excess post-exercise oxygen consumption" (EPOC) depends on exercise intensity and duration as well as other factors, such as the types and durations of activities in a normal living; EPOC has been estimated at about 15 percent of the increment in expenditure that occurs during the exertion itself. The thermic effect of food (TEF), which needs to be consumed to cover the expenditure associated with a given activity, must also be taken into account. The TEF dissipates about 10 percent of the food energy consumed. Thus, energy expenditure (EE) of a given activity on daily energy expenditure under conditions of energy balance in terms of METS, the EPOC, and the TEF, can be expressed as:

EE = # of METs × min × 0.022 kcal/kg/min × kg body weight × time (min)

where 0.022 kcal/kg/min = 0.0175 kcal/kg/min × 1.15 percent (EPOC) ÷ 0.9 percent (TEF).

In addition, the impact of various activities on an adult's physical activity level (PAL), also referred to as the change in a physical activity level (ΔPAL), is listed in Table 7-5. The PAL value for various activities performed throughout the day can be determined by adding the ΔPAL for each activity, basal energy expenditure (BEE = 1.0) and thermic energy of foods (TEF = 0.1), i.e.,

$$PAL = 1.1 + \Delta PAL_1 + \Delta PAL_2 + \Delta PAL_3 + \ldots$$

For example, given that an adult walks for 1 hour at 4 mph and then swims for 1 hour, the PAL value is 1.1 + 0.20 + 0.34 = 1.64

**Table 7-5 Intensity and impact of various activities
on physical activity level in adults**

Activity	Metabolic Equivalents (METs)*	ΔPAL/10 min**	ΔPAL/h**
Leisure			
Billiards	2.4	0.013	0.08
Canoeing (leisurely)	2.5	0.014	0.09
Dancing (ballroom)	2.9	0.018	0.11
Golf (with cart)	2.5	0.014	0.09
Horseback riding (walking)	2.3	0.012	0.07
Playing accordion	1.8	0.008	0.05
Playing cello	2.3	0.012	0.07
Playing flute	2.0	0.010	0.06
Playing piano	2.3	0.012	0.07
Playing violin	2.5	0.014	0.09
Volleyball (noncompetitive)	2.9	0.018	0.11
Walking (2 mph)	2.5	0.014	0.09
Calisthenics (no weight)	4.0	0.029	0.17
Cycling (leisurely)	3.5	0.024	0.14
Golf (without cart)	4.4	0.032	0.19
Swimming (slow)	4.5	0.033	0.20
Walking (3 mph)	3.3	0.022	0.13
Walking (4 mph)	4.5	0.033	0.20
Chopping wood	4.9	0.037	0.22

Climbing hills (no load)	6.9	0.056	0.34
Climbing hills (5-kg load)	7.4	0.061	0.37
Cycling (moderately)	5.7	0.045	0.27
Aerobic or ballet	6.0	0.048	0.29
Ballroom (fast) or square	5.5	0.043	0.26
Jogging (10-min miles)	10.2	0.088	0.53
Rope skipping	12.0	0.105	0.63
Ice skating	5.5	0.043	0.26
Roller skating	6.5	0.052	0.31
Skiing (water or downhill)	6.8	0.055	0.33
Squash	12.1	0.106	0.63
Surfing	6.0	0.048	0.29
Swimming	7.0	0.057	0.34
Tennis (doubles)	5.0	0.038	0.23
Walking (5 mph)	8.0	0.067	0.40
Activities of daily living			
Gardening (no lifting)	4.4	0.032	0.19
Household tasks, moderate effort	3.5	0.024	0.14
Lifting items continuously	4.0	0.029	0.17
Light activity while sitting	1.5	0.005	0.03
Loading/unloading car	3.0	0.019	0.11
Lying quietly	1.0	0.000	0.00
Mopping	3.5	0.024	0.14
Mowing lawn (power mower)	4.5	0.033	0.20
Raking lawn	4.0	0.029	0.17
Riding in a vehicle	1.0	0.000	0.0
Sitting	0.0	0.000	0.00
Taking out trash	3.0	0.019	0.11
Vacuuming	3.5	0.024	0.14
Walking the dog	3.0	0.019	0.11

Walking from house to car or bus	2.5	0.014	0.09
Watering plants	2.5	0.014	0.09

From the Institute of Medicine, Food and Nutrition Board: Dietary reference intakes for energy, carbohydrate, fiber, fat, fatty acids, protein, amino acids, Washington DC, 2002/2005, The National Academies Press.

*METs are multiples of an individual's resting oxygen uptakes, defined as the rate of oxygen (O_2) consumption of 3.5 ml of O_2/min/kg body weight in adults.

** The ΔPAL is an allowance made to include the delayed effect of physical activity in causing excess postexercise O_2 consumption (EPOC) and the dissipation of some of the food energy consumed through the thermic effect of food (TEF).

How to Determine Physical Activity Coefficient (PA). According to the PAL value determined using the above method, find a corresponding PA from the following table. For instance, if in the above example, the PAL =1.64 and the adult is a man, then the PA is 1.25, and if the adult is a woman, then the PA is 1.27.

Table 7-6 Relationship between PAL and PA

Men		Women	
PAL	PA	PAL	PA
≥1.0 < 1.39 (sedentary)	1.00	≥1.0 < 1.39 (sedentary)	1.00
≥1.4 < 1.59 (low active)	1.11	≥1.4 < 1.59 (low active)	1.12
≥1.6 < 1.89 (active)	1.25	≥1.6 < 1.89 (active)	1.27
≥ 1.9 < 2.49 (very active)	1.48	≥ 1.9 < 2.49 (very active)	1.45

Estimated Energy Requirement (EER). The National Academy of Sciences, Institute of Medicine, and Food and Nutrition Board in partnership with Health Canada, developed the estimated energy requirement for men, woman, children, infants, pregnant, and lactating women, including overweight and obese children, and overweight and obese adults based on the measurement results using doubly labeled water (DLW) method in conjunction with indirect calorimetry. The method is accurate and has a precision of 2% to 8%. In this chapter, we only discuss the EER of adults in normal weights with BMIs of 18.5–25 kg/m². The following two equations are for the adult men and women, both of which are suitable for all the races of people.

EER for Men Ages 19 Years and Older:

EER = 662 - (9.53 × age [y]) + PA × (15.91 × Weight [kg] + 539.6 × Height [m])

where PA is the physical activity coefficient:
PA = 1.00 if PAL is estimated to be ≥1.0 < 1.4 (sedentary)
PA = 1.11 if PAL is estimated to be ≥1.4 < 1.6 (low active)
PA = 1.25 if PAL is estimated to be≥ 1.6 < 1.9 (active)
PA = 1.48 if PAL is estimated to be ≥ 1.9 < 2.5 (very active)

EER for Women Ages 19 Years and Older:

EER = 354 - (6.91 × age [y]) + PA × (9.36 × Weight [kg] + 726 × Height [m])

where PA is the physical activity coefficient:
PA = 1.00 if PAL is estimated to be ≥1.0 < 1.4 (sedentary)
PA = 1.12 if PAL is estimated to be ≥1.4 < 1.6 (low active)
PA = 1.27 if PAL is estimated to be ≥1.6 < 1.9 (active)
PA = 1.45 if PAL is estimated to be ≥1.9 < 2.5 (very active)

How to Calculate your Daily Energy Requirements. As long as your BMI is in the range of 18.5 to 25 kg/m^2, you can use the above equations to compute your daily energy requirements. Taking a man with a weight of 70 kg and a height of 1.77 m and a woman with a weight of 59 kg and a height of 1.65 m as examples, I calculated their daily EER at different PAL levels at different ages compared to 120 years old. The results are presented in Table 7-7 and Table 7-8.

Table 7-7 Daily energy requirements (kcal) for a man 19 years old up to 120 years old with a weight of 70 kg and a height of 1.77 m

Age (yrs)	PAL level			
	Sedentary	Low active	Active	Very active
19	2550	2777	3067	3543
20	2540	2768	3057	3533
21	2531	2758	3048	3524
22	2521	2749	3038	3514

23	2512	2739	3029	3505
24	2502	2730	3019	3495
25	2493	2720	3010	3486
26	2483	2711	3000	3476
27	2473	2701	2991	3467
28	2464	2692	2981	3457
29	2454	2682	2972	3447
30	2445	2672	2962	3438
31	2435	2663	2953	3428
32	2426	2653	2943	3419
33	2416	2644	2934	3409
34	2407	2634	2924	3400
35	2397	2625	2914	3390
36	2388	2615	2905	3381
37	2378	2606	2905	3371
38	2369	2596	2886	3362
39	2359	2587	2876	3352
40	2350	2577	2867	3343
41	2340	2568	2857	3333
42	2331	2558	2848	3324
43	2321	2549	2838	3314
44	2311	2539	2829	3304
45	2302	2530	2819	3295
46	2292	2520	2810	3285
47	2283	2510	2800	3376
48	2273	2501	2791	3266
49	2264	2491	2781	3257
50	2254	2482	2771	3247
51	2245	2472	2762	3238
52	2235	2463	2752	3228
53	2226	2453	2743	3219
54	2216	2444	2733	3209

55	2207	2434	2724	3200
56	2197	2425	2714	3190
57	2188	2415	2705	3181
58	2178	2406	2695	3171
59	2169	2396	2686	3162
60	2159	2387	2676	3152
61	2149	2377	2667	3142
62	2140	2367	2657	3133
63	2130	2358	2648	3123
64	2121	2348	2638	3114
65	2111	2339	2629	3104
66	2102	2329	2619	3095
67	2092	2320	2609	3085
68	2083	2310	2600	3076
69	2073	2301	2590	3066
70	2064	2291	2581	3057
72	2045	2272	2562	3038
74	2026	2253	2543	3019
76	2007	2234	2524	3000
78	1987	2215	2505	2980
80	1968	2196	2486	2961
90	1873	2101	2390	2866
100	1778	2005	2295	2771
110	1682	1910	2200	2676
120	1587	1815	2104	2580

Table 7-8 Daily energy requirements (kcal) for a woman 19 years old up to 120 years old with a weight of 59 kg and a height of 1.65 m

Age (yrs)	PAL level			
	Sedentary	Low active	Active	Very active
19	1973	2183	2445	2760
20	1966	2176	2438	2754

21	1959	2169	2432	2747
22	1952	2162	2425	2740
23	1945	2155	2418	2733
24	1938	2148	2411	2726
25	1931	2141	2404	2719
26	1924	2134	2397	2712
27	1918	2128	2390	2705
28	1911	2121	2383	2698
29	1904	2114	2376	2691
30	1897	2107	2369	2684
31	1890	2100	2362	2677
32	1883	2093	2356	2671
33	1876	2086	2349	2664
34	1869	2079	2342	2657
35	1862	2072	2335	2650
36	1855	2065	2328	2643
37	1848	2058	2321	2636
38	1842	2052	2314	2629
39	1835	2045	2307	2622
40	1828	2038	2300	2615
41	1821	2031	2293	2608
42	1814	2024	2286	2601
43	1807	2017	2280	2595
44	1800	2010	2273	2588
45	1793	2003	2266	2581
46	1786	1996	2259	2574
47	1779	1989	2252	2567
48	1772	1982	2245	2560
49	1766	1976	2238	2553
50	1759	1969	2231	2546
51	1752	1962	2224	2539
52	1745	1955	2217	2532

53	1738	1948	2210	2525
54	1731	1941	2204	2519
55	1724	1934	2197	2512
56	1717	1927	2190	2505
57	1710	1920	2183	2498
58	1703	1913	2176	2491
59	1696	1906	2169	2484
60	1690	1900	2162	2477
61	1683	1893	2155	2470
62	1676	1886	2148	2463
63	1669	1879	2141	2456
64	1662	1872	2134	2449
65	1655	1865	2128	2443
66	1648	1858	2121	2436
67	1641	1851	2114	2429
68	1634	1844	2107	2422
69	1627	1837	2100	2415
70	1620	1830	2093	2408
72	1607	1817	2079	2394
74	1593	1803	2065	2380
76	1579	1789	2052	2367
78	1565	1775	2038	2353
80	1551	1761	2024	2339
90	1482	1692	1955	2270
100	1413	1623	1886	2201
110	1344	1554	1817	2132
120	1275	1485	1747	2063

In Table 7-7, I observed that for each year above 19, the man's daily total energy at various PAL levels should subtract 10 kcal/d, whereas in Table 7-8, the woman's daily total energy at various PAL levels should subtract 7 kcal/d.

Anyone who is 19 years or older can obtain a daily energy requirement table like Table 7-7 or Table 7-8 in terms of the calculation method presented here.

2. Human Body Daily Nutrition Requirements

Nutrients include macronutrients and micronutrients. Macronutrients are water, fat, protein, carbohydrate, and fiber. Fat, protein, and carbohydrate provide energy required in our daily life. Micronutrients include vitamins and minerals.

Macronutrient Daily Requirements. The Institute of Medicine, Food and Nutrition Board, National Academy gives recommended Dietary Reference Intakes (DRIs) for macronutrients, which is summarized in Table 7-9, Table 7-10, and Table 7-11. Table 7-12 summarizes recommended daily intakes of essential amino acids for adults from WHO.

Table 7-9 Dietary reference intakes (DRIs) for macronutrients for adults

Life stage	Total water (L/d)	Carbohy-drate (g/d)	Total fiber (g/d)	Fat (g/d)	Linoleic acid (g/d)	α-Linolenic acid (g/d)	Protein (g/d)
Males							
19-30 y	3.7	130	38	ND	17	1.6	56
31-50 y	3.7	130	38	ND	17	1.6	56
51-70 y	3.7	130	30	ND	14	1.6	56
> 70 y	3.7	130	30	ND	14	1.6	56
Females							
19-30 y	2.7	130	25	ND	12	1.1	46
31-50 y	2.7	130	25	ND	12	1.1	46
51-70 y	2.7	130	21	ND	11	1.1	46
> 70 y	2.7	130	21	ND	11	1.1	46

From the Institute of Medicine, Food and Nutrition Board: Dietary reference intakes for energy, carbohydrate, fiber, fat, fatty acids, protein, amino acids, Washington DC, 2002/2005, The National Academies Press.

ND = not determined.

Table 7-10 Dietary reference intakes (DRIs): acceptable macronutrient distribution ranges for adults

Macronutrient	Range (percent of energy)
Fat	20–35
n-6 Polyunsaturated fatty acids*	5–10
n-3 Polyunsaturated fatty acids*	0.6–1.2
Carbohydrate	45–65
Protein	10–35

From the Institute of Medicine, Food and Nutrition Board: Dietary reference intakes for energy, carbohydrate, fiber, fat, fatty acids, protein, amino acids, Washington DC, 2002/2005, The National Academies Press.

*Approximately 10 percent of the total can come from long-chain n-3 or n-6 fatty acid.

Table 7-11 Dietary reference intakes (DRIs): additional macronutrient recommendations

Macronutrient	Recommendation
Dietary cholesterol	As low as possible while consuming a nutritionally adequate diet
Trans fatty acids	As low as possible while consuming a nutritionally adequate diet
Saturated fatty acids	As low as possible while consuming a nutritionally adequate diet
Added sugars	Limit to no more than 25% of total energy

From the Institute of Medicine, Food and Nutrition Board: Dietary reference intakes for energy, carbohydrate, fiber, fat, fatty acids, protein, amino acids, Washington DC, 2002/2005, The National Academies Press.

Table 7-12 Recommended daily intakes: essential amino acids for adults

Amino acid	Per kg (mg)	59 kg weight (g)	70 kg weight (g)
Histidine (H)	10	0.59	0.70
Isoleucine (I)	20	1.18	1.40
Leucine (L)	39	2.30	2.73
Lysine (K)	30	1.77	2.10
Methionine + cysteine (M + C)	15	0.89	1.05
Phenylalanine + tyrosine (F + Y)	25	1.48	1.75

Threonine (T)	15	0.89	1.05
Tryptophan (W)	4	0.24	0.28
Valine (V)	26	1.53	1.82

From FAO/WHO/UNU: Protein and amino acid requirements in human nutrition, WHO Press, 2007.

In Table 7-9, total water includes all water contained in food, beverages, and drinking water. Total fiber includes all fibers contained in complex carbohydrate and other sources. Protein's DRIs for men and women is based on 0.8 g/kg body weight for the reference body weights (men: 70 kg, and women: 58 kg), so different body weights require different protein's DRIs. 130 g/d is the minimum amount of carbohydrate for adults, which only accounts for 26% of a 2000 kcal that is far lower than the acceptable macronutrient distribution range of 45%–65% in Table 7-10. Table 7-11 lists the additional macronutrient DRIs for dietary cholesterol, trans fatty acids, saturated fatty acids, and added sugars. Table 7-12 summarizes the recommended daily intakes of essential amino acids for adults, which is set up by WHO in 2007. I calculated the daily intake amounts for an adult with a weight of 59 kg or 70 kg, which is also presented in Table 7-12.

Micronutrient Daily Requirements. The Institute of Medicine, Food Nutrition Board, National Academies gives recommended Dietary Reference Intakes (DRIs) for micronutrients, which is summarized and reformatted in Table 7-13 (vitamins) and Table 7-14 (minerals).

Table 7-13 Dietary reference intakes (DRIs): recommended intakes for adults, vitamins

Life stage	A µg/d	C mg/d	D µg/d	E mg/d	K µg/d	B1 mg/d	B2 mg/d	B3 mg/d	B5 mg/d	B6 mg/d	B7 µg/d	B9 µg/d	B12 µg/d	Choline mg/d
Males														
19-30y	900	90	5	15	120	1.2	1.3	16	5	1.3	30	400	2.4	550
31-50y	900	90	5	15	120	1.2	1.3	16	5	1.3	30	400	2.4	550
51-70y	900	90	10	15	120	1.2	1.3	16	5	1.7	30	400	2.4	550
> 70y	900	90	15	15	120	1.2	1.3	16	5	1.7	30	400	2.4	550
Females														
19-30y	700	75	5	15	90	1.1	1.1	14	5	1.3	30	400	2.4	425
31-50y	700	75	5	15	90	1.1	1.1	14	5	1.3	30	400	2.4	425
51-70y	700	75	10	15	90	1.1	1.1	14	5	1.5	30	400	2.4	425
> 70y	700	75	15	15	90	1.1	1.1	14	5	1.5	30	400	2.4	425

Note: (1) A = vitamin A, C = vitamin C, D = vitamin D, E = vitamin E, K = vitamin K, B_1 = Thiamin, B_2 = Riboflavin, B_3 = Niacin, B_5 = Pantothenic Acid, B_7 = Biotin, B_9 = Folate, and B_{12} = Vitamin B_{12}.

(2) Vitamin A as retinol activity equivalents (RAEs). 1 RAE = 1µg retinol, 12 µg β-carotene, 24 µg α-carotene, or 24 µg β-cryptoxanthin. The RAE for dietary provitamin A carotenoid is twofold greater than retinol equivalents (RE), whereas the RAE for preformed vitamin A is the same as RE.

(3) Vitamin D as cholecalciferol. 1 µg cholecalciferol = 40 IU vitamin D.

(4) Vitamin E as α-tocopherol. α-tocopherol includes RRR- α-tocopherol, the only form of α-tocopherol that occurs naturally in food, and the 2R-stereoisomeric forms of α-tocopherol (RRR-, RSR-, RRS, and RSS- α-tocopherol) that occur in fortified food and supplements.

(5) Niacin as niacin equivalent (NE). 1 mg of niacin = 60 mg of tryptophan.

(6) Folate as dietary folate equivalents (DFE). 1 DFE = 1µg food folate = 0.6 µg of folic acid from fortified food or as a supplement consumed with food = 0.5 µg of a supplement taken on an empty stomach.

Table 7-14 Dietary reference intakes (DRIs): recommended intakes for adults, minerals

Life stage	Ca mg/d	Cr µg/d	Cu µg/d	F mg/d	I µg/d	Fe mg/d	Mg mg/d	Mn mg/d	Mo µg/d	P mg/d	Se µg/d	Zn mg/d	K g/d	Na g/d	Cl g/d
Males															
19-30y	1000	35	900	4	150	8	400	2.3	45	700	55	11	4.7	1.5	2.3
31-50y	1000	35	900	4	150	8	420	2.3	45	700	55	11	4.7	1.5	2.3
51-70y	1200	30	900	4	150	8	420	2.3	45	700	55	11	4.7	1.3	2.0
> 70y	1200	30	900	4	150	8	420	2.3	45	700	55	11	4.7	1.3	1.8
Females															
19-30y	1000	25	900	3	150	18	310	1.8	45	700	55	8	4.7	1.5	2.3
31-50y	1000	25	900	3	150	18	320	1.8	45	700	55	8	4.7	1.5	2.3
51-70y	1200	20	900	3	150	8	320	1.8	45	700	55	8	4.7	1.3	2.0
> 70y	1200	20	900	3	150	8	320	1.8	45	700	55	8	4.7	1.3	1.8

Note: Ca = Calcium, Cr = Chromium, Cu = Copper, F = Fluoride, I = Iodine, Fe = Iron, Mg = Magnesium, Mn = Manganese, Mo = Molybdenum, P = Phosphorus, Se = Selenium, Zn = Zinc, K = Potassium, Na = Sodium, and Cl = Chloride.

The USDA recommends that Americans consume 3,000 to 5,000 scores of ORAC daily, so I would like to suggest that everyone should daily consume at least **5, 000 scores of ORAC** at a sedentary activity level, at least 7, 500 scores at a low active activity level, at least 10, 000 scores at a active activity level, and at least 12, 500 scores at a very active activity level.

The **American Heart Association** has recommended two fatty fish servings per week for people who are healthy individuals without cardiovascular disease. The **DHA plus EPA** (combined) equivalency of such fish consumption **is approximately 250-300 mg/day.** The National Institute of Health Workshop recommended **a daily intake of 650 mg of DHA plus EPA for**

normal healthy individuals (for overall health and cardiovascular care) with DHA and EPA representing at least one third of the 650 milligram amount. In 2000, the American Heart Association, in its official Dietary Guidelines, recommended that the daily intake of DHA plus EPA in individuals with coronary heart disease should **target 900 mg/day** since this amount has shown to be beneficial in affecting coronary heart disease mortality rates in patients with coronary disease. Therefore, I would like to suggest that everyone should daily intake at least **500 mg of DHA plus EPA.**

From epidemiology studies that showed positive benefits from dietary consumption of lutein and zeaxanthin, it appears as though 6 mg/day of both compounds may be necessary to detect any beneficial effect. The National Eye Institute (NEI) is preparing for clinical studies by doing pre-clinical dosing experiments to determine the appropriate intake level of these nutrients. Based on the information, I would like to suggest that everyone should daily intake at least **10 mg of lutein plus zeaxanthin.**

Like a drug, any micronutrient also has a safe and effective window area. Below the lower window line, a micronutrient is safe but can not play an effective role in optimum health. Above the upper window line, a micronutrient is toxic and has side effects. Most micronutrients are in foods. This is why people often say: foods are drugs and drugs are foods. Relative to drugs, most nutrients have a bigger window area. The Institute of Medicine, Food Nutrition Board, National Academy has determined tolerable upper intake levels (UL) of most vitamins and minerals for all age groups. Table 7-15 and Table 7-16 only presented adult ULs for vitamins and minerals. UL is the highest level of daily nutrient intake that is likely to pose no risk of adverse health effects to almost all individuals in the general population. Unless otherwise specified, the UL represents total intake from food, water, and supplement. Due to lack of suitable data, the ULs for some nutrients have not been determined.

Table 7-15 Dietary reference intakes (DRIs): adult tolerable intake levels (UL), vitamins

Life stage	A µg/d	C mg/d	D µg/d	E mg/d	K µg/d	B_1 mg/d	B_2 mg/d	B_3 mg/d	B_5 mg/d	B_6 mg/d	B_7 g/d	B_9 g/d	B_{12} g/d	Choline g/d
19-70y	3000	2000	50	1000	ND	ND	ND	35	ND	100	ND	1000	ND	3.5
> 70y	3000	2000	50	1000	ND	ND	ND	35	ND	100	ND	1000	ND	3.5

Note: ND = not determined.

Table 7-16 Dietary reference intakes (DRIs): adult tolerable intake levels (UL), minerals

Life stage	Ca g/d	Cr µg/d	Cu mg/d	F mg/d	I mg/d	Fe mg/d	Mg mg/d	Mn mg/d	Mo mg/d	P g/d	Se µg/d	Zn mg/d	K g/d	Na g/d	Cl g/d	As µg/d	B mg/d	Ni mg/d	Va mg/d
19-70y	2.5	ND	10	10	1.1	45	350	11	2.0	4.0	400	40	ND	2.3	3.6	ND	20	1.0	1.8
> 70y	2.5	ND	10	10	1.1	45	350	11	2.0	3.0	400	40	ND	2.3	3.6	ND	20	1.0	1.8

Note: Arsenic = As, Boron = B, Nickel = Ni, and Vanadium = Va.
ND = not determined.

In California, the government has set a law to limit the daily intakes of heavy metals from nutritional supplement: mercury (Hg): 0.3 µg/d, cadmium (Cd), 4.1µg/d, Arsenic (As): 10 µg/d, and lead (Pb): 0.5µg/d. Any supplement manufacturer in California must indicate that the daily ingestion amounts of these heavy metals in its products do not exceed these limits on its product labels. Otherwise, their products are not allowed to be sold on the market.

3. Energy Requirements Versus Nutrition Requirements

Above recommendations for nutrient intakes from the Institute of Medicine, Food and Nutrition Board, National Academy are generally set to provide an ample supply of the various nutrients needed (i.e., enough to meet or exceed the requirements of almost all healthy individuals in a given life stage and gender group). For most nutrients, the recommended intakes are thus set to correspond to the median amounts sufficient to meet a specific criterion of adequacy plus two standard deviations to meet the needs of nearly all healthy individuals. **In short, the above dietary reference intakes (DRIs) for vitamins and minerals can meet almost all healthy adults**. If they do not exceed the ULs, they should be safe and effective. However, there are also no documented benefits.

The situation for energy is quite different. Individuals who consume energy that exceed their requirements will gain weight over time. This difference is reflected in the fact that there are no recommended DRIs for energy, as it would be inappropriate to recommend an intake that exceeded the requirement (which would lead to weight gain) of 97 to 98 percent of individuals. The requirement of energy for adults of normal weight is expressed as Estimated Energy Requirement (EER), which reflects the energy expenditure associated with an individual's sex, age, height, and physical activity level.

There is another fundamental difference between the requirements of energy and those of other nutrients. Body weight provides each individual with a readily monitored indicator of the adequacy or inadequacy of habitual energy intake, whereas a comparably obvious and individualized indicator of inadequate or excessive intake of other nutrients is not usually evident.

Therefore, everyone who wants to maintain an energy balance must know his/her daily energy requirement in terms of the equations presented in the first section. Then, eat enough foods to get the desired energy to keep its balance.

Energy and nutrients come from the foods that we eat. Getting to know the energy and nutrition values of the most common foods is the first step in achieving our daily energy balance and optimum nutrition. So, the next chapter will summarize and discuss energy and nutrition values of selected foods in terms of their types listed in Appendix A.

Chapter Eight
Energy and Nutrition Values of Foods

Our daily required energy and nutrition come from the foods we eat. If we know the energy and nutrition values of all the foods we eat each day, then it is easy for us to calculate if the energy and nutrition obtained from the foods satisfy our daily energy and nutrition requirements discussed in the last chapter. Fortunately, the U.S. Department of Agriculture (USDA) has developed a food database containing about 7,000 foods, in which we can find the energy and nutrition values of each food. From this database, I selected the energy and nutrition values of 379 best foods, which are listed in Appendix A. In this chapter, I will summarize and discuss the energy and nutrition values of these foods.

1. Energy, Macronutrients, and Cholesterol Values of Selected Foods

The values of energy, protein, fat, saturated fat, trans fat, carbohydrate, sugar, fiber, and cholesterol of the selected foods in Appendix A are summarized in Table 8-1 in terms of food categories. Of all the selected foods, oil contains the highest energy due to its 100% fat in content, while vegetables, fruits, and dairy products contain the lowest energy. Legumes, cereal, bread, grain, nuts and seeds, cheese, and meat and poultry have high levels of energy, whereas egg, and fish and shellfish have low levels of energy.

Table 8-1 Summary of energy, macronutrients, and cholesterol contents of different types of the selected foods per 100 grams

Food category	Energy (kcal)	Protein (g)	Fat (g)	Satrd fat (g)	Trans fat (g)	Carbo (g)	Sugar (g)	Fiber (g)	Chol (g)
Vegetables	10-100	0.6-3.3	0.1-0.8	0.01-0.09	0	2.2-15.9	0-6.8	0.5-5.4	0
Fruits	30-167	0.3-2.2	0.1-15.4	0-2.13	0	7.8-33.5	0-14.8	0-6.8	0

Legumes	60-450	3.5-36.5	0.1-19.9	0-2.88	0	2.4-64.2	0.3-10.7	3.4-24.4	0
Cereal	200-490	5.2-14.9	2.0-24.1	0.3-4.1	0	53.2-88.9	0-38.3	3.2-47.3	0
Grain	86-526	2.3-52.2	0.2-20.8	0.1-8.1	0	19.0-83.1	0.2-3.5	0-33.2	0
Bread	250-290	7.9-11.8	1.8-6.0	0.4-1.6	0	40.0-56.4	0-8.1	2.3-6.5	0-51
Dairy	35-108	1.0-34.3	0.2-7.0	0.1-4.6	0	4.5-10.3	0.1-4.6	0-0.8	2-27
Egg	142-185	10.5-15.9	9.9-15.3	3.0-4.3	0	0.4-2.2	0.4-1.7	0	352-1234
Cheese	138-403	11.3-35.8	1.0-33.1	0.6-21.1	0	0.4-4.8	0-7.7	0	4-105
Nuts & Seeds	180-718	4.7-24.5	1.0-75.8	0.2-12.1	0	13.1-64.5	0-6.2	0-27.3	0
Fish & Shellfish	70-200	15.5-23.3	0.8-13.8	0.1-3.3	0	0-0.9	0	0	30-370
Meat & Poultry	100-800	3.0-20.8	2.5-89.0	0.9-32.2	0-0.8	0-15.0	0-2.0	0-1.2	33-3010
Oil	862-884	0	100	9.6-86.5	0	0	0	0	0

Note: Satrd = Saturated, Carbo = Carbohydrate, and Chol = Cholestrol

The source of the richest protein is cheese, legumes, nuts and seeds, eggs, and meat and poultry. Cereal, grain, and bread are the richest source of carbohydrate in our daily foods, whereas fruits and cereal contain the highest sugar contents.

Vegetables, fruits, legumes, cereal, grain, bread, and nuts and seeds are a good source of fiber for our daily requirements. Egg, and meat and poultry contain the highest cholesterol contents. Each Table in the following lists 10 foods containing the richest protein, fat, saturated fat, carbohydrate, fiber, and cholesterol.

Table 8-2 Ten foods containing the richest protein

Food name	Protein (g /100g)	Category
Peanut flour, defatted	52.2	Grain
Seeds, sesame flour, low fat	50.1	Grain
Seeds, sunflower flour, partially defatted	48.1	Grain
Tofu, dried-frozen (kayatofu)	47.9	Legumes

Soybeans, mature seeds, raw	36.5	Legumes
Cheese, parmesan, hard	35.8	Cheese
Soy flour, full-fat, raw	34.5	Grain
Milk, buttermilk, dried	34.3	Dairy
Seeds, watermelon seed kernels, dried	28.3	Nuts & seeds
Cheese, Monterey, low fat	28.2	Cheese

Table 8-3 Ten foods containing the richest fat

Food name	Fat (g /100g)	Category
Oil	100	Oil
Pork, fresh, backfat, raw	88.7	Meat & poultry
Nuts, macadamia nuts, raw	75.8	Nuts & seeds
Nuts, pecans	72.0	Nuts & seeds
Pork, fresh, separable fat, raw	71.0	Meat & poultry
Nuts, pine nuts, dried	68.4	Nuts & seeds
Nuts, walnuts, English	65.2	Nuts & seeds
Nuts, hazelnuts or filberts	60.8	Nuts & seeds
Pork, fresh, belly, raw	53.0	Meat & poultry
Seeds, sunflower kernels, dried	51.5	Nuts & seeds

Table 8-4 Ten foods containing the richest saturated fat

Food name	Saturated fat (g /100g)	Category
Coconut oil	86.5	Oil
Palm kernel oil	81.5	Oil
Palm oil	49.3	Oil
Pork, fresh, backfat, raw	32.2	Meat & poultry
Cottonseed oil	25.9	Oil
Pork, fresh, separable fat, raw	25.1	Meat & poultry
Cheese, cheddar	21.1	Cheese
Cheese colby	20.2	Cheese
Cheese, cheshire	19.5	Cheese
Cheese, Monterey	19.1	Cheese

Table 8-5 Ten foods containing the richest carbohydrate

Food name	Carbohydrate (g /100g)	Category
Cereals ready-to-eat, corn & oat flour, puffed presweetened, single brand	88.9	Cereal
Cereals ready-to-eat, GENERAL MILLS, Cinnamon Grahams	86.0	Cereal
Cereals ready-to-eat, GENERAL MILLS, FIBER ONE	83.3	Cereal
Potato flour	83.1	Grain
Cereals ready-to-eat, Malt-O-Meal, High Fiber Bran Flakes	80.8	Cereal
Cereals ready-to-eat, bran flakes, single brand	80.4	Cereal
Rye flour , light	80.2	Grain
Rice, white, long-grain, regular, raw	80.0	Grain
Rice, white, medium-grain, regular, raw	79.3	Grain
Rice, white, short-grain, regular, raw	79.2	Grain

Table 8-6 Ten foods containing the richest fiber

Food name	Fiber (g /100g)	Category
Cereals ready-to-eat, GENERAL MILLS, FIBER ONE	47.3	Cereal
Coca, dry powder, unsweetened	33.2	Grain
Lentils, raw	30.5	Legumes
Cereals ready-to-eat, bran, malted flour, single brand	28.6	Cereal
Peas, split, mature seeds, raw	25.5	Legumes
Beans, navy, mature seeds, raw	24.4	Legumes
Rye flour, dark	22.6	Grain
Rice bran, crude	21.0	Grain
Cereals ready-to-eat, bran flakes, single brand	17.6	Cereal
Chickpeas, mature seeds, raw	17.4	Legumes

Table 8-7 Ten foods containing the richest cholesterol

Food name	Cholesterol (mg /100g)	Category
Beef, brain, raw	3010	Meat & poultry
Pork, fresh, brain, raw	2195	Meat & poultry
Lamb, brain, raw	1352	Meat & poultry
Egg, yolk, raw, fresh	1234	Egg
Egg, turkey, whole, fresh, raw	933	Egg
Egg, duck, whole, fresh, raw	884	Egg
Egg, goose, whole, fresh, raw	852	Egg
Egg, quail, whole, fresh, raw	844	Egg
Egg, whole, cooked, fried	457	Egg
Egg, whole, raw, fresh	423	Egg

2. Mineral Values of Selected Foods

The value of minerals of the selected foods in Appendix A is summarized in Table 8-8 in terms of food categories. Legumes, cereal, and cheese contain the highest contents of calcium, while vegetables, fruits, meat and shellfish, and oil contain the lowest contents of calcium.

Table 8-8 Summary of mineral contents of different types of the selected foods per 100 grams

Food category	Ca (mg)	Fe (mg)	Mg (mg)	P (mg)	K (mg)	Na (mg)	Zn (mg)	Cu (mg)	Mn (mg)	Se (µg)	Cr (µg)
Vegetables	1-81	0.2-6.2	7-60	20-164	136-584	2-213	0.1-1.1	0.1-0.4	0.1-0.8	0.1-11.0	0-21
Fruits	3-61	0-2.5	3-32	3-54	77-507	0-18	0-0.68	0-0.3	0-0.7	0-1.0	0-9
Legumes	31-2134	1.0-15.7	25-280	38-704	20-1797	1-2873	1.0-4.9	0.1-0.8	0.2-3.6	0.6-54.3	0-11
Cereal	17-1091	2.2-62.0	27-278	67-813	120-947	1-789	2.4-52.5	0.1-0.9	0.2-9.0	4.4-70.7	0-38
Grain	1-474	1.3-18.5	22-781	43-1580	35-2515	1-182	0.4-11.6	0.1-3.8	0.1-14.2	0.6-70.7	5-11
Bread	43-151	1.8-3.7	23-54	99-178	100-227	390-681	0.7-1.5	0.1-0.3	0.5-1.5	17.3-30.0	0
Dairy	32-193	0-0.2	3-18	14-158	51-204	17-105	0-0.5	0-0.1	0-0.1	1.8-3.7	0
Egg	50-99	1.2-4.1	10-17	170-226	114-222	132-294	1.0-1.6	0-0.1	0	20.0-36.9	8-22
Cheese	61-1146	0.1-0.8	5-44	134-694	62-256	125-1602	0.4-4.4	0-0.1	0-0.1	9.0-22.5	0-56

Food	Ca	Fe	Mg	P	K	Na	Zn	Cu	Mn	Se	Cr
Nuts & Seeds	2-264	1.0-6.7	62-515	79-593	329-1025	0-31	0.5-5.8	0.4-4.1	0.1-8.8	0-25.4	0-7
Fish & Shellfish	3-110	0.1-1.8	20-83	133-402	173-490	43-296	0.3-5.9	0-1.7	0-0.8	12.6-43.3	0-12
Meat & Poultry	2-36	0.6-45.0	13-27	132-364	185-297	42-518	0.7-4.8	0-9.8	0-0.3	13.1-190.0	0-11
Oil	0-1	0-0.6	0	0	0-1	0-2	0	0	0	0	0-47

Note: Ca = Calcium, Fe = Iron, Mg = Magnesium, P = Phosphorus, K = Potassium, Na = Sodium, Zn = Zinc, Cu = Copper, Mn = Manganese, Se = Selenium, and Cr = Chromium.

The richest source of iron in our daily foods is cereal, and meat and poultry. Legumes, cereal, grain, and nuts and seeds contain the highest contents of magnesium, and also have the highest phosphorus level. All types of foods, except oil, contain rich contents of potassium. Cheese contains the highest contents of sodium.

Cereal contains the highest contents of zinc in all types of the selected foods, and grain contains the next highest contents of zinc. In meat and poultry, copper contents are higher than in other types of foods, while manganese contents in grain are higher than in other foods. Meat and poultry contains the highest contents of selenium, and cereal and grain contain the next highest content of selenium after meat and poultry. Cheese possesses the richest chromium.

The Tables shown below list 10 foods containing the richest calcium, iron, magnesium, phosphorus, potassium, sodium, zinc, copper, manganese, and selenium.

Table 8-9 Ten foods containing the richest calcium

Food name	Calcium (mg /100g)	Category
Tofu, dried-frozen (kayatofu), prepared with calcium sulfate	2134	Legumes
Tofu, salted & fermented (fuyu), prepared with calcium sulfate	1229	Legumes
Milk, buttermilk, dried	1184	Dairy
Cheese, parmesan	1184	Cheese
Cheese, Mexican, blend, reduced fat	1146	Cheese
Cereals ready-to-eat, GERNERAL MILLS, HARMONY	1091	Cereal
Seeds, sesame seeds, whole, dried	975	Nuts & seeds
Milk, dry, whole	912	Dairy

Cheese, Mozzarella, part skim	782	Cheese
Cheese, cheddar	721	Cheese

Table 8-10 Ten foods containing the richest iron

Food name	Iron (mg /100g)	Category
Cereals ready-to-eat, KELLOGG, KEL-LOGG'S Complete Wheat Bran Flakes	62.0	Cereal
Beef, spleen, raw	44.6	Meat & poultry
Lamb, spleen, raw	41.9	Meat & poultry
Cereals ready-to-eat, CERNERAL MILLS, CHEERIOS	40.0	Cereal
Cereals ready-to-eat, Malt-O-Meal, High Fiber Bran Flakes	35.2	Cereal
Cereals ready-to-eat, malted flour, single brand	27.9	Cereal
Pork, liver, raw	23.3	Meat & poultry
Pork, spleen, raw	22.3	Meat & poultry
Soybean, mature seeds, raw	15.7	Legumes
Seeds, sesame flour, high fat	15.2	Grain

Table 8-11 Ten foods containing the richest magnesium

Food name	Magnesium (mg /100g)	Category
Rice bran, crude	781	Grain
Cocoa, dry powder, unsweetened	499	Grain
Soy flour, full-fat, raw	429	Grain
Seeds, watermelon seeds kernels, dried	515	Nuts & seeds
Seeds, flaxseed	392	Nuts & seeds
Seeds, sesame flour, high-fat	361	Grain
Seeds, sunflower, partially defatted	346	Grain
Seeds, sesame flour, low-fat	338	Grain
Nuts, cashew nuts, raw	292	Nuts & seeds
Soybeans, mature seeds, raw	280	Legumes

Table 8-12 Ten foods containing the richest phosphorus

Food name	Phosphorus (mg /100g)	Category
Rice bran, crude	1677	Grain
Seeds, cottonseed flour, low fat (glandless)	1587	Grain
Cereals ready-to-eat, malted flour, single brand	813	Cereal
Seeds, sesame flour, high-fat	807	Grain
Peanut flour, defatted	760	Grain
Seeds, sesame flour, low-fat	757	Grain
Cocoa, dry powder, unsweetened	734	Grain
Soybeans, mature seeds, raw	704	Legumes
Seeds, sunflower flour, partially defatted	689	Grain
Wheat flour, white, all-purpose, self-rising, enriched	595	Grain

Table 8-13 Ten foods containing the richest potassium

Food name	Potassium (mg /100g)	Category
Soy flour, full-fat, raw	2515	Grain
Soybeans, mature seeds, raw	1797	Legumes
Seeds, cottonseed flour, low fat (glandless)	1761	Grain
Cocoa, dry powder, unsweetened	1524	Grain
Rice bran, crude	1485	Grain
Beans, black, mature seeds, raw	1483	Legumes
Beans, pink, mature seeds, raw	1464	Legumes
Beans, pinto, mature seeds, raw	1393	Legumes
Beans, kidney, red mature seeds, raw	1359	Legumes
Peanut flour, low fat	1358	Grain

Table 8-14 Ten foods containing the richest sodium

Food name	Sodium (mg /100g)	Category
Tofu, salted & fermented (fuyu), prepared with calcium sulfate	2873	Legumes
Cheese, parmesan, hard	1602	Cheese
Cheese, blue	1395	Cheese
Cheese, America cheddar, imitation	1345	Cheese
Wheat flour, white, all-purpose, self-rising, enriched	1270	Grain
Cheese, Mexican, queso anejo	1131	Cheese
Cheese, feta	1116	Cheese
Cheese, edam	965	Cheese
Cheese, provolone, reduced fat	876	Cheese
Crustaceans, crab, Alaska king, raw	836	Fish & shellfish

Table 8-15 Ten foods containing the richest zinc

Food name	Zinc (mg /100g)	Category
Cereals ready-to-eat, KELLOGG, KELLOGG'S Complete Wheat Bran Flakes	52.5	Cereal
Cereals ready-to-eat, CERNERAL MILLS, CHEE-RIOS	27.8	Cereal
Cereals ready-to-eat, GERNERAL MILLS, HAR-MONY	13.6	Cereal
Cereals ready-to-eat, Malt-O-Meal, High Fiber Bran Flakes	13.4	Cereal
Cereals ready-to-eat, malted flour, single brand	12.9	Cereal
Cereals ready-to-eat, CERNERAL MILLS, Cinnamon Grahams	12.5	Cereal
Cereals ready-to-eat, CERNERAL MILLS, FIBER ONE	12.5	Cereal
Seeds, cottonseed flour, low fat (glandless)	11.6	Grain
Seeds, sesame flour, high-fat	10.7	Grain
Seeds, sesame flour, high-fat	10.0	Grain

Table 8-16 Ten foods containing the richest copper

Food name	Copper (mg /100g)	Category
Beef, liver, raw	9.8	Meat & poultry
Lamb, liver, raw	7.0	Meat & poultry
Seeds, sesame seeds, whole, dried	4.1	Nuts & seeds
Coca, dry powder, unsweetened	3.8	Grain
Soy flour, full-fat, raw	2.9	Grain
Seeds, breadnut tree seeds, dried	2.5	Nuts & seeds
Seeds, cashew nuts, raw	2.2	Nuts & seeds
Seeds, sunflower kernels, dried	1.8	Nuts & seeds
Peanut flour, defatted	1.8	Grain
Nuts, hazelnuts or filberts	1.7	Nuts & seeds

Table 8-17 Ten foods containing the richest manganese

Food name	Manganese (mg /100g)	Category
Rice bran, crude	14.2	Grain
Cereals ready-to-eat, malted flour, single brand	9.0	Cereal
Nuts, pine nuts, dried	8.8	Nuts & seeds
Rye flour, dark	6.7	Grain
Cereals ready-to-eat, Malt-O-Meal, High Fiber Bran Flakes	6.5	Cereal
Rye flour, medium	5.5	Grain
Peanut flour, defatted	4.9	Grain
Nuts, pecans	4.5	Nuts & seeds
Cereals ready-to-eat, KELLOGG, KELLOGG'S Complete Wheat Bran Flakes	4.2	Cereal
Rice flour, brown	4.0	Grain

Table 8-18 Ten foods containing the richest selenium

Food name	Selenium (µg /100g)	Category
Pork, kidneys, raw	190.0	Meat & poultry
Beef, kidneys, raw	141.0	Meat & poultry
Lamb, kidneys, raw	126.9	Meat & poultry
Lamb, liver, raw	82.4	Meat & poultry
Wheat flour, whole-grain	70.7	Grain
Cereals ready-to-eat, Malt-O-Meal, High Fiber Bran Flakes	63.2	Cereal
Seeds, sunflower flour, partially defatted	58.2	Grain
Chicken, liver, raw	54.6	Meat & poultry
Tofu, dried-frozen (koyatofu)	54.3	Legumes
Seeds, sunflower kernels, dried	53.0	Nuts & seeds

3. Vitamin Values of Selected Foods

The value of vitamins of the selected foods in Appendix A is summarized in Table 8-19 in terms of food categories.

Table 8-19 Summary of vitamin contents of different types of the selected foods per 100 grams

Food category	A (µg)	C (mg)	D (µg)	E (mg)	K (µg)	B_1 (mg)	B_2 (mg)	B_3 (mg)	B_5 (mg)	B_6 (mg)	B_7 (µg)	B_9 (µg)	B_{12} (µg)	Choline (mg)
Vegetables	0-835	2.8-184	0	0-2.9	0-1640	0-0.3	0-0.5	0.1-6.5	0.1-1.5	0.1-1.2	0-17	3-194	0-0.1	0-36.2
Fruits	1-38	2.0-92.5	0	0.1-2.7	0-40	0-0.2	0-0.3	0-1.9	0.1-1.5	0-.1-0.4	0.1-5	0-89	0	0-14.2
Legumes	0-35	0-16.3	0	0-0.9	0-47	0.1-0.9	0-0.9	0.1-2.9	0-2.1	0.1-0.5	0-60	27-633	0	0-115.9
Cereal	0-1294	0-207.0	0-6.2	0-26.6	0-9	0.1-5.4	0.3-5.9	2.1-69.0	0-34.9	0.2-9.7	0	30-1390	0-28.3	0-54.2
Grain	0-22	0-6.8	0	0-4.9	0-70	0.1-3.2	0.1-0.5	0.1-34.0	0.1-7.4	0.1-4.1	0-31	3-345	0	0-190.6
Bread	0-63	0-0.4	0-0.4	0-0.5	0-5	0.2-0.5	0.2-0.4	1.5-5.2	0.2-0.8	0-0.3	0-2	34-191	0	0-84.0
Dairy	2-257	0-8.6	0-7.8	0-0.5	0-2	0-0.4	0.2-1.6	0-0.9	0.2-3.1	0-0.3	0-2	1-47	0-3.8	0-118.7
Egg	0-381	0-0.2	0-2.7	0-2.6	0-6	0-0.2	0.4-0.8	0-0.2	0.2-2.9	0-0.4	7-52	4-146	0.1-5.4	0-682.3
Cheese	11-298	0	0-0.9	0-0.4	0.1-3	0-0.2	0.2-0.8	0.1-1.0	0-1.7	0-0.4	0-4	1-65	0.3-2.1	0-27.2
Nuts & Seeds	0-28	0-46.6	0	0-33.2	0-54	0.1-1.6	0.1-1.0	0.8-5.3	0.2-1.9	0.1-1.7	0-27	10-227	0	0-63.0

Fish & Shellfish	2-655	0-16.0	0-40.7	0-7.0	0-5	0-0.4	0-0.5	1.1-14.0	0.1-1.6	0.1-0.8	0-18	2-80	0.2-15.6	0-335.4
Meat & Poultry	0-7391	0-45.5	0-0.8	0-1.2	0-15	0.1-1.0	0.1-3.6	0-15.3	0-7.1	0-1.1	0-11	0-290	0-90.1	0-333.3
Oil	0	0	0	0-41.1	0-71	0	0	0	0	0	0	0	0	0-0.3

Note: A = vitamin A, C = vitamin C, D = vitamin D, E = vitamin E, K = vitamin K, B_1 = Thiamin, B_2 = Riboflavin, B_3 = Niacin, B_5 = Pantothenic Acid, B_7 = Biotin, B_9 = Folate, and B_{12} = Vitamin B_{12}.

The richest source of vitamin A in our daily foods is vegetables, cereal, fish and shellfish, and meat and poultry, while vitamin C mainly comes from cereal, vegetables, and fruits. Fish and shellfish possess the richest contents of vitamin D, whereas oil has the highest contents of vitamin E, and vegetables have much higher contents of vitamin K than the other kinds of foods.

Cereal and grain contain the richest contents of vitamins B_1, B_2, B_3, B_5, and B_6, whereas legumes and egg possess the richest contents of vitamin B_7, and legumes and cereal have the highest contents of vitamin B_9. Meat and poultry is the richest source of vitamin B_{12}. The richest source of choline in our daily foods is egg, fish and shellfish, and meat and poultry.

The following tables present 10 foods containing the richest contents of each vitamin, separately.

Table 8-20 Ten foods containing the richest vitamin A

Food name	Vitamin A (mg /100g)	Category
Lamb, liver, raw	7391	Meat & poultry
Pork, liver, raw	6502	Meat & poultry
Beef, liver, raw	4968	Meat & poultry
Chicken, liver, raw	3296	Meat & poultry
Cereals ready-to-eat, Malt-O-Meal, High Fiber Bran Flakes	1771	Cereal
Cereals ready-to-eat, KELLOGG, KELLOGG'S Complete Wheat Bran Flakes	1294	Cereal
Cereal, oats, instant, fortified, plain, dry	1072	Cereal
Cereals ready-to-eat, CERNERAL MILLS, CHEERIOS	867	Cereal
Carrots, raw	835	Vegetables

Kale, raw	769	Vegetables

Table 8-21 Ten foods containing the richest vitamin C

Food name	Vitamin C (mg /100g)	Category
Peppers, sweet, yellow, raw	183.5	Vegetables
Parsley, raw	133.0	Vegetables
Peppers, sweet, red, raw	127.7	Vegetables
Kale, raw	120.0	Vegetables
Kiwi fruit, fresh, raw	92.5	Fruits
Broccoli, raw	89.2	Vegetables
Peppers, sweet, green, raw	80.4	Vegetables
Lemon, raw, with peel	77.0	Fruits
Persimmon, native, raw	66.0	Fruits
Turnip green, raw	60.0	Vegetables

Table 8-22 Ten foods containing the richest vitamin D

Food name	Vitamin D (µg /100g)	Category
Fish, herring, Atlantic, raw	40.7	Fish & shellfish
Fish, sardine, Pacific, canned in tomato sauce, drained solids with bone	12.0	Fish & shellfish
Fish, mackerel, Atlantic, raw	9.0	Fish & shellfish
Fish, herring, Pacific, raw	7.9	Fish & shellfish
Milk, dry, whole	7.8	Dairy
Cereals ready-to-eat, Malt-O-Meal, High Fiber Bran Flakes	6.2	Cereal
Crustaceans, shrimp, mixed species, raw	3.8	Fish & shellfish
Cereals ready-to-eat, corn & oat flour, Puffed presweetened, single brand	3.5	Cereal
Cereals ready-to-eat, bran flakes, single brand	3.3	Cereal

Egg, yolk, raw, fresh	2.7	Egg

Table 8-23 Ten foods containing the richest vitamin E

Food name	Vitamin E (mg /100g)	Category
Cottonseed oil	35.3	Oil
Seeds, sunflower kernels, dried	33.2	Nuts & seeds
Grapeseed oil	28.8	Oil
Cereals ready-to-eat, Malt-O-Meal, High Fiber Bran Flakes	26.6	Cereal
Nuts, almonds	26.2	Nuts & seeds
Cereals ready-to-eat, GERNERAL MILLS, HARMONY	24.5	Cereal
Canola oil	17.6	Oil
Flaxseed oil	17.5	Oil
Palm oil	15.9	Oil
Nuts, hazelnuts or filberts	15.0	Nuts & seeds

Table 8-24 Ten foods containing the richest vitamin K

Food name	Vitamin K (µg /100g)	Category
Parsley, raw	1640	Vegetables
Chard, Swiss, raw	830	Vegetables
Kale, raw	817	Vegetables
Spinach, raw	483	Vegetables
Turnip greens, raw	251	Vegetables
Broccoli, raab, raw	224	Vegetables
Brussels sprouts, raw	177	Vegetables
Lettuce, green leaf, raw	174	Vegetables
Broccoli, raw	102	Vegetables
Cabbage, raw	76	Vegetables

Table 8-25 Ten foods containing the richest vitamin B$_1$

Food name	Vitamin B$_1$ (mg /100g)	Category
Cereals ready-to-eat, KELLOGG, KELLOGG'S Complete Wheat Bran Flakes	5.4	Cereal
Seeds, sunflower flour, partially defatted	3.2	Grain
Rice bran, crude	2.8	Grain
Cereals ready-to-eat, GERNERAL MILLS, HARMONY	2.7	Cereal
Seeds, sesame flour, high fat	2.7	Grain
Seeds, sesame flour, low fat	2.7	Grain
Seeds, cottonseed flour, low fat	2.1	Grain
Cereal, oats, instant, fortified, plain, dry	2.1	Cereal
Cereals ready-to-eat, CERNERAL MILLS, CHEERIOS	1.9	Cereal
Cereals ready-to-eat, Malt-O-Meal, High Fiber Bran Flakes	1.6	Cereal

Table 8-26 Ten foods containing the richest vitamin B$_2$

Food name	Vitamin B$_2$ (mg /100g)	Category
Cereals ready-to-eat, KELLOGG, KELLOGG'S Complete Wheat Bran Flakes	5.9	Cereal
Cereals ready-to-eat, Malt-O-Meal, High Fiber Bran Flakes	2.0	Cereal
Cereals ready-to-eat, CERNERAL MILLS, CHEERIOS	1.6	Cereal
Dairy, buttermilk, dried	1.6	Dairy
Cereals ready-to-eat, GERNERAL MILLS, HARMONY	1.6	Cereal
Cereals ready-to-eat, bran, malted flour, Single brand	1.5	Cereal
Cereals ready-to-eat, GENERAL MILLS, FIBER ONE	1.4	Cereal
Milk, dry, whole	1.2	Dairy
Soy flour, full-fat, raw	1.2	Grain

Cereal, oats, instant, fortified, plain, dry	1.2	Cereal

Table 8-27 Ten foods containing the richest vitamin B₃

Food name	Vitamin B$_3$ (mg /100g)	Category
Cereals ready-to-eat, KELLOGG, KELLOGG'S Complete Wheat Bran Flakes	69.0	Cereal
Rice bran, crude	34.0	Grain
Cereals ready-to-eat, Malt-O-Meal, High Fiber Bran Flakes	30.3	Cereal
Peanut flour, defatted	27.0	Grain
Cereals ready-to-eat, CERNERAL MILLS, CHEERIOS	19.1	Cereal
Cereals ready-to-eat, GERNERAL MILLS, HARMONY	18.2	Cerea
Cereals ready-to-eat, bran, malted flour, single brand	17.2	Cerea
Cereals ready-to-eat, GENERAL MILLS, FIBER ONE	16.7	Cerea
Lamb, liver, raw	16.1	Meat & poultry
Pork, flesh, liver, raw	15.3	Meat & poultry

Table 8-28 Ten foods containing the richest vitamin B₅

Food name	Vitamin B$_5$ (mg /100g)	Category
Cereals ready-to-eat, KELLOGG, KELLOGG'S Complete Wheat Bran Flakes	34.9	Cereal
Rice bran, crude	7.4	Grain
Beef, liver, raw	7.2	Meat & poultry
Pork, fresh, liver, raw	6.7	Meat & poultry
Seeds, sunflower, partially defatted	6.6	Grain
Chicken, liver, raw	6.2	Meat & poultry
Lamb, liver, raw	6.1	Meat & poultry
Lamb, kidneys, raw	4.2	Meat & poultry

| Beef, kidneys, raw | 4.0 | Meat & poultry |
| Pork, fresh, liver, raw | 3.1 | Meat & poultry |

Table 8-29 Ten foods containing the richest vitamin B$_6$

Food name	Vitamin B$_6$ (mg /100g)	Category
Cereals ready-to-eat, Malt-O-Meal, High Fiber Bran Flakes	9.7	Cereal
Cereals ready-to-eat, KELLOGG, KELLOGG'S Complete Wheat Bran Flakes	7.0	Cereal
Rice bran, crude	4.1	Grain
Cereals ready-to-eat, GERNERAL MILLS, HARMONY	1.8	Cereal
Cereals ready-to-eat, CERNERAL MILLS, CHEERIOS	1.8	Cereal
Cereals ready-to-eat, bran, malted flour, single brand	1.7	Cereal
Cereals ready-to-eat, GENERAL MILLS, FIBER ONE	1.7	Cereal
Nuts, pistachio nuts, raw	1.7	Nuts & seeds
Beef, liver, raw	1.1	Meat & poultry
Pork, flesh, liver, raw	0.9	Meat & poultry

Table 8-30 Ten foods containing the richest vitamin B$_7$

Food name	Vitamin B$_7$ (μg /100g)	Category
Soybeans, mature seeds, raw	60.0	Legumes
Egg, yolk, raw, fresh	52.0	Egg
Barley, pearled, raw	31.0	Grain
Nuts, pecans	27.0	Nuts & seeds
Egg, whole, raw, fresh	23.0	Egg
Cowpeas, common, mature seeds, raw	21.0	Legumes
Fish, mackerel, Atlantic, raw	18.0	Fish & shellfish

Cauliflower, raw	17.0	Vegetables
Mushrooms, white, raw	16.0	Vegetables
Chicken, broiler or fryer, light meat, meat & skin, raw	11.0	Meat & poultry

Table 8-31 Ten foods containing the richest vitamin B_9

Food name	Vitamin B_9 (µg /100g)	Category
Cereals ready-to-eat, KELLOGG, KELLOGG'S Complete Wheat Bran Flakes	1390	Cereal
Cereals ready-to-eat, Malt-O-Meal, High Fiber Bran Flakes	1290	Cereal
Cereals ready-to-eat, CERNERAL MILLS, CHEERIOS	975	Cereal
Cereals ready-to-eat, GERNERAL MILLS, HARMONY	727	Cereal
Cowpeas, common, mature seeds, raw	633	Legumes
Chickpeas, mature seeds, raw	557	Legumes
Beans, pinto, mature seeds, raw	525	Legumes
Lentils, raw	479	Legumes
Beans, pink, mature seeds, raw	463	Legumes
Beans, black, mature seeds, raw	444	Legumes

Table 8-32 Ten foods containing the richest vitamin B_{12}

Food name	Vitamin B_{12} (µg /100g)	Category
Lamb, liver, raw	90.1	Meat & poultry
Beef, liver, raw	59.3	Meat & poultry
Lamb, kidneys, raw	52.4	Meat & poultry
Cereals ready-to-eat, Malto-O-Meal, High Fiber Bran Flaks	28.3	Cereal
Beef, kidneys, raw	27.5	Meat & poultry

Pork, fresh, liver, raw	26.0	Meat & poultry
Cereals ready-to-eat, KELLOGG, KELLOGG'S Complete Wheat Bran Flakes	20.7	Cereal
Chicken, liver, raw	16.6	Meat & poultry
Fish, mackerel, king, raw	15.6	Fish & shellfish
Fish, herring, Atlantic, raw	13.7	Fish & shellfish

Table 8-33 Ten foods containing the richest choline

Food name	Choline (mg /100g)	Category
Egg, yolk, raw, fresh	682.3	Egg
Fish, roe, mixed species, raw	335.4	Fish & shellfish
Beef, liver, raw	333.3	Meat & poultry
Egg, whole, cooked, fried	272.6	Egg
Egg, duck, whole, fresh, raw	263.4	Egg
Egg, goose, whole, fresh, raw	263.4	Egg
Egg, quail, whole, fresh, raw	263.4	Egg
Egg, whole, fresh, raw	251.1	Egg
Pork, fresh, stomach, raw	194.8	Meat & poultry
Chicken, liver, raw	194.4	Meat & poultry

4. Values of Essential Amino Acids, EPA, DHA, and Lutein plus Zeaxanthin of Selected Foods

The values of essential amino acids, EPA, DHA, and lutein plus zeaxanthin of the selected foods in Appendix A are summarized in Table 8-34, in terms of food categories

Table 8-34 Summary of important amino acids, EPA, DHA, lutein, and zeaxanthin contents of different types of the selected foods per 100 grams

Food category	W (mg)	T (mg)	I (mg)	L (mg)	K (mg)	M+C (mg)	F+Y (mg)	V (mg)	H (mg)	EPA (mg)	DHA (mg)	L+Z (µg)
Vegetables	0-159	0-503	0-508	0-938	0-752	0-295	0-1118	0-620	0-348	0	0	0-39550

	W	T	I	L	K	M	C	F	Y	V	H	EPA	DHA	L+Z
Fruits	0-50	0-82	0-167	0-359	0-162	0-137	0-322	0-282	0-333	0	0			0-271
Legumes	0-747	0-1956	0-2376	0-3644	0-3157	0-1276	0-3938	0-2418	0-1394	0	0			0-640
Cereal	0-192	0-506	0-586	0-498	0-1050	0-675	0-1173	0-931	0-753	0	0			0-782
Grain	0-1091	0-2081	0-2157	0-3841	0-2298	0-2668	0-4827	0-2800	0-1570	0	0			0-1355
Bread	78-131	172-306	217-399	388-692	181-297	208-413	403-842	260-461	126-225	0	0			0-72
Dairy	17-484	46-1548	56-2075	95-3360	68-2720	92-1177	99-3302	63-2296	23-930	0	0			0
Egg	136-282	468-797	565-866	854-1399	768-1217	642-933	992-1574	678-985	264-416			0-11	0-114	0-1094
Cheese	0-482	0-1038	0-1894	0-3452	0-3306	0-1193	0-3917	0-2454	0-1384	0	0			0
Nuts & Seeds	32-390	90-1112	314-1342	563-2149	18-1833	29-1272	641-3047	363-1556	195-775	0	0			0-651
Fish & Shellfish	161-283	630-1017	662-1142	1332-1956	1330-2142	615-952	1054-2213	746-1307	382-687			0-1086	0-1401	0
Meat & Poultry	0-301	0-977	0-1091	0-1910	0-1983	0-1826	0-1891	0-1260	0-905			0-220	0-490	0
Oil	0	0	0	0	0	0	0	0	0	0	0	0	0	0

Note: W = Tryptophan, T = Threonine, I = Isoleucine, L = Leucine, K = Lysine, M = Methionie, C = Cystine, F = Phenylalanine, Y = Tyrosine, V = Valine, H = Histidine, EPA = Eicosapentaenoic acid, DHA = Docosahexaenoic acid, and L+Z = Lutein + Zeaxanthin.

In Table 8-34, I found that legumes, grain, dairy products, and cheese contain the richest various amino acids, while fish and shellfish, meat and poultry, nuts and seeds have moderate amounts of these amino acids, and vegetables, fruits, and cereal possess the lowest contents of these amino acids.

Fish and shellfish contain the richest EPA and DHA, meat and poultry contain the next richest, and eggs contain the next richest after meat and poultry, while vegetables, fruits, legumes, cereal, grain, bread, dairy products, cheese, nuts and seeds, and oil do not contain any EAP or DHA. Table 8-35 and Table 8-36 show 10 foods containing the richest EPA and DHA.

Table 8-35 Ten foods containing the richest EPA

Food name	EPA (mg /100g)	Category
Fish, shad, America, raw	1086	Fish & shellfish
Fish, salmon, chinook, raw	1008	Fish & shellfish
Fish, roe, mixed species, raw	983	Fish & shellfish
Fish, herring, Pacific, raw	969	Fish & shellfish
Fish, mackerel, Atlantic, raw	898	Fish & shellfish
Fish, herring, Atlantic, raw	709	Fish & shellfish
Fish, sablefish, raw	677	Fish & shellfish

Fish, salmon, Atlantic, farmed, raw	618	Fish & shellfish
Fish, anchovy, European, raw	538	Fish & shellfish
Fish, halibut, Greenland, raw	526	Fish & shellfish

Table 8-36 Ten foods containing the richest DHA

Food name	DHA (mg /100g)	Category
Fish, mackerel, Atlantic, raw	1401	Fish & shellfish
Fish, roe, mixed species, raw	1363	Fish & shellfish
Fish, shad, America, raw	1321	Fish & shellfish
Fish, salmon, Atlantic, farmed, raw	1293	Fish & shellfish
Fish, salmon, Atlantic, wild, raw	1115	Fish & shellfish
Fish, mackerel, Spanish, raw	1012	Fish & shellfish
Fish, salmon, chinook, raw	944	Fish & shellfish
Fish, anchovy, European, raw	911	Fish & shellfish
Fish, tuna, bluefin, raw	890	Fish & shellfish
Fish, herring, Atlantic, raw	862	Fish & shellfish

Vegetables contain the richest lutein and zeaxanthin, and grains and eggs contain the next richest lutein and zeaxanthin. Fruits, legumes, cereal, grain, bread, and nuts and seeds possess some of them, but dairy products, fish and shellfish, meat and poultry, and oil do not have any of them. Ten foods that contain the richest lutein and zeaxanthin are listed in Table 8-37.

Table 8-37 Ten foods containing the richest lutein and zeaxanthin

Food name	Lutein + Zeaxanthin (µg /100g)	Category
Kale, raw	39550	Vegetables
Turnip greens, raw	12825	Vegetables
Spinach, raw	12198	Vegetables
Chard, Swiss, raw	11000	Vegetables
Parsley, raw	5561	Vegetables
Lettuce, cos or romaine, raw	2312	Vegetables
Squash, summer, zucchini, includes skin, raw	2125	Vegetables

Leeks (bulb & lower leaf-portion), raw	1900	Vegetables
Lettuce, green leaf, raw	1730	Vegetables
Lettuce, red leaf, raw	1724	Vegetables

Chapter Nine
Human Nutrition Optimization

1. Optimization and Its Application in Industry

Optimization problems are made up of three basic ingredients:

(1) An **objective function** that we want to minimize or maximize. For instance, in a manufacturing process, we might want to maximize the profit or minimize the cost. In designing an automobile panel, we might want to maximize the strength. In our life, we would like to maximize our longevity with optimum health.

(2) A set of **unknowns** or **variables** which affect the value of the objective function. In the manufacturing problem, the variables might include the amounts of different resources used or the time spent on each activity. In the panel design problem, the variables used define the shape and dimensions of the panel. In our longevity, the variables might include genetics, exercise, spirituality, and human nutrition.

(3) A set of **constraints** that allow the unknowns to take on certain values but exclude others. For the manufacturing problem, it does not make sense to spend a negative amount of time on any activity, so we constrain all the "time" variables to be non-negative. In the panel design problem, we would probably want to limit the weight of the product and to constrain its shape. In our longevity, we would exclude the factors of genetics, exercise, and spirituality, and focus on the variables of human nutrition.

Optimization is finding values of the variables that minimize or maximize the objective function while satisfying the constraints.

Optimization has been widely used in many industries such as chemical, petrochemical, material, metallurgical, pharmaceutical, biopharmaceutical, and agricultural. Optimization has resulted in billions of benefits each year with the best product quality and minimum cost. For example, enterprise optimization in the pharmaceutical industry can produce 28 billion dollars of value.

Based on the same rationale, if we can optimize the variables that affect our health, then we will be able to maximize our longevity. Besides genetics, exercise, and spirituality, our optimum health depends on human nutrition: what we breathe, what we drink, and what we eat. So, in this chapter, I will discuss how to optimize human nutrition, including macronutrients: oxygen, water, protein, fat, carbohydrate, and fiber, and micronutrients: vitamins and minerals.

2. The Most Important Nutrient—Oxygen Optimization

As discussed in Chapter Two, oxygen is the most vital nutrient because our life can only sustain for a few minutes without it. A normal human would utilize about 3.5 ml of oxygen/kg/min. By calculation, a normal 70 kg human breathes in 352.8 liters (504 g) of oxygen each day (24 hours) from air that is equivalent to 1680 liters of air, based on the 21% of oxygen in the air. Daily requirements of oxygen and air amounts for adults with a body weight of 44 kg–90 kg have been computed, which is presented in Table 9-1.

Table 9-1 Daily human body requirements of oxygen and air amounts

Body weight (kg [lb])	Oxygen volume (L)	Oxygen weight (g)	Air volume (L)
44 [97]	222	317	1056
46 [101]	232	331	1104
48 [106]	242	346	1152
50 [110]	252	360	1200
52 [115]	262	374	1248
54 [119]	272	389	1296
56 [124]	282	403	1344
58 [128]	292	418	1392
60 [132]	302	432	1440
62 [137]	312	446	1488
64 [141]	323	461	1536
66 [146]	333	475	1584
68 [150]	343	490	1632
70 [154]	353	504	1680

72 [159]	363	518	1728
74 [163]	373	533	1776
76 [168]	383	547	1824
78 [172]	393	562	1872
80 [176]	403	576	1920
82 [181]	413	590	1968
84 [185]	423	605	2016
86 [189]	433	619	2064
88 [194]	444	634	2112
90 [198]	454	648	2160

Table 9-1 shows us that each person must breathe enough oxygen from air based on his/her body weight to meet his/her physiological needs. Therefore, the most important nutrient—oxygen optimization is actually the optimization of air quality, which can be divided into outdoor air quality optimization and indoor air quality optimization. First, let's see the original air composition, and then discuss air quality optimization.

Air Composition. The sea-level composition of air in percent by volume at the temperature of 15°C and the pressure of 101325 Pa is shown in Table 9-2.

Table 9-2 Air composition by volume

Name	Symbol	Percentage by volume
Nitrogen	N_2	78.084%
Oxygen	O_2	20.9476%
Argon	Ar	0.934%
Carbon Dioxide	CO_2	0.0314%
Neon	Ne	0.001818%
Methane	CH_4	0.0002%
Helium	He	0.000524%
Krypton	Kr	0.000114%
Hydrogen	H_2	0.00005%
Xenon	Xe	0.0000087%

From CRC Handbook of Chemistry and Physics by David R. Lide, Editor-in-Chief, 1997 Edition

The air composition in Table 9-2 is an optimal composition in which oxygen concentration is the best for our health. However, air pollution is getting more and more serious these days, and it is lowering oxygen concentration and raising carbon dioxide concentration, and increasing hazardous chemicals and particulate matters in the air. Atmospheres with oxygen concentrations below 19.5 percent can have adverse physiological effects, and atmospheres with less than 16 percent oxygen can become life threatening. Therefore, the objective of air quality optimization is to eliminate hazardous compositions in the air and to achieve the optimal air composition.

Outdoor Air Quality Optimization. With economic development, air pollution is getting more and more serious, especially in developing countries. It has been recognized that outdoor air pollution can play a large role in exacerbating cardiopulmonary diseases and shortening life. The most dramatic evidence of this was given by a series of major pollution incidents in London, England in the 1950s and 1960s, where deaths and hospital admissions clearly increased in the days following the elevated pollution levels. Several countries, including the United States and Canada, have set more stringent standards for pollution emissions in an attempt to reduce ambient concentrations.

A number of studies conducted worldwide have linked daily variations in the number of deaths to daily fluctuations in ambient pollution levels. These studies indicate that the daily number of deaths increases as outdoor pollution concentrations increase. Our health and longevity are related to outdoor air quality. In the world, most of the people who are more than 100 years old live in the suburban areas, where there is good air quality, whereas the people who live in areas with heavy air pollution have shortened lives with various diseases.

Reducing air pollution and optimizing outdoor air quality is the responsibility of every government in the world. Every government must protect our environment at the time of developing the economy. Before undertaking a new project, the related experts must first evaluate its effect on the air quality. If the health cost caused by the new project is larger than the investment, then the government should stop the project. The leaders in every government in the world should cooperate to take action together to help control air pollution and optimize outdoor air quality. For example, establishing a worldwide air optimization organization to help monitor the global air quality and set up some rules that every country must abide by, would help optimize the air quality quickly and efficiently. In addition, each person should reduce his/her contribution to air pollution as less as possible by, for example, driving less, and walking and bicycling more.

Indoor Air Quality Optimization. Most people are aware that outdoor air pollution can damage their health, but may not know that indoor air pollution can also have significant effects. The Environmental Protection Agency (EPA) studies of human exposure to air pollutants indicate that indoor air levels of many pollutants may be 2–5 times, and occasionally more than 100 times, higher than outdoor levels. These levels of indoor air pollutants are of particular concern because it is estimated that most people spend as much as 90% of their time indoors.

Over the past several decades, our exposure to indoor air pollutants is believed to have increased due to a variety of factors, including the construction of more tightly sealed buildings, reduced ventilation rates in order to save energy, the use of synthetic building materials and furnishings, and the use of chemically formulated personal care products, pesticides, and household cleaners.

Health effects from indoor air pollutants may be experienced soon after exposure, or possibly, years later. Immediate effects may show up after a single exposure or repeated exposures. These can include irritation of the eyes, nose, and throat, headaches, dizziness, and fatigue. Such immediate effects are usually short-term and treatable. Sometimes the treatment is simply eliminating the person's exposure to the source of the pollution, if it can be identified. Symptoms of some diseases, including asthma, hypersensitivity pneumonitis, and humidifier fever, may also show up soon after exposure to some indoor air pollutants.

Other health effects may show up either years after the exposure has occurred or only after long or repeated periods of exposure. These effects, which include some respiratory diseases, heart disease, and cancer, can be severely debilitating or fatal. It is prudent to try to improve or optimize the indoor air quality in our home even if symptoms are not noticeable.

There are three basic strategies to optimize indoor air quality: source control, improved ventilation, and the use of air cleaners.

Usually the most effective way to optimize indoor air quality is to eliminate individual sources of pollution or to reduce their emissions. Some sources, like those that contain asbestos, can be sealed or enclosed; others, like gas stoves, can be adjusted to decrease the amount of emissions. In many cases, source control is also a more cost-efficient approach to protecting indoor air quality than increasing ventilation because increasing ventilation can increase energy costs.

For most indoor air quality problems at home, source control is the most effective solution.

Another approach to lowering the concentrations of indoor air pollutants in your home is to increase the amount of outdoor air coming indoors.

Most home heating and cooling systems, including forced air heating systems, do not mechanically bring fresh air into the house. Opening windows and doors, operating windows or attic fans, when the weather permits, or running a window air conditioner with the vent control open increases the outdoor ventilation rate. Local bathroom or kitchen fans that exhaust outdoors remove contaminants directly from the room where the fan is located and also increase the outdoor air ventilation rate. It is particularly important to take as many of these steps as possible while you are involved in short-term activities that can generate high levels of pollutants, for example, painting, paint stripping, heating with kerosene heaters, cooking, or engaging in maintenance and hobby activities such as welding, soldering, or sanding. If you can, you might want to do some of these activities outdoors.

The use of air cleaner is the last method that can be used for optimizing indoor air quality. There are many different types and sizes of air cleaners on the market, ranging from relatively inexpensive table-top models to sophisticated and expensive whole-house systems. Some air cleaners are highly effective at particle removal, while others, including most table-top models, are much less so. Air cleaners are generally not designed to remove gaseous pollutants.

3. The Second Most Important Nutrient—Water Optimization

As discussed in Chapter Two, water is the second most important nutrient, because life can only sustain for a few days without it. The body weight of a normal adult is composed of about 65% water. Homeostatic regulation by the gastrointestinal tract, kidneys, and the brain keeps the water content of the body fairly constant. The body has no provision for water storage, thus the amount of water lost every 24 hours must be replaced in order to maintain a good health and body efficiency.

How many milliliters (ml) of water a day do we need to consume under "average conditions of energy expenditure and environmental conditions" to maintain the water balance in our bodies? The National Research Council recommends 1 ml/kcal/day energy expenditure for adults. This translates into approximately 35 ml/kg/day for adults with normal body weights. From our food intake, we can obtain about 27% water, and about 9% water from oxidative metabolism of the food we eat each day. By calculation, the daily required water amounts for different body weights under normal temperatures are presented in Table 9-3. In hot weather, daily water intake will be increased by about 44%. During prolonged exercise, daily water intake will be increased by about 187%.

Table 9-3 Daily human body water requirements

Body weight (kg [lb])	Total required water (ml)	Water to be drunk (ml)	*Cups to be drunk
44 [97]	1540	986	4.1
46 [101]	1610	1030	4.3
48 [106]	1680	1075	4.5
50 [110]	1750	1120	4.7
52 [115]	1820	1165	4.9
54 [119]	1890	1210	5.0
56 [124]	1960	1254	5.2
58 [128]	2030	1299	5.4
60 [132]	2100	1344	5.6
62 [137]	2170	1389	5.8
64 [141]	2240	1434	6.0
66 [146]	2310	1478	6.2
68 [150]	2380	1523	6.3
70 [154]	2450	1568	6.5
72 [159]	2520	1613	6.7
74 [163]	2590	1658	6.9
76 [168]	2660	1702	7.1
78 [172]	2730	1747	7.3
80 [176]	2800	1792	7.5
82 [181]	2870	1837	7.7
84 [185]	2940	1882	7.8
86 [189]	3010	1926	8.0
88 [194]	3080	1971	8.2
90 [198]	3150	2016	8.4

*1 cup = 240 ml of water

From Table 9-3, we know that under normal conditions, different body weights require different amounts of water in order to keep the water at equilibrium in the body. An adult with a body weight of 88 kg (194 lb) needs to drink about 8 cups of water a day, which is twice the amount an adult with a body weight of 44 kg (97 lb) needs. So, the recommendation of 8 glasses of water per day to everyone is not correct. You should drink an amount of water according to your body weight, weather conditions, and exercise strength and time.

Besides the water from the food and the metabolism, we need to drink about 1000 ml to 2000 ml of water every day in terms of our body weights. So, the quality of the water we drink each day is of vital importance to our health. However, water pollution is a major problem in our world. It has been suggested that it is the leading worldwide cause of deaths and diseases, and that it accounts for the deaths of more than 14,000 people daily. Each year, about 1.1 billion people lack proper drinking water. In addition to the acute problems of water pollution in developing countries, industrialized countries continue to struggle with pollution problems as well. In the most recent national report on water quality in the United States, 45 percent of assessed stream miles, 47 percent of assessed lake acres, and 32 percent of assessed bay and estuarine square miles were classified as polluted.

Therefore, controlling water pollution and optimizing water quality is the responsibility of every government in the world. Every government should provide high quality drinking water for their people. In addition, each person should reduce his/her contributions to water pollution as well, like not littering in lakes, rivers, or the ocean.

Drinking Water Standards. The World Health Organization (WHO) set up the latest drinking water standards in Geneva in 1993. The European Union (EU) drew up the Council Directive 98/83/EC on the quality of water intended for human consumption, adopted by the Council on November 3rd, 1998. The U.S. Environmental Protection Agency (EPA) and the U.S. Food and Drug Administration (FDA) set drinking water standards in 1996. The EPA sets standards for tap water, while the FDA regulates bottled water as a packaged food under the Federal Food, Drug and Cosmetic Act and has established standards of identifications and qualifications for bottled water. The FDA has also established good manufacturing practice requirements for processing and bottling drinking water.

The drinking water standards from WHO, EU, EPA, and FDA are mostly similar, some of which are listed in Table 9-4.

Table 9-4 Some drinking water standards

Substance/attribute	Standard	Potential health effects from ingestion of water
Arsenic	0.01 mg/L	Skin damage or problems with circulatory systems, and may increase the risk of getting cancer

Cadmium	0.03 mg/L	Kidney damage
Cyanide	0.07 mg/L	Nerve damage or thyroid problems
Lead	0.01 mg/L	Infants and children: delays in physical or mental development; children could show slight deficits in attention span and learning ability Adults: kidney problems; high blood pressure
Mercury	0.001 mg/L	Kidney damage
Benzene	0.005 mg/L	Anemia; decrease in blood platelets; increased risk of cancer
Alpha particles	15 picocuries/L	Increased risk of cancer
Cryptoporidium	Zero	Gastrointestinal illness, e.g., diarrhea, vomiting, and cramps
pH	6.5–8.5	Long term drinking water with high or low pH values causes various diseases, e.g., high blood pressure, diabetes, and cancer

In some developing countries, due to economic development, water pollution has been getting more and more serious. Some villages have become "cancer village", which is caused by drinking the arsenic contaminated water that contains about 3.0 mg/L of arsenic, which is about 300 times the standard set by WHO. Leaders of a responsible government should take an effective measure to solve the problem of water pollution at the time of developing the economy and optimize the quality of drinking water using advanced technology to reach the standards set by WHO for human health.

In addition, in order to maintain our health and longevity, we ourselves can optimize the water we drink everyday by choosing different types of drinking water. All Americans can learn about the quality of their drinking water, both tap water and bottled water, before deciding to drink tap water, bottled water, or both. If your water comes from a public water system, the best way to learn about tap water is to read your water supplier's annual water quality report. If your water comes from a household well, the EPA recommends testing the water regularly for bacteria, nitrates, and other contaminants. The best way to learn more about bottled water is to read its label or contact the producer directly. Bottled water is more expensive than tap water. If you drink tap water, I suggest that you boil the water for a full minute, which can kill cryptosporidium that can cause illness.

Natural mineral water with no pollution is the best drinking water for our optimum heath. Most people over 100 years old live in the mountain areas of the world, where natural mineral water and fresh air can be found. One of the longest-living races of people in the world is called the Hunza. These people, living in northern Pakistan, are found in several high-altitude mountain valleys. Many Hunzas are documented centenarians (over age one hundred). Researchers believe that the Hunza miracle derives from the water that they drink. The mountain water that flows into the Hunza villages comes from the surrounding glaciers. Structured hexagonally, this water is filled with mineral solutes, and it tests out as highly alkaline.

Drinking Water and Beverages. Drinking water is the best kind of water for daily water intake. However, most people like to drink coffee, tea, et al. But these beverages can not replace water completely, because most of beverages are acidic, which influences equilibrium in the body, which could cause various diseases. Table 9-5 is the recommended daily intake of beverages for a 70-kg adult modified from Popkin et al. If this person drinks 200 ml of coffee, then he/she needs to drink 1300 ml of water to reach one day's total water intake of 1500 ml. If your weight is more or less than 70 kg, then you should make adjustments for the daily intake of beverages and drinking water according to your actual weight.

Table 9-5 Recommended daily intake of beverage for a 70-kg adult

Type	Suggested amount*	Acceptable range*
Drinking water	1500 ml/day	600–1500 ml/day
Tea (unsweetened)	600 ml/day	0–800 ml/day
Coffee (unsweetened)	200 ml/day	0–400 ml/day
Non-calorically sweetened soft drinks	0 ml/day	0–900 ml/day
Caloric beverages with nutrients		
–fruit juice, vegetable juice, full fat milk, sports drinks	120 ml/day	120 ml/day
–alcoholic beverages	0 ml/day	0–2 drinks/day
Calorically sweetened soft drinks	0 ml/day	0–250 ml/day

Modified from Popkin et al. America Journal Clinical Nutrition 2006, 83: 529-542.

4. Daily Energy and Other Macronutrients and Micronutrients Optimization

Save for oxygen and water, our daily energy and other nutrients come from the foods we eat. So, determining the different amounts of various types of foods to meet our daily requirements of energy and nutrition is the objective of this section. In Chapter Eight, I have discussed energy and nutrition values of different types of the selected 379 best foods listed in Appendix A. In Chapter Seven, I discussed and summarized the human body's daily energy and nutrition requirements for different ages at different body weights at different physical activity levels. Now, I take a 40-year-old woman with a weight of 59 kg and a height of 1.65 m at a sedentary activity level as an example to help instruct the procedure of optimizing daily energy and nutrition from the foods we eat.

Step One: List the daily energy and nutrition requirements (objective functions) for this woman. From Chapter Seven, we can find the data and I organized them in Table 9-6.

The daily energy required by a woman with a weight of 59 kg and a height of 1.65 m at a sedentary activity level, as presented in Table 7-8 of Chapter Seven, is 1828 kcal. Dr. Walford found that minimal caloric intake with high nutrients can extend our life span based on his clinical studies on animals. So, I reduce 10% of her daily energy to 1645 kcal, which is her minimal daily energy requirement. Thus, her daily energy intake range in Table 9-6 is 1645–1828 kcal/d.

Her daily protein reference intake of 46–160 g/d is calculated based on a recommendation from the Institute of Medicine, Food and Nutrition Board, Washington DC, 2002/2005 that the percent of energy provided by protein should account for 10%–35% of the total energy.

Her daily fat reference intake of 41–71 g/d is calculated based on the recommendation that the percent of energy provided by fat should account for 20%–35%.

Her daily carbohydrate reference intake of 205–297 g/d is also calculated based on the recommendation that the percent of energy provided by carbohydrate should account for 45%–65%.

In addition, her daily sugar reference intake of not more that 114 g/d is calculated based on the recommendation that the percent of energy provided by added sugar should be no more than 25%. Patients with diabetes should choose food combinations to meet their daily energy and nutrition requirements with as less sugar as possible.

Table 9-6 Daily energy and nutrition requirements of a 40-year-old woman with a weight of 59 kg and a height of 1.65 m at a sedentary activity level

Objective function	Reference intake	Tolerable intake limit (UL)
Energy	1645–1828 kcal/d	ND
Protein	46–160 g/d	ND
Fat	41–71 g/d	ND
Saturated fat	as low as possible	ND
Trans fat	as low as possible	ND
Carbohydrate	205–297 g/d	ND
Sugar	≤ 114 g/d	ND
Fiber	≥ 25 g/d	ND
Cholesterol	as low as possible	ND
ORAC	≥ 5000 μmol TE/d	ND
Calcium	≥ 1000 mg/d	2.5 g/d
Iron	≥ 18 mg/d	45 mg/d
Magnesium	≥ 320 mg/d	ND
Phosphorus	≥ 700 mg/d	4.0 g/d
Potassium	≥ 4.7 g/d	ND
Sodium	≥ 1.5 g/d	2.3 g/d
Zinc	≥ 8 mg/d	40 mg/d
Copper	≥ 900 μg/d	10000 μg/d
Manganese	≥ 1.8 mg/d	11 mg/d
Selenium	≥ 55 μg/d	400 μg/d
Chromium	≥ 25 μg/d	ND
Vitamin A	≥ 700 μg/d	3000 μg/d
Vitamin C	≥ 75 mg/d	2000 mg/d
Vitamin D	≥ 5 μg/d	50 μg/d
Vitamin E	≥ 15 mg/d	1000 mg/d
Vitamin K	≥ 90 μg/d	ND
Vitamin B_1	≥ 1.1 mg/d	ND

Vitamin B$_2$	≥ 1.1 mg/d	ND
Vitamin B$_3$	≥ 14 mg/d	35 mg/d
Vitamin B$_5$	≥ 5 mg/d	ND
Vitamin B$_6$	≥ 1.3 mg/d	100 mg/d
Vitamin B$_7$	≥ 30 µg/d	ND
Vitamin B$_9$	≥ 400 µg/d	1000 µg/d
Vitamin B$_{12}$	≥ 2.4 µg/d	ND
Choline	≥ 425 mg/d	3.5 g/d
Tryptophan	≥ 0.24 g/d	ND
Threonine	≥ 0.89 g/d	ND
Isoleucine	≥ 1.18 g/d	ND
Leucine	≥ 2.30 g/d	ND
Lysine	≥ 1.77 g/d	ND
Methionine + cysteine	≥ 0.89 g/d	ND
Phenylalanine + tyrosine	≥ 1.48 g/d	ND
Valine	≥ 1.53 g/d	ND
Histidine	≥ 0.59 g/d	ND
Eicosapentaenoic acid (EPA) + Docosahexaenoic acid (DHA)	≥ 500 mg/d	ND
Lutein + zeaxanthin	≥ 10 mg/d	ND

Note: ND = not determined.

Step Two: From Appendix A, find some foods and list all their nutrients shown in Table 9-6. Unavailable data are replaced with zeros. By optimizing amounts of various foods, this woman can obtain a menu to meet her daily energy and nutrition requirements. An optimized menu is as follows:

1 medium raw egg 100g
2 slices wheat bread 50 g
1 glass 1% milk with added vitamin A 244 g
Atlantic farmed raw salmon 50 g
Raw kale 100g
1 medium apple with skin 150 g
Dried sunflower kernels 25 g
1 medium raw red tomato 100 g
Raw broccoli raab 100 g

Corn oil 10 g

1 medium raw banana 150 g

Step Three: Calculate the total amounts and %DRI (Dietary Reference Intake) of each nutrient. The results are shown in Table 9-7.

Table 9-7 Total amounts and %DRI of each nutrient from the optimized menu for the 40-year-old woman

Energy/Nutrient	Amount	%DRI
Energy	1692 kcal	NA
Protein	91.97 g	NA
Fat	66.15 g	NA
Saturated fat	12.15 g	NA
Trans fat	0	NA
Carbohydrate	205.47 g	NA
Sugar	75.43 g	NA
Fiber	39.25 g	156%
Cholesterol	464.7 mg	NA
ORAC	15578.5 µmol TE	312%
Calcium	1028.4 mg	103%
Iron	44.4 mg	247%
Magnesium	713.6 mg	223%
Phosphorus	2069.3 mg	296%
Potassium	4.77 g	102%
Sodium	1.17 g	78%
Zinc	14.6 mg	182%
Copper	3.37 mg	374%
Manganese	8.0 mg	446%
Selenium	114.7 µg	209%
Chromium	68.5 µg	274%
Vitamin A	1805.0 µg	258%
Vitamin C	181.3 mg	242%
Vitamin D	6.5 µg	131%
Vitamin E	14.9 mg	99.3%

Vitamin K	1101.2 µg	1227%
Vitamin B$_1$	3.0 mg	276%
Vitamin B$_2$	3.6 mg	327%
Vitamin B$_3$	26.8 mg	191%
Vitamin B$_5$	6.2 mg	125%
Vitamin B$_6$	3.7 mg	285%
Vitamin B$_7$	96.9 µg	323%
Vitamin B$_9$	957.7 µg	239%
Vitamin B$_{12}$	3.8 µg	157%
Choline	548.0 mg	129%
Tryptophan	1.21 g	504%
Threonine	3.71 g	416%
Isoleucine	4.40 g	373%
Leucine	7.28 g	316%
Lysine	6.07 g	343%
Methionine + cysteine	3.29 g	369%
Phenylalanine + tyrosine	7.65 g	517%
Valine	4.83 g	316%
Histidine	2.40 g	406%
Eicosapentaenoic acid (EPA) + Docosa-hexaenoic acid (DHA)	996.5 mg	199%
Lutein + zeaxanthin	41.2 mg	412%

Note: NA = not applicable.

Table 9-7 shows that the optimized menu for a 40-year-old woman with a weight of 59 kg and a height of 1.65 m at a sedentary activity level containing all 50 nutrients, including energy and ORAC, meets her daily nutrition requirements except sodium, and all the nutrients are not beyond their tolerable intake limits. Also, energy, protein, fat, and carbohydrates are all in the range of the recommended values. In addition, based on the weights of vegetables and fruits, the pH of this menu is estimated to be about 6.5–7.5.

Following the same procedure as above, I obtained an optimized menu for a 40-year-old man with a weight of 70 kg and a height of 1.77 m at a sedentary activity level:

American cheddar imitation cheese 50 g

2 slices wheat bread 50 g
1 glass 1% milk with added vitamin A 244 g
Raw Atlantic farmed herring fish 50 g
1 medium raw apple with skin 150 g
Raw white medium-grain rice 150 g
Raw full-fat soy flour 100 g
1 raw medium red tomato 100 g
Single brand bran flakes cereals ready-to-eat 80 g
Raw breast chicken (meat & skin) 100 g
Raw turnip green 100 g
Raw broccoli raab 100 g
Corn oil 15 g
Dried sunflower kernels 10 g
1 medium raw bananas 150 g

More data are summarized in Table 9-8 and Table 9-9.

Table 9-8 Daily energy and nutrition requirements of a 40-year-old man with a weight of 70 kg and a height of 1.77 m at a sedentary activity level

Objective function	Reference intake	Tolerable intake limit (UL)
Energy	2115–2350 kcal/d	ND
Protein	59–206 g/d	ND
Fat	52–91 g/d	ND
Saturated fat	as low as possible	ND
Trans fat	as low as possible	ND
Carbohydrate	264–381 g/d	ND
Sugar	≤ 147 g/d	ND
Fiber	≥ 38 g/d	ND
Cholesterol	as low as possible	ND
ORAC	≥ 5000 μmol TE/d	ND
Calcium	≥ 1000 mg/d	2.5 g/d
Iron	≥ 8 mg/d	45 mg/d
Magnesium	≥ 420 mg/d	ND
Phosphorus	≥ 700 mg/d	4.0 g/d
Potassium	≥ 4.7 g/d	ND

Sodium	≥ 1.5 g/d	2.3 g/d
Zinc	≥ 11 mg/d	40 mg/d
Copper	≥ 900 µg/d	10000 µg/d
Manganese	≥ 2.3 mg/d	11 mg/d
Selenium	≥ 55 µg/d	400 µg/d
Chromium	≥ 35 µg/d	ND
Vitamin A	≥ 900 µg/d	3000 µg/d
Vitamin C	≥ 90 mg/d	2000 mg/d
Vitamin D	≥ 5 µg/d	50 µg/d
Vitamin E	≥ 15 mg/d	1000 mg/d
Vitamin K	≥ 120 µg/d	ND
Vitamin B_1	≥ 1.2 mg/d	ND
Vitamin B_2	≥ 1.3 mg/d	ND
Vitamin B_3	≥ 16 mg/d	35 mg/d
Vitamin B_5	≥ 5 mg/d	ND
Vitamin B_6	≥ 1.3 mg/d	100 mg/d
Vitamin B_7	≥ 30 µg/d	ND
Vitamin B_9	≥ 400 µg/d	1000 µg/d
Vitamin B_{12}	≥ 2.4 µg/d	ND
Choline	≥ 550 mg/d	3.5 g/d
Tryptophan	≥ 0.28 g/d	ND
Threonine	≥ 1.05 g/d	ND
Isoleucine	≥ 1.40 g/d	ND
Leucine	≥ 2.73 g/d	ND
Lysine	≥ 2.10 g/d	ND
Methionine + cysteine	≥ 1.05 g/d	ND
Phenylalanine + tyrosine	≥ 1.75 g/d	ND
Valine	≥ 1.82 g/d	ND
Histidine	≥ 0.70 g/d	ND
Eicosapentaenoic acid (EPA) + Docosahexaenoic acid (DHA)	≥ 500 mg/d	ND

| Lutein + zeaxanthin | ≥ 10 mg/d | ND |

Note: ND = not determined.

Table 9-9 Total amounts and %DRI of each nutrient from the optimized menu for the 40-year-old man

Energy/nutrient	Amount	%DRI
Energy	2264 kcal	NA
Protein	108.64 g	NA
Fat	69.11 g	NA
Saturated fat	14.52 g	NA
Trans fat	0.11 g	NA
Carbohydrate	332.82 g	NA
Sugar	78.16 g	NA
Fiber	42.54 g	112%
Cholesterol	132.4 mg	NA
ORAC	10906.5 µmol TE	218%
Calcium	1244.9 mg	125%
Iron	41.1 mg	514%
Magnesium	1135.8 mg	270%
Phosphorus	2318.6 mg	331%
Potassium	6.32 g	134%
Sodium	1.51 g	101%
Zinc	16.9 mg	154%
Copper	5.0 mg	551%
Manganese	13.9 mg	603%
Selenium	86.2 µg	157%
Chromium	59.5 µg	170%
Vitamin A	2040.4 µg	227%
Vitamin C	141.5 mg	157%
Vitamin D	26.2 µg	524%
Vitamin E	16.9 mg	111%
Vitamin K	1044.5 µg	870%

Vitamin B$_1$	2.6 mg	217%
Vitamin B$_2$	3.9 mg	299%
Vitamin B$_3$	39.5 mg	247%
Vitamin B$_5$	8.3 mg	166%
Vitamin B$_6$	4.3 mg	332%
Vitamin B$_7$	22.6 µg	75%
Vitamin B$_9$	1233.2 µg	308%
Vitamin B$_{12}$	8.3 µg	347%
Choline	433.0 mg	79%
Tryptophan	1.27 g	453%
Threonine	3.98 g	379%
Isoleucine	4.74 g	338%
Leucine	7.85 g	288%
Lysine	6.68 g	318%
Methionine + cysteine	3.61 g	344%
Phenylalanine + tyrosine	8.03 g	459%
Valine	5.12 g	282%
Histidine	2.69 g	384%
Eicosapentaenoic acid (EPA) + Docosahexaenoic acid (DHA)	815.5 mg	163%
Lutein + zeaxanthin	26.4 mg	264%

Note: NA = not applicable.

In Table 9-9, I observed that, except for vitamin B$_7$ (78%DRI) and choline (79%DRI), all the other nutrients in the optimized menu for a 40-year-old man with a weight of 70 kg and a height of 1.77 m at a sedentary activity level meet his daily nutrition requirements, but are not beyond their tolerable intake limits. A lower amount of vitamin B$_7$ and choline may be caused by unavailable data when calculating the total amount. Also, energy, protein, fat, and carbohydrates are all in the range of recommended values. In addition, based on the weights of vegetables and fruits, the pH of this menu is estimated to be about 6.5–7.5.

The foods in the above two menus are cheap and easy to get at any supermarkets. For the woman menu, the cost is about 2.5 to 3 dollars, and for the man menu, the cost is about 3 to 3.5 dollars. Therefore, we adults cost about only 2.5 to 3.5 dollars every day and can obtain enough energy and nutrition though optimizing the different types of foods. In the time of economic crisis, most people like to cook for themselves. As long as we learn to optimize nutrition by following the above procedure, we can not only save a lot of money, but also, we can achieve optimum health, thereby extending our longevity.

Using the selected energy and nutrition values of the 379 best foods in Appendix A, we can create hundreds of menus that satisfy our daily energy and nutrition requirements. If you take time to familiarize yourself with the data by reading Chapter Eight, you can easily optimize your daily menu to meet your daily energy and nutrition requirements.

If you buy a food from a supermarket that is not in Appendix A, you can use the energy and nutrition values on its label to do the calculation, or maybe you can find these values for it in SR20 Search, a database of USDA. I believe that in the future, all foods sold in supermarkets should be labeled with energy and nutrition values. Also, all foods sold in restaurants should be marked with these values. Thus, everyone will know how to balance his/her energy and nutrition by optimizing the foods they eat.

Chapter Ten
Dietary Supplements and their Energy and Nutrition Values

In Chapter Nine, we learned that everyone can obtain enough energy and nutrition from optimized daily menus. Thus, we do not need to take any dietary supplements. However, most of us do not have them, and it is reported that half of Americans take dietary supplements everyday, so in this chapter, I will make a brief introduction to dietary supplements and their energy and nutrition values.

1. Dietary Supplements

Dietary supplements (also called nutritional supplements, or supplements) were defined in a law passed by the U.S. Congress in 1994 (see the box below).

About Dietary Supplements

A dietary supplement must meet all of the following conditions:

- It is a product (other than tobacco) that is intended to supplement the diet and that contains one or more of the following: vitamins, minerals, herbs or other botanicals, amino acids, or any combination of the above ingredients.
- It is intended to be taken in tablet, capsule, powder, softgel, gelcap, or liquid form.
- It is not represented for use as a conventional food or as a sole item of a meal or the diet.
- It is labeled as being a dietary supplement.

Dietary supplements are sold in grocery, health food, drug, and discount stores, as well as through mail-order catalogs, TV programs, the Internet, and direct sales.

There are many kinds of dietary supplements on the market, such as B-vitamins, vitamin C, calcium, selenium, or multivitamins and multiminerals. If you want to know how to choose what kind of products you need, you must be familiar with the nutritional facts on the label.

2. Energy and Nutrition Values of Dietary Supplements

In order to understand the energy and nutrition values of dietary supplements, we must know how to read a supplement label. I will use two different types of labels (Label A and Label B) as two examples to explain these values from the existing products on the market.

Table 10-1 Label A supplement facts

Serving Size 4 Tablets
Servings per Bottle 30

	Amount per 4 Tablets	%Daily Value
Vitamin A (as retinyl acetate and 75% as beta-carotene)	14,000 IU	280%
Vitamin C (as ascorbic acid)	535 mg	890%
Vitamin D (as cholecalciferol)	400 IU	100%
Vitamin E (as –d-alpha tocopheryl acetate)	176 IU	586%
Thiamin (as thiamin mononitrate)	1.728 mg	115%
Riboflavin	2.367 mg	192%
Niacin (as miacinamide)	20 mg	100%
Vitamin B_6 (as pyridoxine hydro-chloride)	6.9 mg	345%
Folate (as folic acid)	0.4 mg	100%
Vitamin B_{12} (as cyanocolalamin)	6 mcg	100%
Biotin	0.3 mg	100%
Pantothenic acid (as d-calcium pantothenate)	10 mg	100%
Calcium (as di-calcium phosphate and 75% as calcium carbonate)	250 mg	25%
Iron (as ferric phosphate)	18 mg	100%
Phosphorus (as di-calcium phosphate)	50 mg	5%
Iodine (as potassium iodine)	150 mcg	100%
Magnesium (as magnesium oxide)	104.27 mg	26%
Zinc (as zinc oxide)	15 mg	100%
Selenium (as selenium yeast)	100 mcg	143%

Copper (as copper gluconate)	2 mg	100%
Manganese (as manganese gluconate)	2.5 mg	125%
Chromium (as chromium yeast)	120 mcg	100%
Molybdenum (as molybdenum yeast)	75 mcg	100%
Choline (as choline bitartrate)	11.752 mg	*

Daily value not established.

Table 10- 2 Label B supplement facts

Serving Size 32 g (2 scoops)
Servings per Container 11

Calories 110		Calories from Fat 0	
	Amount per Serving	**%Daily Value***	
Total Fat	0 g	0%	
Saturated Fat	0 g	0%	
Cholesterol	0 mg	0%	
Sodium	135 mg	6%	
Total Carbohydrate	10 g	3 %	
Dietary Fiber	0 g	0%	
Sugars	9 g		
Protein	18g	36%	
Vitamin A	0%		
Vitamin C	0%		
Calcium	0%		
Iron	0%		

*Percent Daily Values are based on a 2,000 calorie diet. Your daily values may be higher or lower depending on your calorie needs.

		Calories:	2,000	2,500
Total Fat		Less than	65 g	80 g
Saturated Fat		Less than	20 g	25g
Cholesterol		Less than	300 mg	300 mg
Sodium		Less than	2,400 mg	2,400 mg

Total Carbohydrate			300 g	375 g
Dietary Fiber			25 g	30 g
Calories per gram: Fat 9 Carbohydrate 4 Protein 4				
Amino acid profile (mg per serving):				
Alanine	436	Histidine*	482	Proline	860
Arginine	706	Isoleucine*	862	Serine	632
Aspartic acid	1116	Leucine*	1498	Threonine*	760
Crysteine*	214	Lysine*	1197	Tryptophan*	209
Glutamic acid	2264	Methionine*	314	Tyrosine*	721
Glycine	389	Phenylalanine*	912	Valine*	947
*Essential amino acids				

Note: The values on the two labels exceed the newer recommended levels. 100% of the daily values on the labels were last updated in 1968.

Label A Supplement Facts in Table 10-1 shows that this is a multi-vitamins and minerals product (referred to as product A), while Label B Supplement Facts in Table 10-2 shows that this is a product for supplementing proteins (amino acids) and carbohydrates (referred to as product B).

"% Daily Value" or "% DV" on the label in Table 10-1 or Table 10-2 is the percentage of the Daily Value, a value created by the FDA for food and supplement labeling. It's based on and is a simplification of the DRI, but it doesn't take into account age or gender as the DRIs do. If the "% Daily Value" noted is 50%, then you will receive half of the FDA's recommendation of the daily dosage of that supplement contained in one serving.

Serving Size shows you how many tablets, capsules, softgels, or grams of powder you need to take in order to reach the recommended Daily Value percentage or the amounts represented on the label. People often assume that by taking one supplement a day, they are satisfying the recommended Daily Value. This is not always the case; consumers should read the labels carefully to find the percentage of the Daily Value they are getting from one serving. Serving size of product A is 4 tablets, not one tablet, and serving size of product B is 32 g (2 scoops), not one scoop.

Scientific units such as "I.U.", "mg" and "mcg" are different ways of measuring the amounts of vitamins and minerals in each tablet, capsule, or softgel. "I.U." or "International Unit" is the global standard for measuring fat-soluble vitamins (e.g. vitamins A, D and E). Both water-soluble vitamins, such as the B vitamins, vitamin C, and minerals, are measured in milligrams (mg) and micrograms (mcg, or μg). One milligram (1/1000 of a gram) is equal to 1000 micrograms. Conversion Factors from IU to mg or μg for vitamin A, vitamin E, and vitamin D are recorded in Table 10-3 for your reference.

Table 10-3 Conversion factors from IU to mg or µg

Vitamin A	1 IU = 0.344 µg all-trans retinyl acetate = 0.550 µg all-trans retinyl palmitate = 0.600 µg all-trans β-carotene North America = 1.800 µg all-trans β-carotene Europe = 0.300 (RE) retinol equivalent
Vitamin E	1 IU = 0.735 mg d-alpha-tocopheryl acetate Natural = 0.671 mg d-alpha-tocopheryl Natural = 0.826 mg d-alpha-tocopheryl succinate Natural = 1 mg dl-alpha-tocopheryl acetate Synthetic = 0.909 mg dl-alpha-tocopheryl Synthetic = 1.124 mg dl-alpha-tocopheryl succinate Synthetic
Vitamin D	1 IU = 0.025 µg calciferol

For example, vitamin A in product A is 14,000 IU per serving (4 tablets), composed of 25% retinyl acetate and 75% beta-carotene. Amount of vitamin A in micrograms = 14,000 × 25% × 0.344 + 14,000 × 75% × 0.6 = 1,204 + 6,300 = 7504 µg.

Now, you should familiarize yourself with the energy and nutrition values of dietary supplements by reading their labels. But how do you know what kinds and amounts of dietary supplements you need to take?

3. How to determine your daily requirements of dietary supplements

If you optimize your daily menu to meet your daily energy and nutrition requirements, then you do not need to take any dietary supplements. However, if you cannot optimize your daily menu, then you should first evaluate or ask a nutritionist to evaluate your nutrition status based on your existing diet to see if you lack any kinds of nutrients. After evaluation, you can take the dietary supplements you need. For instance, if you find that you only have 600 mg of calcium from your daily diet, you should take 400 mg of calcium from dietary supplements to meet the daily calcium requirement of 1,000 mg.

Please do not take any supplements at will or only by following the instructions on the labels, because it is not only a waste of your money, but it will also harm your health—exceeding the tolerable intake level (UL) of daily nutrition intake poses a risk of adverse health effects. Let's take a 40-year-old woman with a weight of 59 kg and a height of 1.65 m at a sedentary activity level as an example to help explain this situation. As discussed in Chapter Nine, we have obtained an optimized menu for her. Assuming that after eating meals following the optimized menu, she takes one serving (4 tablets) of product A and one serving (two scoops) of product B, in terms of their label instructions. The energy and nutrition from the optimized menu and the supplements are summarized in Table 10-4.

Table 10-4 Amounts and %DRI
of each nutrient for a 40-year-old woman

Energy/Nutrient	Amount from menu	Amount from supplement	Total amount	%DRI
Energy	1692 kcal	110 kcal	1802 kcal	NA
Protein	91.97 g	18 g	119.97g	NA
Fat	66.15 g	0	66.15 g	NA
Saturated fat	12.15 g	0	12.15 g	NA
Trans fat	0	0	0	NA
Carbohydrate	205.47 g	10 g	215.47 g	NA
Sugar	75.43 g	9 g	84.43 g	NA
Fiber	39.25 g	0	39.25g	156%
Cholesterol	464.7 mg	0	464.7 mg	NA
ORAC	15578.5 µmol TE	0	15578.5 µmol TE	312%
Calcium	1028.4 mg	250 mg	1278.4 mg	128%
Iron	44.4 mg	18 mg	62.4 mg	347%
Magnesium	713.6 mg	104.3 mg	817.9 mg	256%
Phosphorus	2069.3 mg	50 mg	2119.3 mg	303%
Potassium	4.77 g	0	4.77 g	102%
Sodium	1.17 g	0.14 g	1.31 g	87%
Zinc	14.6 mg	15 mg	29.6 mg	370%
Copper	3.37 mg	2 mg	5.37 mg	597%
Manganese	8.0 mg	2.5 mg	10.5 mg	583%
Selenium	114.7 µg	100 µg	214.7 µg	390%
Chromium	68.5 µg	120 µg	188.5µg	752%

Vitamin A	1805.0 µg	7504 µg	9309 µg	1330%
Vitamin C	181.3 mg	535 mg	716.3 mg	955%
Vitamin D	6.5 µg	10 µg	16.5 µg	330%
Vitamin E	14.9 mg	129.4 mg	144.3 mg	962%
Vitamin K	1101.2 µg	0	1101.2 µg	1227%
Vitamin B_1	3.0 mg	1.7 mg	4.7 mg	427%
Vitamin B_2	3.6 mg	2.4 mg	6.0 mg	545%
Vitamin B_3	26.8 mg	20 mg	46.8 mg	334%
Vitamin B_5	6.2 mg	10 mg	16.2 mg	324%
Vitamin B_6	3.7 mg	6.9 mg	10.6 mg	815%
Vitamin B_7	96.9 µg	300 µg	369.9 µg	1323%
Vitamin B_9	957.7 µg	400 µg	1357.7 µg	339%
Vitamin B_{12}	3.8 µg	6 µg	9.8 µg	408%
Choline	548.0 mg	11.8 mg	559.8 mg	132%
Tryptophan	1.21 g	0.21 g	1.42 g	592%
Threonine	3.71 g	0.76 g	4.47 g	502%
Isoleucine	4.40 g	0.86 g	5.26 g	446%
Leucine	7.28 g	1.50 g	8.78 g	382%
Lysine	6.07 g	1.20 g	7.27 g	411%
Methionine + cysteine	3.29 g	0.53 g	3.82 g	429%
Phenylalanine + tyrosine	7.65 g	1.63 g	9.28 g	627%
Valine	4.83 g	0.95 g	5.78 g	378%
Histidine	2.40 g	0.48 g	2.88 g	488%
Eicosapentaenoic acid (EPA) + Docosahexaenoic acid (DHA)	996.5 mg	0	996.5 mg	153%
Lutein + zeaxanthin	41.2 mg	0	41.2 mg	412%

Note: NA = not applicable.

Table 10-4 clearly indicates that the amount of iron (62.4 mg), vitamin A (9309 µg), vitamin B_3 (46. 8 mg), and vitamin B_9 (1357.7 µg) exceeds their respective upper tolerable intake level (iron: 45 mg/d, vitamin A: 3000 µg/d, vitamin B_3: 35 mg/d, and vitamin B_9: 1000 µg/d). Like a drug, these molecules, due to excess amounts in homeostasis can cause toxicity that can lead some diseases, if in excess for a long time. This is why some people can not obtain good health even by taking a lot of supplements every day.

In fact, it is so difficult for each one of us to gain just enough energy and nutrition from our conventional diet, if we're not optimizing what we eat. This is why there are more overweight and obese people (including adults and children) in many countries in the world, because they gain too much calories from the foods they eat.

Chapter Eleven
Achieve Optimum Health and Longevity through Human Nutrition Optimization

1. Human Longevity

Since the 1900s, human longevity has been remarkably increasing, with an existing Guinness's record of 113. This record almost reaches God's order, as the LORD says, "*My Spirit will not content with man forever, for his mortal; his days will be a hundred and twenty years.*" (Genesis 6: 3).

Man includes all of us regardless of sex and race, so each of us could live up to 120 years as long as we keep optimum health. Humans currently have the potential to live 120 years, but few actually do. The average life expectancy today is around 80 years, which is impressive but nowhere near our full potential.

2. Factors Affecting Human Longevity

Research has found that the following factors affect human longevity:

- Genetics

- Exercise

- Spirituality

- Nutrition

In 1997, Finch and Tanzi published their research achievements about the influence of genetics on longevity in the journal *Science*, finding that the heritability of life spans is small. Studies of twins have suggested that genetics accounts for up to 30 percent of the variance in human longevity. An even stronger relationship between genetics and longevity was observed by analyzing the genetics of centenarians and their families. In one study, the siblings of centenarians were three to four times more likely to reach the age of 100 than the siblings of non-centenarians. Another study showed that the immediate ancestors of Jeanne Calment of France (who died at the age of 122, after breaking the record for human life span) were ten times more likely to reach the age of 80 than the ancestral cohort. So far, the effect of genetics on human longevity is paradox.

It was found that simply engaging in physical activity will improve health and life expectancy. Physical activity is the main group in which exercise and physical fitness are subgroups of. Exercise is the most important of the five components of a healthy lifestyle. A healthy lifestyle is defined as: eating a healthy diet, maintaining a healthy weight, exercising regularly, quitting (or not starting) smoking, and minimizing stress.

At any age or level of ability, our bodies all need regular physical activity in order to function well. Here are just a few of the major benefits of exercise:

- Increased muscle mass, strength, and flexibility

- Lower body fat, especially in the abdomen

- Higher metabolic rate and less tendency to gain weight

- Improved ability to perform everyday tasks like lifting or cleaning

- Better balance and less risk of falls or fractures

- Increased joint mobility and less arthritic pain

- Decreased risk of many chronic diseases, including heart disease, high blood pressure, diabetes, depression, memory problems, osteoporosis, and cancers

- Increased longevity

- Improved quality of life

One 1999 study, published in the journal *Demography,* tracked 20,000 Americans and found that white people **who regularly attended church lived an average 7 years longer than their nonchurchgoing counterparts, and black people lived a remarkable 14 years longer**. People who believe in God often feel more peaceful and less stressful than people who don't believe in God. As discussed in Chapter Five, stress can produce free radicals in our bodies, which can lead to many diseases that shorten our longevity, if the free radicals cannot be eliminated in time. Explorer and National Geographic writer Dan Buettner has studied the so-called Blue Zones of the world, areas where people have much greater longevity than the normal, many living active lives at ages beyond one hundred. Faith is among the consistent characteristics of centenarians in the Blue Zones. In an article carried by the Bowling Green Student Magazine, Spring 2002, Dr. Pargament noted that many studies have shown that religious involvement can help extend life expectancy.

As discussed previously in this book, human nutrition plays a key role in our health and longevity. Without oxygen—the most important nutrient, our life can only sustain for a few minutes, and without water—the second most important nutrient, our life can only sustain for a few days. If air and water are polluted, our health and longevity will be greatly affected. If we lack other nutrients (malnutrition), such as vitamins and minerals, we will have various diseases that shorten our longevity. If we have over-nutrition, we will also have many problems with our health, such as obesity and chronic diseases.

The World Health Organization (WHO) estimated that one billion adults are overweight and obese worldwide, however, the number of the starving and undernourished individuals remains steady at 600 million.

In summary, genetics, exercise, spirituality, and nutrition together determine our longevity. However, the effect of genetics on human longevity is paradox, and we cannot choose our genes. How to exercise and how to practice spirituality to extend our longevity are beyond the scope of this book. Hence, I will only discuss how to achieve optimal health and longevity through human nutrition optimization in the next section.

3. Achieve Optimum Health and Longevity through Human Nutrition Optimization

In Chapter Nine, we have detailed the optimization of oxygen and water, so here, I will only discuss other nutrition optimization for different types of persons.

(1) Normal Weight People

For normal weight people with a body mass index (BMI) of between 18.5 and 25, you only need to follow the procedure discussed in Chapter Nine to optimize the amounts of food you want to eat to satisfy your daily energy and nutrition requirements at different physical activity levels.

To determine our daily energy intake, we can all obtain a value by using the equation listed in Chapter Seven based on age, weight, and physical activity level, which should meet the energy requirements of our absolute majority. But, different people have different metabolic efficiency, which refers to the percentage of your caloric intake that goes into making usable energy. Normally, metabolic efficiency is about 33 percent, while the highest efficiency that we can possibly reach is 50 percent. So, some of us should make some adjustments to our calculated energy values in order to maintain a constant body weight, because body weight provides each individual with a readily monitored indicator of the adequacy or inadequacy of habitual energy intake.

To determine our daily nutrition intakes, we can find these values in Chapter Seven, according to life stage and gender. These dietary reference intakes (DRIs) for vitamins and minerals can meet almost all healthy adults with normal weights. If these nutrients do not exceed their ULs, they should be safe and effective.

For normal weight people, keep optimizing your nutrition and you will maintain optimum health, which leads to longevity. The earlier you start, the better.

(2) Overweight or Obese People

The World Health Organization (WHO) has called the worldwide rise in obesity a global epidemic. One billion adults are overweight, of which 300 million are obese, which is due to over-nutrition. On average, each of them has at least 50 pounds more than his/her ideal body weight. According to the American Diabetes Association, approximately 64% of American adults are overweight or obese, due mostly to poor eating habits and a lack of exercise. The 1999–2000 Australian Diabetes, Obesity and Lifestyle Study estimated that 60% of Australians aged 25 years or older are overweight or obese. The data from WHO (2000) shows that the prevalence of obesity in most European countries has increased by about 10%–40% in the past 10 years, ranging from 10% to 20% in men and 10% to 25% in women. The most alarming increase has been observed in the Great Britain, where nearly two thirds of adult men and over half of adult women are overweight or obese. Even in developing countries, more and more people are getting overweight or obese.

BMIs of overweight people are between 25 and 30, while BMIs of obese persons are 30 or over. Overweight and obesity is caused by accumulation of fat in the body, whereas accumulation of fat in the body is attributed to an imbalance of energy in which energy intake from the diet exceeds energy expenditure from physical activity and metabolic processes over a considerable period. Even a slight imbalance over a long term can result in increased weight. The result of excess energy intake relative to energy expenditure is the storage of unused energy as body fat. If overweight or obese people want to maintain their existing weight, they must intake enough energy from their diet in terms of their body weights. The following two equations are for overweight or obese adult men and women to compute their estimated energy requirement (EER).

For overweight and obese women 19 years and older (BMI ≥ 25 kg/m²),

EER = 448 -7.95 × age (y) + PA × (11.4 × Weight [kg] + 619 × Height [m])

where PA is the physical activity coefficient:
PA = 1.00 if PAL is estimated to be ≥1.0 < 1.4 (sedentary)
PA = 1.16 if PAL is estimated to be ≥1.4 < 1.6 (low active)
PA = 1.27 if PAL is estimated to be ≥1.6 < 1.9 (active)
PA = 1.44 if PAL is estimated to be ≥1.9 < 2.5 (very active)

For overweight and obese men 19 years and older (BMI ≥ 25 kg/m²),

EER = 1086 -10.1 × age (y) + PA × (13.7 × Weight [kg] + 416 × Height [m])

where PA is the physical activity coefficient:
PA = 1.00 if PAL is estimated to be ≥1.0 < 1.4 (sedentary)
PA = 1.12 if PAL is estimated to be ≥1.4 < 1.6 (low active)
PA = 1.29 if PAL is estimated to be ≥ 1.6 < 1.9 (active)
PA = 1.59 if PAL is estimated to be ≥ 1.9 < 2.5 (very active)

What we put in our mouths has a tremendous effect on our health. A 2006 study published in *Neurology* that tracked 2,223 healthy workers ages 32 to 62 years old for five years found that a higher BMI is associated with lower cognitive scores. In a study that tracked over 10,000 men and women ages from 40 to 45 years old at outset for an average of 27 years, obesity was found to be linked with dementia. Obese women were 200% more likely to have dementia than women with normal weight, while obese men had a 30% increase in dementia. Recent research has shown that those with a high body weight, a high cholesterol level, and a high blood pressure are 600% more likely to lose healthy brain function and be diagnosed with Alzheimer's than people who maintain a healthy body weight. Also, there is good evidence of an association between overweight and obesity and cardiovascular disease, coronary heart disease, hart failure, stroke, osteoporosis, type 2 diabetes, and some cancers. Obviously, overweight and obesity largely influence our health, thereby shortening our longevity. Statistics has shown that obese people have never lived up to 80 years.

Therefore, how to optimize what overweight and obese people eat in order to lose weight is of global significance. Here, I take a 40-year-old obese woman with a weight of 89 kg (196 lb) and a height of 1.65 m (65 in) at a sedentary activity level as an example to help instruct overweight and obese people to achieve a normal weight by optimizing their daily energy and nutrition from the foods they eat.

Step one: Calculate her estimated energy requirement (EER) for maintaining her existing energy balance. From the above prediction equation, her EER is computed as: 2166 kcal/d. From Chapter Nine, obtain her EER as: 1828 kcal/d for keeping a normal weight (59kg) (130 lb). This woman who is obese requires 338 kcal/d more energy than in her status of a normal weight.

Step two: Design a reasonable weight loss and maintenance schedule for her energy requirement. Researchers at the University of California in Los Angeles found that body weight should be lost very gradually because our body needs time to adapt to a new homeostasis, even to a healthier lifestyle. Imposing severe caloric restriction too rapidly leads to health problems, thereby shortening life span. So, it is reasonable to design a 10-month weight loss plan for her to lose 30 kg (66 lb), i.e., 3 kg per month. 3 kg of fat is equivalent to 27,000 kcal of energy, which means that if she wants to lose 3 kg of her body weight per month, then she should reduce her intake of energy by 900 kcal each day from each start point weight. After losing 30 kg, she should gradually increase her energy intake to reach 1828 kcal/d to keep a normal weight. Her weight loss and maintenance schedule for her energy requirement each month is shown in Table 11-1.

Table 11-1 A 40-year-old woman's weight loss and maintenance schedule for her energy requirement each month

Month	Weight to be lost	Start point weight [lb]	Start point energy	Energy to be required
1st	3 kg	89 kg [196]	2166 kcal/d	1266 kcal/d
2nd	3 kg	86 kg [190]	2132 kcal/d	1232 kcal/d
3rd	3 kg	83 kg [183]	2098 kcal/d	1198 kcal/d
4th	3 kg	80 kg [176]	2063 kcal/d	1163 kcal/d
5th	3 kg	77 kg [170]	2029 kcal/d	1129 kcal/d
6th	3 kg	74 kg [163]	1995 kcal/d	1095 kcal/d
7th	3 kg	71 kg [157]	1961 kcal/d	1061 kcal/d
8th	3 kg	68 kg [150]	1927 kcal/d	1027 kcal/d
9th	3 kg	65 kg [143]	1892 kcal/d	992 kcal/d
10th	3 kg	62 kg [137]	1858 kcal/d	958 kcal/d
11th	0	59 kg [130]	1828 kcal/d	1248 kcal/d
12th	0	59 kg [130]	1828 kcal/d	1538 kcal/d

| 13th | 0 | 59 kg [130] | 1828 kcal/d | 1828 kcal/d |

Anyone who wants to lose weight can design his/her own weight loss and maintenance schedule for his/her energy requirement in terms of the above calculation. You can make adjustments in accordance with your actual needs.

Step three: Optimize the food menus for each month. Following the procedure presented in Chapter Nine together with the energy and nutrition data listed in Appendix A, we can obtain many menus for each month in Table 11-1 to meet each month's energy and nutrition requirements. Due to energy reduction of 900 kcal each day in ten months, the foods will be decreased by about 40%. If she reduces about 40% of foods relative to the same types of foods she eats in the obese status, she will feel very hungry. As we know, eating foods containing high fat, high protein, and high fiber makes us not feel hungry for a longer time. So, we may determine a ratio of fat: protein: carbohydrate as 30%: 30%: 40% of total energy to satisfy the energy requirements for the first month to the eleventh month with ± 5% error for each one. And the fiber amount is set up to be no less than 35 g/d for these months.

Once optimized, we can obtain a first-month menu for her:

1 raw fresh egg 100 g
1 glass 1% milk with added vitamin A 244 g
Atlantic raw herring fish 50 g
Raw spinach 100g
Dried sunflower kernels 25 g
1 medium raw red tomato 100 g
General Mills, fiber one cereals ready-to-eat 40 g
Raw broccoli raab 100 g
1 large raw banana 200 g

Step four: Calculate the total amounts and %DRI of each nutrient. The results are shown in Table 11-2.

Table 11-2 Total amounts and %DRI of each nutrient of the optimized first-month menu for a 40-year-old obese woman

Energy/Nutrient	Amount	%DRI
Energy	1271 kcal	NA
Protein	94.68 g	NA
Fat	61.92 g	NA
Saturated fat	13.02 g	NA

Trans fat	0	NA
Carbohydrate	121.71 g	NA
Sugar	50.82 g	NA
Fiber	38.97 g	156%
Cholesterol	465.2 mg	NA
ORAC	7146 μmol TE	143%
Calcium	1114.6 mg	112%
Iron	25.1 mg	140%
Magnesium	414.3 mg	130%
Phosphorus	1578.8 mg	226%
Potassium	2.79 g	59%
Sodium	0.60g	37%
Zinc	15.6 mg	195%
Copper	2.3 mg	254%
Manganese	7.0 mg	388%
Selenium	133.2 μg	242%
Chromium	60.8 μg	243%
Vitamin A	971.1 μg	139%
Vitamin C	87.8 mg	117%
Vitamin D	24.4 μg	488%
Vitamin E	15.0 mg	100%
Vitamin K	716.7 μg	796%
Vitamin B_1	1.9 mg	170%
Vitamin B_2	2.5 mg	228%
Vitamin B_3	15.7 mg	112%
Vitamin B_5	4.8 mg	96%
Vitamin B_6	2.9 mg	219%
Vitamin B_7	45.1 μg	150%
Vitamin B_9	678.2 μg	170%
Vitamin B_{12}	11.2 μg	467%
Choline	412.8 mg	97%
Tryptophan	1.31 g	544%

Threonine	3.67 g	412%
Isoleucine	4.52 g	384%
Leucine	6.86 g	298%
Lysine	6.82 g	385%
Methionine + cysteine	3.24 g	364%
Phenylalanine + tyrosine	7.62 g	515%
Valine	5.02 g	328%
Histidine	2.63 g	446%
Eicosapentaenoic acid (EPA) + Docosahexaenoic acid (DHA)	862.5 mg	165%
Lutein + zeaxanthin	14.1 mg	141%

Note: NA = not applicable.

Table 11-2 shows that the optimized first-month menu containing all 50 nutrients, including energy and ORAC, meets her daily nutrition requirements except for sodium and potassium, and all the nutrients are not beyond their tolerable intake limits. Also, energy, protein, fat, and carbohydrate are all in the range of recommended values. In addition, based on the weights of vegetables and fruits, the pH of this menu is estimated to be about 7.0–8.5.

In light of the above procedures, we can obtain many menus for this obese woman for each month starting with the first month to the eleventh month. For the twelfth and thirteenth months, we may adjust the ratio of fat: protein: carbohydrate to 25%: 25%: 50% of the total energy to satisfy the energy requirements with ± 5% error for each one. And the fiber amount is set to be no less than 25 g/d for the last two months.

(3) People with Diabetes

Diabetes is a chronic disease that occurs when the pancreas does not produce enough insulin, or alternatively, when the body cannot effectively use the insulin it produces. Insulin is a hormone that regulates blood sugar. Hyperglycaemia, or raised blood sugar, is a common effect of uncontrolled diabetes and over time, it leads to serious damage to many of the body's systems, especially the nerves and blood vessels. Type I diabetes (previously known as insulin-dependent or childhood-onset) is characterized by a lack of insulin production. Without daily administration of insulin, Type I diabetes can be rapidly fatal. Type II diabetes (formerly called non-insulin-dependent or adult-onset) results from the body's ineffective use of insulin. Type II diabetes comprises of 90% of the people with diabetes around the world.

The World Health Organization (WHO) estimates that more than 180 million people worldwide have diabetes. This number is likely to more than double by 2030. 18 million people in the United States have diabetes and it will probably reach up to 30 million by 2030. In China, 21 million people have diabetes and this number most likely will double by 2030. In Canada, there are 2 million people with diabetes, and will probably be 3.5 million by 2030. In 2005, an estimated 2.9 million people died from diabetes. Almost 80% of diabetes deaths occur in low and middle-income countries. Almost half of diabetes deaths occur in people under the age of 70 years; 55% of diabetes deaths are in women. WHO projects that diabetes deaths will increase by more than 50% in the next 10 years without urgent action. Most notably, diabetes deaths are projected to increase by over 80% in upper-middle income countries between 2006 and 2015.

The leading causes of Type II diabetes are obesity, an unhealthy diet, high stress levels, not exercising regularly or at all, and also the increase in old age. Acidic foods are the main reason why body tissues are over-stimulated and in turn, this can lead to a lot of damage in the body. Type II diabetes are one of the symptoms of an acidic lifestyle. To counteract the effects of acid foods on the pH levels, it is necessary to include a lot of alkalizing vegetables, especially green varieties, green juices, and good fats in your daily diet. If you eat plant proteins that can be found in grains and legumes, your body will be able to restore the balance levels.

In a 2000 study published in the *Journal of Nutritional Sciences* entitled, "Correlation between Blood Chromium (III) Level, Blood Glucose and Lipid Concentrations in Diabetes", researchers looked at the measurement of blood glucose and serum lipids (cholesterols) in diabetics and healthy subjects and the effect of chromium yeast on these parameters. The study showed that people with increased blood glucose levels and serum lipids, which are common in diabetics, may experience deficiencies of chromium in the blood.

Eating food raises blood-sugar levels. Foods containing high sugar contents, as shown in Appendix A, affect blood sugar the fastest. So, people with diabetes should optimize the foods they eat to make sure that the daily energy provided by the sugar is not more than 10% of the total energy.

Therefore, if people with diabetes optimize the foods they eat every day to keep the pH of their diets in the range of 7.0–8.5, the chromium content in the range of 150–350 µm, and the energy from the sugar not more than 10 percent of the total energy, while at the same time meeting the daily energy and other nutrition requirements, they will be able to control diabetes or even get rid of it. This will greatly prolong their longevity.

(4) People with Alzheimer's disease

Alzheimer's disease (AD) is an irreversible, progressive brain disease that slowly destroys memory and thinking skills, and eventually even the ability to carry out the simplest tasks. In most people with AD, symptoms first appear after age 60. Dementia is a progressive cognitive decline with symptoms like disorientation, personality change, inattentiveness, and poor reasoning ability. AD is the most common cause of dementia and accounts for 50%–60% of all cases.

A 2005 study published in *Lancet*, the world's leading independent general medical journal, revealed disturbing figures about the progression of dementia on a global scale. It showed that 24.3 million people suffer from dementia today, 4.6 million new cases of dementia occur every year, or one new case every 7 seconds, and on a global scale, the number of people affected by dementia doubles every 20 years to roughly 81.1 million by 2040. So, about 13.5 million people suffer from AD worldwide. In light of a recent estimate, as many as 5.3 million people in the United States are living with Alzheimer's.

It has been observed that the levels of brain monoamine oxidase B (MAO-B) increase during aging. Several neurodegenerative diseases, such as Parkinson's and Alzheimer's, reveal high MAO-B in the brain. A 2008 study published in *British Journal of Nutrition* found that both inorganic and organic selenium supplements can decrease brain MAO-B enzyme activity. Selenium supplements, such as Viva Selenium Yeast, have been applied to Alzheimer's patients, in whom improvements have been observed.

Accordingly, if people with Alzheimer's disease optimize the foods they eat every day to make the selenium content in the range of 150–300 µm, while at the same time meeting their daily energy and other nutrition requirements, they will be able to control their Alzheimer's conditions. If we can increase selenium intake to about 200 µm per day in optimized menus starting at 55 years old, we will be able to greatly decrease the chances of getting Alzheimer's disease or even prevent it.

Summary

Now, it is my great pleasure to summarize the main points of this book as follows:

- Everybody is composed of 59 different chemical elements. Of the 59 elements in our bodies, almost 30 elements have been found to have a key function in helping us live and be healthy.

- A normal adult is composed of approximately 60% water, 17% protein, 17% fat, 3% minerals, and 1% carbohydrate. Due to metabolism, our bodies lose all of these compositions in different amounts every day. So, we must supplement these compositions daily to meet the needs of our metabolisms.

- Human nutrition—macronutrients include oxygen, water, protein, fat, carbohydrate, and fiber. Each of them has very important functions in our bodies. Oxygen is the most important nutrient because our lives can sustain for only a few minutes without it. Water is the second most important nutrient because our lives can sustain for only a few days without it.

- Human nutrition—micronutrients include vitamins and minerals. Vitamins are a group of organic compounds distinct from protein, fat, and carbohydrate, which neither provide energy nor serve as structural components of tissue, but are essential for life in minute amount for normal physiological functions, such as maintenance, growth, development, and reproduction. Similar to vitamins, minerals are also essential for life in minute amount for normal physiological function.

- Free radicals produced in our bodies can cause many diseases that accelerate our aging. Metabolic processes, cigarette-smoking, exposure to electromagnetic radiation such as copy machines, computer monitors, cell phones, and television sets, exposure to free radicals in the air that we breathe and in the water that we drink, processed foods that have many added chemicals, smog, pesticides, drugs, and/ or emotional stress all contribute to manufacturing free radicals in our bodies. In order to reduce the free radical amounts, we should pay much attention to all of these factors, except for the factor of metabolic processes.

• Our bodies' weights of 44 kg to 90 kg produce about 11g to 23 g of free radicals every day under normal condition. The higher the ORAC score, the more powerful the food is as an antioxidant. High ORAC foods are critical for your health, as they help eliminate free radicals that contribute to or cause cancer, aging, heart disease, and other diseases and conditions. By eating a diet with a minimum of 5,000 ORAC values per day, you can increase your blood plasma level of antioxidants by more than 25%.

• Our bodies' weights of 44 kg to 90 kg contain about 3.3 kg (3.1 liters) to 6.8 kg (6.4 liters) of blood, which flows into 60, 000 miles of veins and arteries. Blood is the river of life and has many vital functions, particularly in our immune system because it helps prevent diseases. The pH in our blood controls various functions of blood and must be kept in a very narrow range of 7.35–7.45 in order to ensure its normal functions. Below or above this range means symptoms and diseases.

• Most diseases are acid related. The underlying causes of cancer, heart disease, arteriosclerosis, high blood pressure, diabetes, arthritis, gout, kidney disease, asthma, allergies, psoriasis and other skin disorders, indigestion, diarrhea, nausea, obesity, tooth and gum diseases, osteo- porosis, eye diseases, etc., are the accumulation of acids in tissues and cells. Poor blood and lymph circulation, and poor cell activity are due to toxic acidic residues accumulating around the cell mem- brane which prevent nutritional elements from entering the cells. The accumulation of toxic acids is caused by the low pH of blood that leads to a lack of oxygen in cells and tissues. All these diseases accelerate the aging process.

• Foods and drinks that you ingest, metabolic activities, and stress can all affect the pH of your blood. Although your body is already designed to keep the pH of your body fluids in a tight, slightly alka- line range by five major mechanisms at work at all times to prevent these forces from shifting the pH of your blood to outside of the 7.35–7.45 range, what you eat and drink has a big influence on the pH of your blood. So, we should optimize what we drink and eat to meet the requirements of our blood pH.

- Life requires energy to grow and sustain. How do you know how much energy you need daily? The following two equations are used to calculate the estimated energy requirement (EER) for the adult men and women in normal weights with BMIs of 18.5–25 kg/m².

EER for Men Ages 19 Years and Older:

EER = 662 - (9.53 × age [y]) + PA × (15.91 × Weight [kg] + 539.6 × Height [m])

EER for Women Ages 19 Years and Older:

EER = 354 - (6.91 × age [y]) + PA × (9.36 × Weight [kg] + 726 × Height [m])

- Overweight and obese people need more energy to maintain their weights. The following two equations are for overweight or obese adult men and women to compute their estimated energy requirement (EER).

For overweight and obese women 19 years and older (BMI ≥ 25 kg/m²),

EER = 448 - 7.95 × age (y) + PA × (11.4 × Weight [kg] + 619 × Height [m])

For overweight and obese men 19 years and older (BMI ≥ 25 kg/m²),

EER = 1086 - 10.1 × age (y) + PA × (13.7 × Weight [kg] + 416 × Height [m])

- Individuals who consume energy that exceed their requirements, they will gain weight over time. So, there are no recommended dietary reference intakes (DRIs) for energy.

- The dietary reference intakes (DRIs) of vitamins and minerals almost can meet all healthy adults. If they do not exceed ULs, they should be safe and effective.

- UL is the highest level of daily nutrient intake that is likely to pose no risk of adverse health effects to almost all individuals in the general population. Due to a lack of suitable data, ULs for some nutrients have not been determined.

- The energy and nutrition values of 379 best foods are listed in Appendix A. These foods can satisfy the daily needs of our absolute majority.

- Our bodies' weights of 44 kg to 90 kg require 317g (222 liters) to 648 g (454 liters) of oxygen, daily, i.e. 1056 liters to 2160 liters of air. Air pollution plays a large role in exacerbating cardiopulmonary diseases and shortening life.

- Reducing air pollution and optimizing air quality are the responsibility of every government in the world. Leaders of every government in the world should cooperate to take action together to help control air pollution and optimize air quality.

- Indoor air levels of many pollutants may be 2–5 times, and occasionally more than 100 times, higher than outdoor levels. It is prudent to try to improve or optimize the indoor air quality in our home even if symptoms are not noticeable. There are three basic strategies to optimize indoor air quality: source control, improved ventilation, and the use of air cleaners.

- Our bodies' weights of 44 kg to 90 kg daily need 4.1 cups to 8.4 cups of water under normal conditions. Water quality plays a key role in our health and longevity. Controlling water pollution and optimizing water quality is also the responsibility of every government in the world. Every government should provide high quality drinking water for their people.

- Our daily energy and nutrition come from the foods we eat. We can optimize the different amounts of various types of foods to meet our daily energy and nutrition requirements, as demonstrated in this book by two examples. The optimization results indicate that for a normal adult, he/she only needs about three U.S. dollars a day to buy the optimized foods that will meet his/her daily energy and nutrition requirements.

- Everyone can obtain enough energy and nutrition from optimized daily menus. However, if you cannot optimize your daily menu, then you should first evaluate or ask a nutritionist to evaluate your nutrition status based on your existing diet to see if you lack any kinds of nutrients. After evaluation, you can take the dietary supplements you need.

- Research found that white people who regularly attend church live an average of 7 years longer than their nonchurchgoing counterparts, and black people live a remarkable 14 years longer. People who believe in God often feel more peaceful and less stressful than people who don't believe in God. As discussed in this book, stress can produce free radicals and acids in our bodies, which can lead to many diseases that shorten our longevity, if the free radicals and acids are not eliminated in time.

- Normal weight people can keep their weights and optimum health through optimizing the foods they eat, which will lead to longevity.

- Overweight or obese people can lose weight and improve their health through optimizing the foods they eat, which will prolong their longevity.

- People with diabetes can control or even get rid of diabetes through optimizing what they eat, which will prolong their longevity.

- People with Alzheimer's disease can control their Alzheimer's conditions through optimizing what they eat, which will also prolong their longevity.

- Our health and longevity lies in the optimization of what we breathe, drink, and eat!

The World Health Organization (WHO) has called the worldwide rise in obesity a global epidemic. One billion adults are overweight, of which 300 million are obese, which is caused due to over-nutrition. On average, each of them has at least 50 pounds more than his/her ideal body weight. However, the number of the starving and undernourished individuals remains steady at 600 million. If we learn to optimize the nutrition we need, we will be able to solve the worldwide problem of over-nutrition and malnutrition.

Overweight and obesity and their associated health problems have a significant economic impact on the global health care system. According to a study of national costs attributed to both overweight (BMI 25–30) and obesity (BMI greater than 30), medical expenses accounted for 9.1 percent of total U.S. medical expenditures and have reached as high as $147 billion in 2008: an extra $1,429 per year for each obese person, from $78.5 billion in 1998. Approximately half of these costs were paid by Medicaid and Medicare.

In 2001, Canada's economic burden in terms of overweight and obesity was estimated at $4.3 billion ($1.6 billion in direct costs and $2.7 billion in indirect costs). Furthermore, the economic burden of physical inactivity is estimated at $5.3 billion dollars ($1.6 billion in direct costs and $3.7 billion in indirect costs). The economic costs of physical inactivity and obesity represent 2.6% and 2.2% of all health care costs in Canada, respectively.

In other countries, the medical cost for treating the related diseases associated with overweight and obese has been largely increased. Therefore, if we learn to optimize the nutrition we need, we will be able to greatly reduce the medical expenditures.

I hope people in every country will benefit from reading this book. And, I wish all of you will live longer with optimum health.

Appendix A: Energy and Nutrition Values of Selected Foods

Table A-1 Energy, macronutrients, cholesterol, and ORAC values per 100 grams of selected foods

Food category and name	Energy (kcal)	Water (g)	Protein (g)	Fat (g)	Carbohy- drate (g)	Fiber (g)	Sugar (g)	Satd. Fat (g)	Trans Fat (g)	Choles- terol (mg)	ORAC (µmol TE)
Vegetables											
Artichoke, raw	47	84.94	3.27	0.15	10.51	5.4	0.99	0.036	0	0	6552
Asparagus, raw	20	99.22	2.20	0.12	3.88	2.1	1.88	0.040	0	0	2150
Beets, raw	43	87.58	1.61	0.17	9.56	2.8	6.76	0.027	0	0	1945
Broccoli, raw	34	89.30	2.82	0.37	6.64	2.6	1.70	0.039	0	0	1362
Broccoli, cooked, boiled, drained, without salt	35	89.25	2.38	0.41	7.18	3.3	1.39	0.079	0	0	2386
Broccoli raab, raw	22	92.55	3.17	0.49	2.85	2.7	0.38	0.050	0	0	3083
Broccoli raab, cooked	33	91.41	3.83	0.52	3.12	2.8	0.62	0.057	0	0	1552
Broccoli, frozen, spears, unprepared	29	90.55	3.06	0.34	5.35	3.0	1.47	0.052	0	0	1352
Brussels sprouts, raw	43	86	3.38	0.30	8.95	3.8	2.20	0.062	0	0	NA
Cabbage, raw	25	92.18	1.28	0.10	5.80	2.5	3.20	0.034	0	0	508
Cabbage, Chinese(pe-tsai), raw	16	94.39	1.20	0.20	3.23	1.2	1.41	0.043	0	0	NA
Cabbage, red, raw	31	90.39	1.43	0.16	7.37	2.1	3.83	0.021	0	0	2252

Carrots, baby, raw	35	90.35	0.64	0.13	8.24	2.9	4.76	0.023	0	0	436
Carrots, raw	41	88.29	0.93	0.24	9.58	2.8	4.74	0.037	0	0	666
Cauliflower, raw	25	91.91	1.98	0.10	5.30	2.5	2.40	0.015	0	0	829
Celery, raw	16	95.43	0.69	0.17	2.97	1.6	1.83	0.042	0	0	497
Chard, Swiss, raw	19	92.66	1.80	0.20	3.74	1.6	1.10	0.030	0	0	NA
Corn, sweet, yellow, raw	86	75.96	3.22	1.18	19.02	2.7	3.22	0.182	0	0	728
Cucumber, peeled, raw	12	96.73	0.59	0.16	2.16	0.7	1.38	0.013	0	0	126
Cucumber, with peel, raw	15	95.23	0.65	0.11	3.63	0.5	1.67	0.037	0	0	214
Eggplant, raw	24	92.41	1.01	0.19	5.70	3.4	2.35	0.034	0	0	933
Garlic, raw	149	58.58	6.36	0.50	33.06	2.1	1.00	0.089	0	0	5346
Kale, raw	50	84.46	3.30	0.70	10.01	2.0	0	0.091	0	0	NA
Leeks (bulk & lower leaf-portion), raw	61	83	1.50	0.30	14.15	1.8	3.90	0.040	0	0	490
Lettuce, butterhead (includes boston & bibb types), raw	13	95.63	1.35	0.22	2.23	1.1	0.94	0.029	0	0	1423
Lettuce, cos or romaine, raw	17	94.61	1.23	0.30	3.29	2.1	1.19	0.039	0	0	963
Lettuce, green leaf, raw	15	95.07	1.36	0.15	2.79	1.3	0.78	0.020	0	0	1447
Lettuce, iceberg (includes crisphead types), raw	14	95.64	0.90	0.14	2.97	1.3	1.97	0.018	0	0	438

Lettuce, red leaf, raw	16	95.64	1.33	0.22	2.26	0.9	0.48	0	0	0	2380
Mushrooms, brown, Italian or Crimini, raw	27	92.30	2.50	0.10	4.12	0.6	1.72	0.014	0	0	NA
Mushrooms, enoki, raw	44	88.54	2.56	0.32	7.68	2.7	0.22	0.028	0	0	NA
Mushrooms, Maitake, raw	37	90.53	1.94	0.19	6.81	2.7	2.07	0.030	0	0	NA
Mushrooms, portabella, raw	26	91.20	2.50	0.20	5.07	1.5	1.80	0.026	0	0	NA
Mushrooms, Shiitake, dried	296	9.50	9.58	0.99	75.37	11.5	2.21	0.225	0	0	NA
Mushrooms, white, raw	22	92.43	2.18	0.34	3.28	1.0	1.65	0.043	0	0	NA
Onions, raw	40	89.11	1.10	0.10	9.34	1.7	4.24	0.042	0	0	1034
Onions, sweet, raw	32	91.24	0.80	0.08	7.55	0.9	5.02	0	0	0	614
Parsley, raw	36	87.71	2.97	0.79	6.33	3.3	0.85	0.132	0	0	1301
Peppers, sweet, green, raw	20	93.89	0.86	0.17	4.64	1.7	2.40	0.058	0	0	923
Peppers, sweet, red, raw	31	92.21	0.99	0.30	6.03	2.1	4.20	0.027	0	0	791
Peppers, sweet, yellow, raw	27	90.02	1.00	0.21	6.31	0.9	4.35	0.031	0	0	965
Potatoes, red, flesh & skin, raw	70	80.96	1.89	0.14	15.90	1.7	1.00	0.034	0	0	1098
Potatoes, white, flesh & skin, raw	69	81.58	1.68	0.10	15.71	2.4	1.15	0.025	0	0	2036
Radishes, raw	16	95.27	0.68	0.10	3.40	1.6	1.86	0.032	0	0	1736
Spinach, raw	23	91.40	2.86	0.39	3.63	2.2	0.42	0.063	0	0	1515

Squash, summer, zucchini, includes skin, raw	16	94.64	1.21	0.18	3.35	1.1	1.73	0.037	0	0	180
Squash, winter, butternut, raw	45	86.41	1.00	0.10	11.69	2.0	2.20	0.021	0	0	396
Soybean, mature seeds, sprouted, raw	122	69.05	13.09	6.70	9.57	1.1	847	0.929	0	0	962
Tomato, red, ripe, raw, year round average	18	94.50	0.88	0.20	3.92	1.2	2.63	0.028	0	0	367
Turnip greens, raw	32	89.67	1.50	0.30	7.13	3.2	0.81	0.070	0	0	NA
Waterchestnut, Chinese, (matai), raw	97	73.46	1.40	0.10	23.94	3.0	4.80	0.026	0	0	NA
Fruits											
Apples, raw, with skin	52	85.56	0.26	0.17	13.81	2.4	10.39	0.028	0	0	3082
Apples, raw, without skin	48	86.67	0.27	0.13	12.76	1.3	10.10	0.021	0	0	2573
Applesauce, canned, unsweetened, without added ascorbic acid	43	88.35	0.17	0.05	11.29	1.2	10.09	0.008	0	0	1965
Apricots, raw	48	86.35	1.40	0.39	11.12	2.0	9.24	0.027	0	0	1115
Avocados, raw, all commercial varieties	160	73.23	2.00	14.66	8.53	6.7	0.66	2.126	0	0	1933
Avocados, raw, California	167	72.33	1.96	15.41	8.64	6.8	0.30	2.126	0	0	NA

Avocados, raw, Florida	120	78.81	2.23	10.06	7.82	5.6	2.42	1.960	0	0	NA
Bananas, raw	89	74.91	1.09	0.33	22.84	2.6	12.23	0.112	0	0	879
Bananas, dehydrated, banana powder	346	3.00	3.89	1.81	88.28	9.9	47.30	0.698	0	0	NA
Blackberries, raw	43	88.15	1.39	0.49	9.61	5.3	4.88	0.014	0	0	5347
Blueberries, raw	57	84.21	0.74	0.33	14.49	2.4	9.96	0.028	0	0	6554
Cranberries, raw	46	87.13	0.39	0.13	12.20	4.6	4.04	0.011	0	0	9584
Elderberries, raw	73	79.80	0.66	0.50	18.40	7.0	0	0.023	0	0	14697
Figs, raw	74	79.11	0.75	0.30	19.18	2.9	16.26	0.060	0	0	3383
Grapefruit, raw, pink & red, all areas	42	88.06	0.77	0.14	10.66	1.6	6.89	0.021	0	0	1548
Grapes, American style (slip skin), raw	67	81.30	0.63	0.35	17.15	0.9	16.25	0.114	0	0	1118
Grapes, red & green, seedless, raw	69	80.54	0.72	0.14	18.10	0.9	15.48	0.054	0	0	1126
Honeydew melons, raw	36	89.82	0.54	0.14	9.09	0.8	8.12	0.038	0	0	241
Lemon, raw, with peel	20	87.40	1.20	0.30	10.70	4.7	0	0.039	0	0	NA
Limes, raw	30	88.26	0.70	0.20	10.54	2.8	1.69	0.022	0	0	82
Kiwi fruit (Chinese gooseberries), fresh, raw	61	83.07	1.14	0.52	14.66	3.0	8.99	0.029	0	0	882

Mangos, raw	65	81.71	0.51	0.27	17.00	1.8	14.80	0.066	0	0	1002
Nectarine, raw	44	87.59	1.06	0.32	10.55	1.7	7.89	0	0	0	750
Oranges, raw, navels	49	85.97	0.91	0.15	12.54	2.2	8.50	0.019	0	0	1819
Oranges, mandarin, tangerines, raw	53	85.17	0.81	0.31	13.34	1.8	10.58	0.039	0	0	1620
Peaches, raw	39	88.87	0.91	0.25	9.54	1.5	8.39	0.019	0	0	1814
Pears, raw	58	83.71	0.38	0.12	15.46	3.1	9.80	0.006	0	0	2941
Persimmon, native, raw	127	64.40	0.80	0.40	33.50	0	0	0	0	0	NA
Pineapple, raw, all varieties	50	86.00	0.54	0.12	13.12	1.4	9.85	0.009	0	0	385
Plums, raw	46	87.23	0.70	0.28	11.42	1.4	9.92	0.017	0	0	6259
Raisins, seedless	299	15.43	3.07	0.46	79.18	3.7	59.19	0.058	0	0	3037
Raspberries, raw	52	85.75	1.20	0.64	11.94	6.5	4.42	0.019	0	0	4482
Strawberries, raw	32	90.95	0.67	0.30	7.68	2.0	4.89	0.015	0	0	3577
Watermelon, raw	30	91.45	0.61	0.15	7.55	0.4	6.20	0.016	0	0	142
Apple juice, canned or bottled	47	87.93	0.06	0.11	11.68	0.1	10.90	0.019	0	0	408
Cranberry juice, cocktail, bottled	54	86.17	0	0.10	13.52	0	11.87	0.009	0	0	NA
Grape juice drink, canned	57	85.30	0	0	14.55	0.1	14.11	0	0	0	NA
Grapefruit juice, pink, raw	39	90.00	0.50	0.10	9.20	0	9.10	0.014	0	0	1548

Grapefruit juice, white, raw	39	90.00	0.50	0.10	9.20	0.1	9.10	0	0	0	793
Lemon juice, raw	25	90.73	0.38	0	8.63	0.4	2.40	0	0	0	1225
Lime juice, raw	25	90.79	0.42	0.07	8.42	0.4	1.69	0.008	0	0	823
Orange juice, raw	45	88.30	0.70	0.20	10.40	0.2	8.40	0.024	0	0	726
Prune juice, canned	71	81.24	0.61	0.03	17.45	1.0	16.45	0	0	0	2034
Legumes										
Beans, black, mature seeds, raw	341	11.02	21.60	1.42	62.36	15.2	2.12	0	0	0	8040
Beans, kidney, red mature seeds, raw	337	11.75	22.53	1.06	61.29	15.2	2.10	0.154	0	0	8454
Beans, navy, mature seeds, raw	337	12.10	22.33	1.50	60.75	24.4	3.88	0.170	0	0	1530
Beans, pink, mature seeds, raw	343	10.06	20.96	1.13	64.19	12.7	2.14	0.292	0	0	8320
Beans, pinto, mature seeds, raw	347	11.33	21.42	1.23	62.55	15.5	2.11	0.235	0	0	7779
Beans, pinto, mature seeds, cooked	143	62.95	9.01	0.65	26.22	9.0	0.34	0.109	0	0	904
Beans, snap, green, raw	31	90.27	1.82	0.12	7.13	3.4	1.40	0.026	0	0	759
Chickpeas (garbanzo beans), mature seeds, raw	364	11.53	19.30	6.04	60.65	17.4	10.70	0.626	0	0	847

Cowpeas, common, mature seeds, raw	336	11.95	23.52	1.26	60.03	10.6	6.90	0.331	0	0	4347
Lentils, raw	353	10.40	25.80	1.06	60.08	30.5	2.03	0.156	0	0	7282
Peas, split, mature seeds, raw	341	11.27	24.55	1.16	60.37	25.5	8.00	0.161	0	0	524
Soybeans, mature seeds, raw	446	8.54	36.49	19.94	30.16	9.3	7.33	2.884	0	0	5764
Tofu, silken, firm (MURI-NU)	62	87.40	6.90	2.70	2.40	0.1	1.27	0.406	0	0	NA
Tofu, silken, soft (MURI-NU)	55	89.00	4.80	2.70	2.90	0.1	1.31	0.357	0	0	NA
Tofu, yogurt	94	77.50	3.50	1.80	15.96	0.2	1.24	0.259	0	0	NA
Tofu, dried-frozen (koy-atofu)	480	5.78	47.94	30.34	14.58	7.2	7.38	4.388	0	0	NA
Tofu, dried-frozen (koy-atofu), prepared with calcium sulfate	472	5.78	47.94	30.34	12.79	1.2	11.59	4.388	0	0	NA
Tofu, fried	271	50.52	17.19	20.18	10.49	3.9	2.72	2.918	0	0	NA
Tofu, fried, prepared with calcium sulfate	271	50.52	17.19	20.18	10.50	3.9	3.72	2.918	0	0	NA
Tofu, hard, prepared with nigari	146	71.12	12.68	9.99	4.39	0.6	4.33	1.445	0	0	NA

Tofu, regular, prepared with calcium sulfate	76	84.55	8.08	4.78	1.88	0.3	1.85	0.691	0	0	NA
Tofu, salted and fermented (fuyu), prepared with calcium sulfate	116	70.01	8.15	8.00	5.15	NA	NA	1.157	0	0	NA
Cereal											
Buckwheat	343	9.75	13.25	3.40	71.50	10.0	0	0.741	0	0	NA
Buckwheat flour, whole-groat	335	11.15	12.62	3.10	70.59	10.0	2.60	0.677	0	0	NA
Cereals ready-to-eat, granola, homemade	489	5.40	14.85	24.06	53.25	9.0	20.00	4.058	0	0	2294
Cereals ready-to-eat, bran flakes, single brand	320	3.70	9.40	2.20	80.40	17.6	18.90	0.400	0	0	NA
Cereals ready-to-eat, bran, malted flour, single brand	287	2.80	12.70	2.10	78.20	28.6	24.40	0.300	0	0	NA
Cereals ready-to-eat, corn & oat flour, puffed presweetened, single brand	395	1.50	5.20	2.10	88.90	2.5	38.30	0.600	0	0	NA
Cereals ready-to-eat, GERNERAL MILLS, CHEERIOS	367	3.76	11.33	5.90	74.68	10.1	4.02	0.954	0	0	NA

Cereals ready-to-eat, GERNERAL MILLS, Cinnamon Grahams	378	2.63	5.00	2.80	86.00	3.2	38.00	0.500	0	0	NA
Cereals ready-to-eat, GERNERAL MILLS, FIBER ONE	200	3.19	6.67	3.33	83.33	47.3	0	0.379	0	0	NA
Cereals ready-to-eat, GERNERAL MILLS, HARMONY	365	2.83	11.00	2.20	79.00	4.0	24.00	0.500	0	0	NA
Cereals ready-to-eat, Malt-O-Meal, High Fiber Bran Flakes	388	2.50	10.60	2.51	80.80	14.9	19.50	0.588	0	0	NA
Cereal, oats, instant, fortified, plain, dry	375	10.37	12.72	6.25	67.55	10.0	1.51	1.537	0	0	2308
Cereals ready-to-eat, KELLOGG, KELLOGG'S Complete Wheat Bran Flakes	318	3.00	10.00	2.00	79.00	17.5	17.00	0.400	0	0	NA
Cereals, Whole wheat hot, natural cereal, dry	342	9.90	11.20	2.00	75.20	9.5	0.42	0.300	0	0	NA
Grain											
Barley, pearled, raw	352	10.09	9.91	1.16	77.72	15.6	0.80	0.244	0	0	NA
Barley, pearled, cooked	123	68.80	2.26	0.44	28.22	3.8	0.28	0.093	0	0	NA

Barley malt flour	361	8.21	10.28	1.84	78.30	7.1	0.80	0.386	0	0	NA
Cocoa, dry powder, unsweetened	229	3.00	19.60	13.70	54.30	33.2	1.75	8.070	0	0	80933
Cornmeal, whole-grain, white	362	10.26	8.12	3.59	76.89	7.3	0.64	0.505	0	0	NA
Cornmeal, whole-grain, yellow	362	10.26	8.12	3.59	76.89	7.3	0.64	0.505	0	0	NA
Cornmeal, white (Navajo)	398	5.42	10.99	5.04	77.14	10.4	1.46	0.853	0	0	NA
Cornmeal, yellow (Navajo)	384	10.15	9.85	5.88	72.90	9.4	1.56	1.043	0	0	NA
Corn flour, whole-grain, white	361	10.91	6.93	3.86	76.85	7.3	0.64	0.543	0	0	NA
Corn flour, whole-grain, yellow	361	10.91	6.93	3.86	76.85	7.3	0.64	0.543	0	0	NA
Corn, sweet, yellow, raw	86	75.96	3.22	1.18	19.02	2.7	3.22	0.182	0	0	782
Oat flour, partially debranned	404	8.55	14.66	9.12	65.70	6.5	0.80	1.607	0	0	NA
Peanut flour, defatted	327	7.80	52.20	0.55	34.70	15.8	8.22	0.063	0	0	NA
Peanut flour, low fat	428	7.80	33.80	21.90	31.27	15.8	0	3.040	0	0	NA
Popcorn, air-popped	387	3.32	12.94	4.54	77.90	14.50	0.87	0.570	0	0	1743
Potato flour	357	6.52	6.90	0.34	83.10	5.9	3.52	0.090	0	0	NA
Rice bran, crude	316	6.13	13.35	20.85	49.69	21.0	0.90	4.171	0	0	24287

Rice flour, brown	363	11.97	7.23	2.78	76.48	4.6	0.85	0.557	0	0	NA
Rice flour, white	366	11.89	5.95	1.42	80.13	2.4	0.12	0.386	0	0	NA
Rice noodles, cooked	109	73.82	0.91	0.20	24.90	1.0	0	0.023	0	0	NA
Rice noodles, dry	364	11.91	3.44	0.56	83.24	1.6	0	0.153	0	0	NA
Rice, brown, long-grain, cooked	111	73.09	2.58	0.90	22.96	1.8	0.35	0.180	0	0	NA
Rice, brown, long-grain, raw	370	10.37	7.94	2.92	77.24	3.5	0.85	0.584	0	0	NA
Rice, brown, medium-grain, cooked	112	72.96	2.32	0.83	23.51	1.8	0	0.165	0	0	NA
Rice, brown, medium-grain, raw	362	12.37	7.50	2.68	76.17	3.4	0	0.536	0	0	NA
Rice, white, long-grain, regular, cooked	130	68.44	2.69	0.28	28.17	0.4	0.05	0.077	0	0	NA
Rice, white, long-grain, regular, raw	365	11.62	7.13	0.66	79.95	1.3	0.12	0.180	0	0	NA
Rice, white, medium-grain, cooked	130	68.61	2.38	0.21	28.59	0.3	0	0.057	0	0	NA
Rice, white, medium-grain, raw	360	12.89	6.61	0.58	79.34	0	0	0.158	0	0	NA

Rice, white, short-grain, cooked	130	68.53	2.36	0.19	28.73	0	0	0.051	0	0	NA
Rice, white, short-grain, raw	358	13.29	6.50	0.52	79.15	2.8	0	0.140	0	0	NA
Rye flour, dark	324	11.07	14.03	2.69	68.74	22.6	1.04	0.309	0	0	NA
Rye flour, light	367	8.78	8.39	1.36	80.23	14.6	1.04	0.145	0	0	NA
Rye flour, medium	354	9.85	9.39	1.77	77.49	14.6	1.04	0.198	0	0	NA
Seeds, cottonseed flour, low fat (glandless)	332	6.90	49.83	1.41	36.10	0	0	0.310	0	0	NA
Seeds, sesame flour, high fat	526	0.90	30.78	37.10	26.62	0	0	5.196	0	0	NA
Seeds, sesame flour, low fat	333	7.10	50.14	1.75	35.51	0	0	0.201	0	0	NA
Seeds, sunflower flour, partially defatted	326	7.47	48.06	1.61	35.83	5.2	0	0.138	0	0	NA
Soy flour, full-fat, raw	436	5.16	34.54	20.65	35.19	9.6	7.50	2.987	0	0	NA
Wheat flour, white, all-purpose, enriched bleached	364	11.92	10.33	0.98	76.31	2.7	0.27	0.155	0	0	NA
Wheat flour, white, all-purpose, enriched unbleached	364	11.92	10.33	0.98	76.31	2.7	0.27	0.155	0	0	NA
Wheat flour, white, all-purpose, self-rising, enriched	354	10.59	9.89	0.97	74.22	2.7	0.22	0.154	0	0	NA
Wheat flour, whole-grain	339	10.27	13.70	1.87	72.57	12.2	0.41	0.322	0	0	24287

Bread

Bread, cracked-wheat	260	35.80	8.70	3.90	49.50	5.5	0	0.916	0	0	NA
Bread, egg	283	34.70	9.50	6.00	47.80	2.3	1.78	1.593	0	51	NA
Bread, French or Vienna (includes sourdough)	289	27.81	11.75	1.83	56.44	2.4	2.56	0.497	0	0	NA
Bread, Italian	271	35.70	8.80	3.50	50.00	2.7	0.83	0.855	0	0	NA
Bread, oat bran	236	44.00	10.40	4.40	39.80	4.5	7.70	0.697	0	0	NA
Bread, oatmeal	269	36.70	8.40	4.40	48.50	4.0	8.14	0.703	0	0	NA
Bread, pumpernickel	250	37.90	8.70	3.10	47.50	6.5	0.53	0.437	0	0	NA
Bread, raisin	274	33.60	7.90	4.40	52.30	4.3	5.68	1.081	0	0	NA
Bread, rye	258	37.30	8.50	3.30	48.30	5.8	3.85	0.626	0	0	NA
Bread, wheat	266	35.74	10.91	3.64	47.51	3.6	5.75	0.803	0	0	NA
Bread, white, commercially prepared (includes soft bread crumbs)	266	36.44	7.64	3.29	50.61	2.4	4.31	0.717	0	0	NA
Dairy											
Milk, buttermilk, dried	387	2.97	34.30	5.78	49.00	0	49.00	3.598	0	69	NA
Milk, buttermilk, fluid, cultured, low fat	40	90.13	3.31	0.88	4.79	0	4.79	0.548	0	4	NA
Milk, chocolate, fluid, reduced fat	76	82.17	2.99	1.90	12.13	0.7	9.55	1.177	0	8	1263

Milk, chocolate, fluid, whole	83	82.30	3.17	3.39	10.34	0.8	9.54	2.104	0	12	NA
Milk, dry, whole	496	2.47	26.32	26.71	38.42	0	38.42	16.742	0	97	NA
Milk, goat, fluid	69	87.03	3.56	4.14	4.45	0	4.45	2.667	0	11	NA
Milk, human, mature, fluid	70	87.50	1.03	4.38	6.89	0	6.89	2.009	0	14	NA
Milk, fluid, 1% milkfat, with added vitamin A	42	89.92	3.37	0.97	4.99	0	5.20	0.633	0	5	NA
Milk, fluid, nonfat (fat free or skim)	35	90.80	3.41	0.18	4.85	0	5.09	0.117	0	2	NA
Milk, producer, fluid, 3.7% milkfat	64	87.69	3.28	3.66	4.65	0	4.65	2.278	0	14	NA
Milk, fluid, 2% milkfat, with added vitamin A	50	89.33	3.30	1.97	4.68	0	5.06	1.257	0	8	NA
Milk, sheep, fluid	108	80.70	5.98	7.00	5.36	0	5.36	4.603	0	27	NA
Milk, whole, 3.25% milkfat	60	88.32	3.22	3.25	4.52	0	5.26	1.865	0	10	NA
Egg										
Egg, duck, whole, fresh, raw	185	70.83	12.81	13.77	1.45	0	0.93	3.681	0	884	NA
Egg, goose, whole, fresh, raw	185	70.43	13.87	13.27	1.35	0	0.94	3.595	0	852	NA
Egg, quail, whole, fresh, raw	158	74.35	13.05	11.09	0.41	0	0.41	3.557	0	844	NA

Egg, turkey, whole, fresh, raw	171	72.50	13.68	11.88	1.15	0	1.15	3.632	0	933	NA
Egg, white, raw, fresh	48	87.57	10.90	0.17	0.73	0	0.71	0	0	0	NA
Egg, whole, cooked, fried	196	69.13	13.63	15.31	0.88	0	0.83	4.294	0	457	NA
Egg, whole, cooked, hard-boiled	155	74.62	12.58	10.61	1.12	0	1.12	3.267	0	424	NA
Egg, whole, cooked, omelet	157	75.87	10.59	12.03	0.68	0	0.65	3.296	0	356	NA
Egg, whole, cooked, poached	142	75.54	12.53	9.90	0.76	0	0.77	3.087	0	422	NA
Egg, whole, cooked, scrambled	167	73.15	11.09	12.21	2.20	0	1.73	3.679	0	352	NA
Egg, whole, raw, fresh	143	75.84	12.58	9.94	0.77	0	0.77	3.099	0	423	NA
Egg, yolk, raw, fresh	317	52.31	15.86	26.54	3.59	0	0.56	9.551	0	1234	NA
Cheese											
Cheese, America cheddar, imitation	239	53.10	16.70	14.00	11.60	0	7.74	8.790	0	36	NA
Cheese, blue	353	42.41	21.40	28.74	2.34	0	0.50	18.669	0	75	NA
Cheese, brick	371	41.11	23.24	29.68	2.79	0	0.51	18.764	0	94	NA
Cheese, brie	334	48.42	20.75	27.68	0.45	0	0.45	17.410	0	100	NA
Cheese, camembert	300	51.80	19.80	24.26	0.46	0	0.46	15.259	0	72	NA

Food										
Cheese, caraway	376	39.28	25.18	29.20	3.06	0	0.68	18.584	0	93	NA
Cheese, cheddar	403	36.75	24.90	33.14	1.25	0	0.52	21.092	0	105	NA
Cheese, cheshire	387	37.65	23.37	30.60	4.78	0	NA	19.475	0	103	NA
Cheese, Colby	394	38.20	23.76	32.11	2.57	0	0.52	20.218	0	95	NA
Cheese, cottage, 1% milkfat	72	82.48	12.39	1.02	2.72	0	2.72	0.645	0	4	NA
Cheese, cottage, 2% milkfat	90	79.31	13.74	1.93	3.63	0	0.33	1.221	0	8	NA
Cheese, cream, fat free	96	75.53	14.41	1.36	5.80	0	0.40	0.899	0	8	NA
Cheese, edam	357	41.56	24.99	27.80	1.43	0	1.43	17.572	0	89	NA
Cheese, feta	264	55.22	14.21	21.28	4.09	0	4.09	14.946	0	89	NA
Cheese, Mexican, blend, reduced fat	282	48.20	24.69	19.40	3.41	0	0.56	11.580	0	62	NA
Cheese, Mexican, queso anejo	373	38.06	21.44	29.98	4.63	0	4.63	19.033	0	105	NA
Cheese, Monterey	373	41.01	24.48	30.28	0.68	0	0.50	19.066	0	89	NA
Cheese, Monterey, low fat	313	46.00	28.20	21.60	0.70	0	0.56	14.040	0	65	NA
Cheese, Mozzarella, part skim	254	53.78	24.26	15.92	2.77	0	1.13	10.114	0	64	NA
Cheese, muenster	368	41.77	23.41	30.04	1.12	0	1.12	19.113	0	96	NA
Cheese, parmesan, hard	392	29.16	35.75	25.83	3.22	0	0.80	16.410	0	68	NA

Cheese, provolone, reduced fat	274	50.60	24.70	17.60	3.50	0	0.55	11.300	0	55	NA
Cheese, Ricotta, part skim	138	74.41	11.39	7.91	5.14	0	0.31	4.972	0	31	NA
Cheese, Swiss	380	37.12	26.93	27.80	5.38	0	1.32	17.779	0	92	NA
Cheese, tilsit	340	42.86	24.41	25.98	1.88	0	0	16.775	0	102	NA
Nuts and Seeds											
Nuts, acorns, raw	387	27.90	6.15	23.86	40.75	0	0	3.102	0	0	NA
Nuts, almonds	575	4.70	21.22	49.42	21.67	12.2	3.89	3.731	0.017	0	4454
Nuts, cashew nuts, raw	553	5.20	18.22	43.85	30.19	3.3	5.91	7.783	0	0	1948
Nuts, chestnuts, Chinese, raw	224	43.95	4.20	1.11	49.07	0	0	0.164	0	0	NA
Nuts, chestnuts, European, raw	213	48.65	2.42	2.26	45.56	8.1	0	0.452	0	0	NA
Nuts, chestnuts, Japanese, raw	154	61.41	2.25	0.53	34.91	0	0	0.078	0	0	NA
Nuts, coconut meat, raw	354	46.99	3.33	33.49	15.23	9.0	6.23	29.698	0	0	NA
Nuts, ginkgo nuts, raw	182	55.20	4.32	1.68	37.60	0	0	0.319	0	0	NA
Nuts, hazelnuts or filberts	628	5.31	14.95	60.75	16.70	9.7	4.34	4.464	0	0	9645
Nuts, macadamia nuts, dry roasted, without salt added	718	1.61	7.79	76.08	13.38	8.0	4.14	11.949	0	0	1695

Food										
Nuts, macadamia nuts, raw	718	1.36	7.91	75.77	13.82	8.6	4.57	12.061	0	0	NA
Nuts, mixed nuts /w peanuts, dry roasted, with salt added	594	1.75	17.30	51.45	25.35	9.0	4.64	6.899	0	0	NA
Nuts, mixed nuts /w peanuts, dry roasted, without salt added	594	1.75	17.30	51.45	25.35	9.0	4.64	6.899	0	0	NA
Nuts, mixed nuts /w peanuts, oil roasted, with salt added	617	2.03	16.76	56.33	21.41	9.0	4.28	8.725	0	0	NA
Nuts, pecans	691	3.52	9.17	71.97	13.86	9.6	3.97	6.180	0	0	17940
Nuts, pine nuts, dried	673	2.28	13.69	68.37	13.08	3.7	3.59	4.899	0	0	616
Nuts, pistachio nuts, raw	557	3.97	20.61	44.44	27.97	10.3	7.64	5.440	0	0	7983
Nuts, walnuts, English	654	4.07	15.23	65.21	13.71	6.7	2.61	6.126	0	0	13541
Seeds, breadfruit seeds, raw	191	56.27	7.40	5.59	29.24	5.2	0	1.509	0	0	NA
Seeds, breadnut tree seeds, dried	367	6.50	8.62	1.68	79.39	14.9	0	0.454	0	0	NA
Seeds, breadnut tree seeds, raw	217	45.00	5.97	0.99	46.28	0	0	0.267	0	0	NA
Seeds, flaxseed	534	6.96	18.29	42.16	28.88	27.3	1.55	3.663	0	0	NA
Seeds, lotus seeds, dried	332	14.16	15.41	1.97	64.47	0	0	0.330	0	0	NA

Seeds, pumpkin & squash seed kernels, dried	541	6.92	24.54	45.85	17.81	3.9	1.00	8.674	0	0	NA
Seeds, sesame seeds, whole, dried	573	4.69	17.73	49.67	23.45	11.8	0.30	6.957	0	0	NA
Seeds, sunflower kernels, dried	584	4.73	20.78	51.46	20.00	8.6	2.62	4.455	0	0	NA
Seeds, watermelon seed kernels, dried	557	5.05	28.33	47.37	15.31	0	0	9.779	0	0	NA
Fish and Shellfish										
Fish, anchovy, European, raw	131	73.37	20.35	4.84	0	0	0	1.282	0	60	NA
Fish, bass, striped, raw	97	79.22	17.73	2.33	0	0	0	0.507	0	80	NA
Fish, bluefish, raw	124	70.86	20.04	4.24	0	0	0	0.915	0	59	NA
Fish, butterfish, raw	146	74.13	17.28	8.02	0	0	0	3.380	0	65	NA
Fish, catfish, channel, farmed, raw	135	75.38	15.55	7.59	0	0	0	1.768	0	47	NA
Fish, catfish, channel, wild, raw	95	80.36	16.38	2.82	0	0	0	0.722	0	58	NA
Fish, cod, Atlantic, raw	82	81.22	17.81	0.67	0	0	0	0.131	0	43	NA
Fish, cod, Pacific, raw	82	81.28	17.90	0.63	0	0	0	0.081	0	37	NA

Crustaceans, crab, Alaska king, raw	84	79.57	18.29	0.60	0	0	0.090	0	42	NA
Crustaceans, crab, blue, raw	87	79.02	18.06	1.08	0.04	0	0.222	0	78	NA
Crustaceans, crab, queen, raw	90	80.58	18.50	1.18	0	0	0.143	0	55	NA
Fish, drum, freshwater, raw	119	77.33	17.54	4.93	0	0	1.119	0	64	NA
Fish, haddock, raw	87	79.92	18.91	0.72		0	0.130	0	57	NA
Fish, halibut, Atlantic & Pacific, raw	110	77.92	20.81	2.29		0	0.325	0	32	NA
Fish, halibut, Greenland, raw	186	70.27	14.37	13.84	0	0	2.419	0	46	NA
Fish, herring, Atlantic, raw	158	72.05	17.96	9.04	0	0	2.040	0	60	NA
Fish, herring, Pacific, raw	195	71.52	16.39	13.88	0	0	3.257	0	77	NA
Crustaceans, lobster, northern, raw	90	76.76	18.80	0.90	0.50	0	0.180	0	95	NA
Fish, mackerel, Atlantic, raw	205	63.55	18.60	13.89	0	0	3.257	0	70	NA
Fish, mackerel, king, raw	105	75.85	20.28	2.00	0	0	0.363	0	53	NA
Fish, mackerel, Spanish, raw	139	71.67	19.29	6.30	0	0	1.828	0	76	NA
Fish, monkfish, raw	76	83.24	14.48	1.52	0	0	0.340	0	25	NA
Fish, mullet, striped, raw	117	77.01	19.35	3.79	0	0	1.116	0	49	NA

Fish, ocean perch, Atlantic, raw	94	78.70	18.62	1.63	0	0	0	0.244	0	42	NA
Fish, pike, walleye, raw	93	79.31	19.14	1.22	0	0	0	0.249	0	86	NA
Fish, pollock, Atlantic, raw	92	78.18	19.44	0.98	0	0	0	0.135	0	71	NA
Fish, pollock, walleye, raw	81	81.56	17.18	0.80	0	0	0	0.164	0	71	NA
Fish, roe, mixed species, raw	143	67.73	22.32	6.43	0	0	0	1.456	0	374	NA
Fish, sablefish, raw	195	71.02	13.41	15.30	0	0	0	3.201	0	49	NA
Fish, salmon, Atlantic, farmed, raw	183	68.90	19.90	10.85	0	0	0	2.183	0	59	NA
Fish, salmon, Atlantic, wild, raw	142	68.50	19.84	6.34	0	0	0	0.981	0	55	NA
Fish, salmon, chinook, raw	179	71.64	19.93	10.43	0	0	0	3.100	0	50	NA
Fish, salmon, coho, wild, raw	146	72.66	21.62	5.93	0	0	0	1.260	0	45	NA
Fish, salmon, pink, raw	116	76.35	19.94	3.45	0	0	0	0.558	0	52	NA
Fish, sardine, Pacific, canned in tomato sauce, drained solids with bone	186	66.65	20.86	10.46	0.71	0.1	0.43	2.686	0	61	
Fish, shad, America, raw	197	68.19	16.93	13.77	0	0	0	3.126	0	75	NA
Fish, shark, mixed species, raw	130	73.58	20.98	4.51	0	0	0	0.925	0	51	NA

Crustaceans, shrimp, mixed species, raw	106	75.86	20.31	1.73	0.91	0	0.328	0	152	NA
Fish, swordfish, raw	121	75.62	19.80	4.01	0	0	1.097	0	39	NA
Fish, tuna, fresh, bluefin, raw	144	68.09	23.33	4.90	0	0	1.257	0	38	NA
Fish, wolffish, Atlantic, raw	96	79.90	17.50	2.39	0	0	0.365	0	46	NA
Meat and Poultry										
Beef, bottom sirloin, tri-tip, separable lean only, trimmed to 0" fat, select, raw	129	73.48	21.34	4.21	0	0	1.500	0	37	NA
Beef, brisket, flat half, separable lean and fat, trimmed to 1/8" fat, all grades, raw	277	59.07	17.94	22.18	0	0	8.951	0	81	NA
Beef, brisket, point half, separable lean and fat, trimmed to 1/4" fat, all grades, raw	331	53.50	16.12	29.09	0	0	11.840	0	76	NA
Beef, chuck, clod steak, separable lean only, trimmed to 1/4" fat, all grades, raw	129	73.26	21.13	4.24	0	0	1.323	0	59	NA

Food										
Beef, flank, separable lean only, trimmed to 0" fat, all grades, raw	141	72.08	21.57	5.47	0	0	0	2.058	0	33	NA
Beef, ground, 70% lean meat / 30% fat, raw	332	54.38	14.35	30	0	0	0	11.282	1.826	78	NA
Beef, rib, shortribs, separable lean only, choice, raw	173	69.38	19.05	10.19	0	0	0	4.330	0	59	NA
Beef, round, bottom round, separable lean only, trimmed to 1/2" fat, prime, raw	159	70.25	21.87	7.30	0	0	0	2.610	0	59	NA
Beef, tenderloin, separable lean only, trimmed to 1/4" fat, prime, raw	169	69.92	20.78	8.85	0	0	0	3.540	0	62	NA
Beef, brain, raw	143	76.29	10.86	10.30	1.05	0	0	2.300	0.610	3010	NA
Beef, heart, raw	112	77.11	17.72	3.94	0.14	0	0	1.383	0.180	124	NA
Beef, kidneys, raw	103	77.89	17.40	3.09	0.29	0	0	0.868	0.100	411	NA
Beef, liver, raw	135	70.81	20.36	3.63	3.89	0	0	1.233	0.170	275	NA
Beef, lung, raw	92	79.38	16.20	2.50	0	0	0	0.860	0	242	NA
Beef, spleen, raw	105	77.20	18.30	3.00	0	0	0	1.000	0	263	NA
Pork, boneless loin, fresh	145	71.35	19.02	7.18	0.76	0	0.08	2.840	0	49	NA

Food											
Pork, center cut chops, fresh	167	69.17	18.74	9.62	0.84	0	0.28	3.600	0	52	NA
Pork, cured, bacon, raw	458	40.20	11.60	45.04	0.66	0	0	14.993	0	68	NA
Pork, cured, patties, grilled	342	51.35	13.30	30.85	1.70	0	0	11.090	0	72	NA
Pork, fresh, backfat, raw	812	7.69	2.92	88.69	0	0	0	32.210	0	57	NA
Pork, fresh, backribs, separable lean and fat, raw	282	59.39	16.12	23.58	0	0	0	8.730	0	81	NA
Pork, fresh, belly, raw	518	36.74	9.34	53.01	0	0	0	19.330	0	72	NA
Pork, fresh, loin, tenderloin, separable lean only, raw	106	76.91	20.39	2.09	0	0	0	0.673	0.020	48	NA
Pork, fresh, ground, raw	263	61.06	16.88	21.19	0	0	0	7.870	0	72	NA
Pork, fresh, leg(ham), whole, separable lean and fat, raw	245	62.47	17.43	18.87	0	0	0	6.540	0	73	NA
Pork, flesh, loin, country-style ribs, separable lean only, raw	140	72.84	20.76	5.64	0	0	0	2.003	0.045	74	NA
Pork, flesh, separable fat, raw	665	23.97	5.82	70.99	0	0	0	25.082	0.786	77	NA
Pork, flesh, shoulder, arm picnic, separable lean only, raw	140	73.13	19.75	6.16	0	0	0	2.130	0	65	NA

Food											
Pork, flesh, brain , raw	127	78.36	10.28	9.21	0	0	0	2.079	0	2195	NA
Pork, flesh, feet, raw	212	64.99	23.16	12.59	0	0	0	3.570	0	88	NA
Pork, flesh, heart, raw	118	76.21	17.27	4.36	1.33	0	0	1.160	0	131	NA
Pork, flesh, kidneys, raw	100	80.06	16.46	3.25	0	0	0	1.040	0	319	NA
Pork, flesh, liver, raw	134	71.06	21.39	3.65	2.47	0	0	1.170	0	301	NA
Pork, flesh, lung, raw	85	79.52	14.08	2.72		0	0	0.960	0	320	NA
Pork, fresh, spleen, raw	100	78.43	17.86	2.59	0	0	0	0.860	0	363	NA
Pork, fresh, stomach, raw	159	73.50	16.85	10.14	0	0	0	4.025	0.130	223	NA
Chicken breast tender, raw	263	52.74	14.73	15.75	15.01	1.1	0.37	3.260	0	41	NA
Chicken patty, frozen, raw	292	50.04	14.33	20.04	13.61	1.2	0	4.013	0	45	NA
Chicken, broiler or fryer, back, meat only, raw	137	75.31	19.59	5.92	0	0	0	1.520	0	81	NA
Chicken, broiler or fryer, breast, meat & skin, raw	172	69.46	20.85	9.25	0	0	0	2.660	0.115	64	NA
Chicken, broiler or fryer, leg, meat & skin, raw	187	69.91	18.15	12.12	0	0	0	3.410	0.105	83	NA
Chicken, broiler or fryer, leg, meat only, raw	120	76.13	20.13	3.81	0	0	0	0.980	0.104	80	NA
Chicken, broiler or fryer, light meat, meat & skin, raw	186	68.6	20.27	11.07	0	0	0	3.160	0	67	NA

Food										
Chicken, heart, all classes, raw	153	73.56	15.55	9.33	0.71	0	0	2.660	0	136	NA
Chicken, liver, all classes, raw	116	76.46	16.92	4.83	0	0	0	1.563	0.065	345	NA
Chicken, roasting, meat & skin, raw	216	65.50	17.14	15.85	0	0	0	4.530	0	73	NA
Chicken, roasting, meat only, raw	111	74.95	20.33	2.70	0	0	0	0.670	0	65	NA
Chicken, wing, frozen, glazed, barbecue flavored	211	61.79	19.67	12.67	3.34	0.6	2.04	3.321	0	126	NA
Lamb, domestic, shoulder, arm, separable lean & fat, trimmed to 1/4" fat, raw	260	61.76	16.79	20.90	0	0	0	9.150	0	71	NA
Lamb, ground, raw	282	59.47	16.56	23.41	0	0	0	10.190	0	73	NA
Lamb, New Zealand, frozen, shoulder, whole, separable lean & fat, trimmed to 1/8" fat, raw	251	62.00	17.19	19.74	0	0	0	9.900	0	74	NA
Lamb, brain, raw	122	79.20	10.40	8.58	0	0	0	2.190	0	1352	NA
Lamb, heart, raw	122	76.71	16.47	5.68	0.21	0	0	2.250	0	135	NA
Lamb, kidneys, raw	97	79.23	15.74	2.95	0.82	0	0	1.000	0	337	NA
Lamb, liver, raw	139	71.37	20.38	5.02	1.78	0	0	1.940	0	371	NA

Lamb, lungs, raw	95	79.70	16.70	2.60	0	0	0.890	0	0	NA
Lamb, spleen, raw	101	78.15	17.20	3.10	0	0	1.030	0	250	NA
Turkey, dark meat, raw	125	74.48	20.07	4.38	0	0	1.470	0	69	NA
Turkey, leg, meat & skin, raw	144	72.69	19.54	6.72	0	0	2.060	0	71	NA
Turkey, light meat, raw	115	73.82	23.56	1.56	0	0	0.500	0	60	NA
Turkey, meat & skin, raw	160	70.40	20.42	8.02	0	0	2.260	0	68	NA
Turkey, wing, meat & skin, raw	197	66.49	20.22	12.32	0	0	3.280	0	70	NA
Oil										
Avocado oil	884	0	0	100	0	0	11.560	0	0	NA
Canola oil	884	0	0	100	0	0	7.368	0	0	NA
Coconut oil	862	0	0	100	0	0	86.500	0	0	NA
Corn oil	884	0	0	100	0	0	12.948	0	0	NA
Cottonseed oil	884	0	0	100	0	0	25.900	0	0	NA
Flaxseed oil	884	0	0	100	0	0	9.400	0	0	NA
Grapeseed oil	884	0	0	100	0	0	9.600	0	0	NA
Olive oil	884	0	0	100	0	0	13.808	0	0	NA
Palm oil	884	0	0	100	0	0	49.300	0	0	NA

Palm kernel oil	862	0	100	0	0	81.500	0	NA
Peanut oil	884	0	100	0	0	16.900	0	NA
Safflower oil, linoleic (>70%)	884	0	100	0	0	6.203	0	NA
Safflower oil, oleic (>70%)	884	0	100	0	0	6.203	0	NA
Sesame oil	884	0	100	0	0	14.200	0	NA
Sunflower oil, high oleic (>70%)	884	0	100	0	0	9.748	0	NA
Sunflower oil, linoleic (~65%)	884	0	100	0	0	10.300	0	NA

Note: (1) ORAC data are taken from Oxygen Radical Absorbance Capacity (ORAC) of Selected Foods – 2007 published by the U.S. Department of Agriculture.

(2) Other data are taken from SR Search 20 database – 2008 published by the U.S. department of Agriculture.

(3) NA: not available.

Table A-2 Nutrition values per 100 grams of selected foods: minerals

Food category and name	Ca (mg)	Fe (mg)	Mg (mg)	P (mg)	K (mg)	Na (mg)	Zn (mg)	Cu (mg)	Mn (mg)	Se (µg)	Cr* (µg)
Vegetables											
Artichoke, raw	44	1.28	60	90	370	94	0.49	0.231	0.256	0.2	0
Asparagus, raw	24	2.14	14	52	202	2	0.54	0.189	0.158	2.3	4
Beets, raw	16	0.80	23	40	325	78	0.35	0.075	0.329	0.7	4
Broccoli, raw	47	0.73	21	66	316	33	0.41	0.049	0.210	2.5	11
Broccoli, cooked, boiled, drained, without salt	40	0.67	21	67	293	41	0.45	0.061	0.194	1.6	NA
Broccoli raab, raw	108	2.14	22	73	196	33	0.77	0.042	0.395	1.0	NA
Broccoli raab, cooked	118	1.27	27	82	343	56	0.54	0.075	0.380	1.3	NA
Broccoli, frozen, spears, unprepared	41	0.72	16	59	250	17	0.34	0.036	0.256	1.9	NA
Brussels sprouts, raw	42	1.40	23	69	389	25	0.42	0.070	0.337	1.6	10
Cabbage, raw	40	0.47	12	26	170	18	0.18	0.019	0.160	0.3	8
Cabbage, Chinese(pe-tsai), raw	77	0.31	13	29	238	9	0.23	0.036	0.190	0.6	NA
Cabbage, red, raw	45	0.80	16	30	243	27	0.22	0.017	0.243	0.6	NA
Carrots, baby, raw	32	0.89	10	28	237	78	0.17	0.100	0.151	0.9	NA
Carrots, raw	33	0.30	12	35	320	68	0.24	0.045	0.143	0.1	5

Cauliflower, raw	22	0.44	15	44	303	30	0.28	0.042	0.156	0.6	3
Celery, raw	40	0.20	11	24	260	80	0.13	0.035	0.103	0.4	8
Chard, Swiss, raw	51	1.80	81	46	379	213	0.36	0.179	0.366	0.9	6
Corn, sweet, yellow, raw	2	0.52	37	89	270	15	0.45	0.054	0.161	0.6	9
Cucumber, peeled, raw	14	0.22	12	21	136	2	0.17	0.071	0.073	0.1	NA
Cucumber, with peel, raw	16	0.28	13	24	147	2	0.20	0.041	0.079	0.3	1
Eggplant, raw	9	0.24	14	25	230	2	0.16	0.082	0.250	0.3	2
Garlic, raw	181	1.70	25	153	401	17	1.16	0.299	1.672	14.2	4
Kale, raw	135	1.70	34	56	447	43	0.44	0.290	0.774	0.9	4
Leeks (bulk & lower leaf-portion), raw	59	2.10	28	35	180	20	0.12	0.120	0.481	1.0	8
Lettuce, butterhead (includes boston & bibb types), raw	35	1.24	13	33	238	5	0.20	0.016	0.179	0.6	NA
Lettuce, cos or romaine, raw	33	0.97	14	30	247	8	0.23	0.048	0.155	0.4	7
Lettuce, green leaf, raw	36	0.86	13	29	194	28	0.18	0.029	0.250	0.6	NA
Lettuce, iceberg (includes crisp-head types), raw	18	0.41	7	20	141	10	0.15	0.025	0.125	0.1	NA
Lettuce, red leaf, raw	33	1.20	12	28	187	25	0.20	0.028	0.203	1.5	NA
Mushrooms, brown, Italian or Crimini, raw	18	0.40	9	120	448	6	1.10	0.500	0.142	26.0	NA

Mushrooms, enoki, raw	1	1.09	16	109	368	3	0.61	0.091	0.079	2.2	NA
Mushrooms, maitake, raw	1	0.30	10	74	204	1	0.75	0.252	0.059	2.2	NA
Mushrooms, portabella, raw	8	0.60	11	130	484	6	0.60	0.400	0.142	11.0	NA
Mushrooms, Shiitake, dried	11	1.72	132	294	1534	13	7.66	5.165	1.176	46.1	NA
Mushrooms, white, raw	3	0.50	9	86	318	5	0.52	0.318	0.047	9.3	14
Onions, raw	23	0.21	10	29	146	4	0.17	0.039	0.129	0.5	11
Onions, sweet, raw	20	0.26	9	17	119	8	0.13	0.056	0.076	0.5	NA
Parsley, raw	138	6.20	50	58	554	56	1.07	0.149	0.160	0.1	NA
Peppers, sweet, green, raw	10	0.34	10	20	175	3	0.13	0.066	0.122	0	10
Peppers, sweet, red, raw	7	0.43	12	26	211	4	0.25	0.017	0.112	0.1	NA
Peppers, sweet, yellow, raw	11	0.46	12	24	212	2	0.17	0.107	0.117	0.3	NA
Potatoes, red, flesh & skin, raw	10	0.73	22	61	455	6	0.33	0.134	0.141	0.5	NA
Potatoes, white, flesh & skin, raw	9	0.52	21	62	407	6	0.29	0.116	0.145	0.3	21
Radishes, raw	25	0.34	10	20	233	39	0.28	0.050	0.069	0.6	3
Spinach, raw	99	2.71	79	49	558	79	0.53	0.130	0.897	1.0	10
Squash, summer, zucchini, includes skin, raw	15	0.35	17	38	262	10	0.29	0.051	0.175	0.2	1
Squash, winter, butternut, raw	48	0.7	34	33	352	4	0.15	0.072	0.202	0.5	3

Food											
Soybean, mature seeds, sprouted, raw	67	2.10	72	164	484	14	1.17	0.427	0.702	0.6	NA
Tomato, red, ripe, raw, year round average	10	0.27	11	24	237	5	0.17	0.059	0.114	0	9
Turnip greens, raw	190	1.10	31	42	296	40	0.19	0.350	0.466	1.2	5
Waterchestnut, Chinese, (matai), raw	11	0.06	22	63	584	14	0.50	0.326	0.331	0.7	4
Fruits											
Apples, raw, with skin	6	0.12	5	11	107	1	0.04	0.027	0.035	0	2
Apples, raw, without skin	5	0.07	4	11	90	0	0.05	0.031	0.038	0	2
Applesauce, canned, unsweetened, without added ascorbic acid	3	0.012	3	7	72	2	0.03	0.026	0.075	0.3	8
Apricots, raw	13	0.39	10	23	259	1	0.20	0.078	0.077	0.1	0
Avocados, raw, all commercial varieties	12	0.55	29	52	485	7	0.64	0.190	0.142	0.4	0
Avocados, raw, California	13	0.61	29	54	507	8	0.68	0.170	0.149	0.4	0
Avocados, raw, Florida	10	0.17	24	40	351	2	0.40	0.311	0.095	0	0
Bananas, raw	5	0.26	27	22	358	1	0.15	0.078	0.270	1.0	9
Bananas, dehydrated, banana powder	22	1.15	108	74	1491	3	0.61	0.391	0.574	3.9	NA
Blackberries, raw	29	0.62	20	22	162	1	0.53	0.165	0.646	0.4	NA

Blueberries, raw	6	0.28	6	12	77	1	0.16	0.057	0.336	0.1	5
Cranberries, raw	8	0.25	6	13	85	2	0.10	0.061	0.360	0.1	0
Elderberries, raw	38	1.60	5	39	280	6	0.11	0.061	0	0.6	NA
Figs, raw	35	0.37	17	14	232	1	0.15	0.070	0.128	0.2	0
Grapefruit, raw, pink & red, all areas	22	0.08	9	18	135	0	0.07	0.032	0.022	0.1	0.5
Grapes, American style (slip skin), raw	14	0.29	5	10	191	2	0.04	0.040	0.718	0.1	3
Grapes, red & green, seedless, raw	10	0.36	7	20	191	2	0.07	0.127	0.071	0.1	3
Honeydew melons, raw	6	0.17	10	11	228	18	0.09	0.024	0.027	0.7	NA
Lemon, raw, with peel	61	0.70	12	15	145	3	0.10	0.260	0	0	1
Limes, raw	33	0.60	6	18	102	2	0.11	0.065	0.008	0.4	1
Kiwi fruit (Chinese gooseberries), fresh, raw	34	0.31	17	34	312	3	0.14	0.130	0.098	0.2	NA
Mangos, raw	10	0.13	9	11	156	2	0.04	0.110	0.027	0.6	NA
Nectarine, raw	6	0.28	9	26	201	0	0.17	0.086	0.054	0	0
Oranges, raw, navels	43	0.13	11	23	166	1	0.08	0.039	0.029	0	3
Oranges, mandarin, tangerines, raw	37	0.15	12	20	166	2	0.07	0.042	0.039	0.1	3
Peaches, raw	6	0.25	9	20	190	0	0.17	0.068	0.061	0.1	2

Food											
Pears, raw	9	0.17	7	11	119	1	0.10	0.082	0.049	0.1	2
Persimmon, native, raw	27	2.50	0	26	310	1	0	0	0	0	0
Pineapple, raw, all varieties	13	0.29	12	8	109	1	0.12	0.110	0.927	0.1	0
Plums, raw	6	0.17	7	16	157	0	0.10	0.057	0.052	0	2
Raisins, seedless	50	1.88	32	101	749	11	0.22	0.318	0.299	0.6	6
Raspberries, raw	25	0.69	22	29	151	1	0.42	0.090	0.670	0.2	0
Strawberries, raw	16	0.41	13	24	153	1	0.14	0.048	0.386	0.4	3
Watermelon, raw	7	0.24	10	11	112	1	0.10	0.042	0.038	0.4	2
Apple juice, canned or bottled	7	0.37	3	7	119	3	0.03	0.022	0.113	0.1	NA
Cranberry juice, cocktail, bottled	3	0.10	1	1	14	2	0.03	0.010	0.048	0.2	NA
Grape juice drink, canned	7	0.13	6	6	33	9	0.03	0.022	0.200	0.1	NA
Grapefruit juice, pink, raw	9	0.20	12	15	162	1	0.05	0.033	0.020	0	NA
Grapefruit juice, white, raw	9	0.20	12	15	162	1	0.05	0.033	0.020	0.1	NA
Lemon juice, raw	7	0.03	6	6	124	1	0.05	0.029	0.008	0.1	NA
Lime juice, raw	14	0.09	8	14	117	2	0.08	0.027	0.018	0.1	NA
Orange juice, raw	11	0.20	11	17	200	1	0.05	0.044	0.014	0.1	NA
Prune juice, canned	12	1.18	14	25	276	4	0.21	0.068	0.151	0.6	NA
Legumes											
Beans, black, mature seeds, raw	123	5.02	171	352	1483	5	3.65	0.841	1.060	3.2	NA

Beans, kidney, red mature seeds, raw	83	6.69	138	406	1359	12	2.79	0.699	1.111	3.2	NA
Beans, navy, mature seeds, raw	147	5.49	175	407	1185	5	3.65	0.834	1.418	11.0	NA
Beans, pink, mature seeds, raw	130	6.77	182	415	1464	8	2.55	0.810	1.376	13.0	NA
Beans, pinto, mature seeds, raw	113	5.07	176	411	1393	12	2.28	0.893	1.148	27.9	17
Beans, pinto, mature seeds, cooked	46	2.09	50	147	436	1	0.98	0.219	0.453	6.2	NA
Beans, snap, green, raw	37	1.04	25	38	209	6	0.24	0.069	0.214	0.6	4
Chickpeas (garbanzo beans), mature seeds, raw	105	6.24	115	366	875	24	3.43	0.847	2.204	8.2	NA
Cowpeas, common, mature seeds, raw	110	8.27	184	424	1112	16	3.37	0.845	1.528	9.0	NA
Lentils, raw	56	7.54	122	451	955	6	4.78	0.519	1.330	8.3	11
Peas, split, mature seeds, raw	55	4.43	115	366	981	15	3.01	0.866	1.391	1.6	4
Soybeans, mature seeds, raw	277	15.70	280	704	1797	2	4.89	1.658	2.517	17.8	10
Tofu, silken, firm (MURI-NU)	32	1.03	27	90	194	36	0.61	0.203	0	0	0
Tofu, silken, soft (MURI-NU)	31	0.82	29	62	180	5	0.52	0.207	0	0	0
Tofu, yogurt	118	1.06	40	38	47	35	0.31	0.075	0	13.0	0
Tofu, dried-frozen (koyatofu)	363	9.73	59	483	20	6	4.90	1.179	3.689	54.3	0

Tofu, dried-frozen (koyatofu), prepared with calcium sulfate	2134	9.73	181	483	20	6	4.90	1.179	3.689	54.3	0
Tofu, fried	372	4.87	60	287	146	16	1.99	0.398	1.495	28.5	0
Tofu, fried, prepared with calcium sulfate	961	4.87	95	287	146	16	1.99	0.398	1.495	28.5	0
Tofu, hard, prepared with nigari	345	2.75	53	231	146	2	1.66	0.328	1.052	16.8	0
Tofu, regular, prepared with calcium sulfate	350	5.36	30	97	121	7	0.80	0.193	0.605	8.9	0
Tofu, salted and fermented (fuyu), prepared with calcium sulfate	1229	1.98	58	73	75	2873	1.56	0.376	1.174	17.3	0
Cereal											
Buckwheat	18	2.20	231	347	460	1	2.40	1.100	1.300	8.3	38
Buckwheat flour, whole-groat	41	4.06	251	337	577	11	3.12	0.515	2.030	5.7	NA
Cereals ready-to-eat, granola, homemade	78	4.23	175	456	540	25	4.03	0.635	4.053	27.8	NA
Cereals ready-to-eat, bran flakes, single brand	56	27.00	214	508	616	732	5.00	0.642	3.568	10.5	NA
Cereals ready-to-eat, bran, malted flour, single brand	76	27.93	278	813	947	417	12.93	0.918	9.030	8.0	NA

Cereals ready-to-eat, corn & oat flour, puffed presweetened, single brand	17	9.31	37	93	120	743	5.17	0.068	0.152	20.1	NA
Cereals ready-to-eat, GERNERAL MILLS, CHEE-RIOS	370	40.00	59	222	241	667	27.78	0.148	1.483	15.7	NA
Cereals ready-to-eat, GERNERAL MILLS, Cinnamon Grahams	333	15.00	27	67	147	789	12.50	0.087	0	4.4	NA
Cereals ready-to-eat, GERNERAL MILLS, FIBER ONE	333	15.00	133	500	600	350	12.50	0.314	1.985	9.0	NA
Cereals ready-to-eat, GERNERAL MILLS, HAR-MONY	1091	16.40	44	182	166	645	13.60	0.145	1.359	21.8	NA
Cereals ready-to-eat, Malt-O-Meal, High Fiber Bran Flakes	44	35.20	169	484	598	672	13.40	0.519	6.516	63.2	NA
Cereal, oats, instant, fortified, plain, dry	352	29.27	138	424	359	258	3.54	0.374	2.920	26.8	NA
Cereals ready-to-eat, KELLOGG, KELLOGG'S Complete Wheat Bran Flakes	53	62.00	140	540	590	715	52.50	0.500	4.219	10.5	NA

	40	3.39	122	379	389	2	2.66	0.458	3.200	70.70	NA
Cereals, Whole wheat hot, natural cereal, dry	40	3.39	122	379	389	2	2.66	0.458	3.200	70.70	NA
Grain											
Barley, pearled, raw	29	2.50	79	221	280	9	2.13	0.420	1.322	37.7	8
Barley, pearled, cooked	11	1.33	22	54	93	3	0.82	0.105	0.259	8.6	NA
Barley malt flour	37	4.71	97	303	224	11	2.06	0.270	1.193	37.7	NA
Cocoa, dry powder, unsweetened	128	13.86	499	734	1524	21	6.81	3.788	3.873	14.3	NA
Cornmeal, whole-grain, white	6	3.45	127	241	287	35	1.82	0.193	0.498	15.5	NA
Cornmeal, whole-grain, yellow	6	3.45	127	241	287	35	1.82	0.193	0.498	15.5	NA
Cornmeal, white (Navajo)	11	3.79	125	280	443	4	3.24	0.219	0.646	0	10
Cornmeal, yellow (Navajo)	6	2.99	107	225	322	4	3.10	0.242	0.641	6.0	10
Corn flour, whole-grain, white	7	2.38	93	272	315	5	1.73	0.230	0.460	15.4	NA
Corn flour, whole-grain, yellow	7	2.38	93	272	315	5	1.73	0.230	0.460	15.4	NA
Corn, sweet, yellow, raw	2	0.52	37	89	270	15	0.45	0.054	0.161	0.6	NA
Oat flour, partially debranned	55	4.00	144	452	371	19	3.20	0.437	4.019	34.0	NA
Peanut flour, defatted	140	2.10	370	760	1290	180	5.10	1.800	4.900	7.1	NA
Peanut flour, low fat	130	4.74	48	508	1358	1	5.99	2.039	4.231	7.1	NA
Popcorn, air-popped	7	3.19	144	358	329	8	3.08	0.262	1.113	0	9
Potato flour	65	1.38	65	168	1001	55	0.54	0.197	0.313	1.1	NA

Rice bran, crude	57	18.54	781	1677	1485	5	6.04	0.728	14.210	15.6	NA
Rice flour, brown	11	1.98	112	337	289	8	2.45	0.230	4.013	23.4	NA
Rice flour, white	10	0.35	35	98	76	0	0.80	0.130	1.200	15.1	NA
Rice noodles, cooked	4	0.14	3	20	4	19	0.25	0.038	0.114	4.5	NA
Rice noodles, dry	18	0.70	12	153	30	182	0.74	0.078	0.498	15.1	NA
Rice, brown, long-grain, cooked	10	0.42	43	83	43	5	0.63	0.100	0.905	9.8	NA
Rice, brown, long-grain, raw	23	1.47	143	333	223	7	2.02	0.277	3.743	23.4	8
Rice, brown, medium-grain, cooked	10	0.53	44	77	79	1	0.62	0.081	1.097	0	NA
Rice, brown, medium-grain, raw	33	1.80	143	264	268	4	2.02	0.277	3.743	0	NA
Rice, white, long-grain, regular, cooked	10	1.20	12	43	35	1	0.49	0.069	0.472	7.5	NA
Rice, white, long-grain, regular, raw	28	0.80	25	115	115	5	1.09	0.220	1.088	15.1	NA
Rice, white, medium-grain, cooked	3	1.49	13	37	29	0	0.42	0.038	0.377	7.5	NA
Rice, white, medium-grain, raw	9	0.80	35	108	86	1	1.16	0.110	1.100	0	NA
Rice, white, short-grain, cooked	1	1.46	8	33	26	0	0.40	0.072	0.357	7.5	NA
Rice, white, short-grain, raw, unenriched	3	0.80	23	95	76	1	1.10	0.210	1.037	0	NA

Rye flour, dark	56	6.45	248	632	730	1	5.62	0.750	6.730	35.7	9
Rye flour, light	21	1.80	70	194	233	2	1.75	0.250	1.970	35.7	9
Rye flour, medium	24	2.12	75	207	340	3	1.99	0.287	5.460	35.7	9
Seeds, cottonseed flour, low fat (glandless)	474	12.58	716	1587	1761	35	11.61	1.172	2.129	0	NA
Seeds, sesame flour, high-fat	159	15.17	361	807	423	41	10.67	1.520	1.489	0	NA
Seeds, sesame flour, low-fat	149	14.22	338	757	397	39	10.00	1.425	1.396	0	NA
Seeds, sunflower flour, partially defatted	114	6.62	346	689	67	3	4.95	1.713	1.975	58.2	NA
Soy flour, full-fat, raw	206	6.37	429	494	2515	13	3.92	2.920	2.275	7.5	NA
Wheat flour, white, all-purpose, enriched bleached	15	4.64	22	108	107	2	0.70	0.144	0.682	33.9	5
Wheat flour, white, all-purpose, enriched unbleached	15	4.64	22	108	107	2	0.70	0.144	0.682	33.9	5
Wheat flour, white, all-purpose, self-rising, enriched	338	4.67	19	595	124	1270	0.62	0.112	1.00	34.4	11
Wheat flour, whole-grain	34	3.88	138	346	405	5	2.94	0.382	3.799	70.7	11
Bread											
Bread, cracked-wheat	43	2.81	52	153	177	538	1.24	0.222	1.371	25.3	NA
Bread, egg	93	3.04	19	106	115	492	0.79	0.162	0.500	30.1	NA

Bread, French or Vienna (includes sourdough)	44	3.63	28	114	128	650	0.93	0.136	0.524	27.1	NA
Bread, Italian	78	2.94	27	103	110	584	0.86	0.191	0.464	27.2	NA
Bread, oat bran	65	3.12	35	141	147	407	0.89	0.135	0.779	30.0	NA
Bread, oatmeal	66	2.70	37	126	142	599	1.02	0.209	0.940	24.6	NA
Bread, pumpernickel	68	2.87	54	178	208	671	1.48	0.287	1.305	24.5	0
Bread, raisin, unenriched	66	1.83	26	109	227	390	0.72	0.198	0.501	0	NA
Bread, rye	73	2.83	40	125	166	660	1.14	0.186	0.842	30.9	0
Bread, wheat	142	3.46	48	155	184	521	1.21	0.159	1.123	28.8	0
Bread, white, commercially prepared (includes soft bread crumbs)	151	3.74	23	99	100	681	0.74	0.253	0.478	17.3	NA
Dairy											
Milk, buttermilk, dried	1184	0.30	110	933	1592	517	4.02	0.111	0.023	20.3	NA
Milk, buttermilk, fluid, cultured, lowfat	116	0.05	11	89	151	105	0.42	0.011	0.002	2.0	NA
Milk, chocolate, fluid, reduced fat	109	0.24	14	102	169	66	0.39	0.075	0.062	3.4	NA
Milk, chocolate, fluid, whole	112	0.24	13	101	167	60	0.41	0.065	0.077	1.9	NA
Milk, dry, whole	912	0.47	85	776	1330	371	3.34	0.080	0.040	16.3	NA
Milk, goat, fluid	134	0.05	14	111	204	50	0.30	0.046	0.018	1.4	NA

Milk, human, mature, fluid	32	0.03	3	14	51	17	0.17	0.052	0.026	1.8	NA
Milk, fluid, 1% milkfat, with added vitamin A	119	0.03	11	95	150	44	0.42	0.010	0.003	3.3	NA
Milk, fluid, nonfat (fat free or skim)	123	0.04	11	101	166	52	0.40	0.011	0.002	2.1	1.5
Milk, producer, fluid, 3.7% milk-fat	119	0.05	13	93	151	49	0.38	0.010	0.004	2.0	NA
Milk, fluid, 2% milkfat, with added vitamin A	117	0.03	11	94	150	41	0.043	0.012	0.003	2.5	0
Milk, sheep, fluid	193	0.10	18	158	137	44	0.54	0.046	0.018	1.7	NA
Milk, whole, 3.25% milkfat	113	0.03	10	91	143	40	0.40	0.011	0.003	3.7	NA
Egg											
Egg, duck, whole, fresh, raw	64	3.85	17	220	222	146	1.41	0.062	0.038	36.4	NA
Egg, goose, whole, fresh, raw	60	3.64	16	208	210	138	1.33	0.062	0.038	36.9	NA
Egg, quail, whole, fresh, raw	64	3.65	13	226	132	141	1.47	0.062	0.038	32.0	NA
Egg, turkey, whole, fresh, raw	99	4.10	13	170	142	151	1.58	0.062	0.038	34.3	NA
Egg, white, raw, fresh	7	0.08	11	15	163	166	0.03	0.023	0.011	20.0	8
Egg, whole, cooked, fried	59	1.98	13	208	147	204	1.20	0.111	0.041	34.2	NA
Egg, whole, cooked, hard-boiled	50	1.19	10	172	126	124	1.05	0.013	0.026	30.8	NA
Egg, whole, cooked, omelet	47	1.55	10	162	114	161	0.93	0.088	0.032	26.7	NA

Egg, whole, cooked, poached	53	1.83	12	190	133	294	1.10	0.102	0.039	31.6	NA
Egg, whole, cooked, scrambled	71	1.20	12	170	138	280	1.00	0.014	0.022	22.5	NA
Egg, whole, raw, fresh	53	1.83	12	191	134	140	1.11	0.102	0.038	31.7	22
Egg, yolk, raw, fresh	129	2.73	5	390	109	48	2.30	0.077	0.055	56.0	30
Cheese										
Cheese, America cheddar, imitation	562	0.33	29	712	242	1345	2.59	0.033	0	15.2	56
Cheese, blue	528	0.31	23	387	256	1395	2.66	0.040	0.009	14.5	NA
Cheese, brick	674	0.43	24	451	136	560	2.60	0.024	0.012	14.5	NA
Cheese, brie	184	0.50	20	188	152	629	2.38	0.019	0.034	14.5	NA
Cheese, camembert	388	0.33	20	347	187	842	2.38	0.021	0.038	14.5	NA
Cheese, caraway	673	0.64	22	490	93	690	2.94	0.024	0.021	14.5	NA
Cheese, cheddar	721	0.68	28	512	98	621	3.11	0.031	0.010	13.9	29
Cheese, cheshire	643	0.21	21	464	95	700	2.79	0.042	0.012	14.5	NA
Cheese, Colby	685	0.76	26	457	127	604	3.07	0.042	0.012	14.5	NA
Cheese, cottage, 1% milkfat	61	0.14	5	134	86	406	0.38	0.028	0.003	9.0	0
Cheese, cottage, 2% milkfat	69	0.16	6	151	96	406	0.42	0.028	0.003	10.2	NA
Cheese, cream, fat free	185	0.18	14	434	163	545	0.88	0.050	0.050	0.050	NA
Cheese, edam	731	0.44	30	536	188	965	3.75	0.036	0.011	14.5	NA

Cheese, feta	493	0.65	19	337	62	1116	2.88	0.032	0.028	15.0	36
Cheese, Mexican, blend, reduced fat	1146	0.13	35	583	93	776	4.30	0.021	0	15.5	NA
Cheese, Mexican, queso anejo	680	0.47	28	444	87	1131	2.94	0.008	0.037	14.5	NA
Cheese, Monterey	746	0.72	27	444	81	536	3.00	0.032	0.011	14.5	36
Cheese, Monterey, low fat	705	0.72	27	444	81	564	3.00	0.032	0	14.5	36
Cheese, Mozzarella, part skim	782	0.22	23	463	84	619	2.76	0.025	0.010	14.4	36
Cheese, muenster	717	0.41	27	468	134	628	2.81	0.031	0.008	14.5	NA
Cheese, parmesan, hard	1184	0.82	44	694	92	1602	2.75	0.032	0.020	22.5	NA
Cheese, provolone, reduced fat	756	0.52	28	496	138	876	3.23	0.026	0.010	14.5	NA
Cheese, Ricotta, part skim	272	0.44	15	183	125	125	1.34	0.034	0.010	16.7	0
Cheese, Swiss	791	0.20	38	567	77	192	4.36	0.043	0.005	18.2	36
Cheese, tilsit	700	0.23	13	500	65	753	3.50	0.026	0.013	14.5	NA
Nuts and Seeds											
Nuts, acorns, raw	41	0.79	62	79	539	0	0.51	0.621	1.337	0	NA
Nuts, almonds	264	3.72	268	484	705	1	3.08	0.996	2.285	2.5	0
Nuts, cashew nuts, raw	37	6.68	292	593	660	12	5.78	2.195	1.655	19.9	0
Nuts, chestnuts, Chinese, raw	18	1.41	84	96	447	3	0.87	0.363	1.601	0	0
Nuts, chestnuts, European, raw	27	1.01	32	93	518	3	0.52	0.447	0.952	0	0

Nuts, chestnuts, Japanese, raw	31	1.45	49	72	329	14	1.10	0.562	1.591	0	0
Nuts, coconut meat, raw	14	2.43	32	113	356	20	1.10	0.435	1.500	10.1	NA
Nuts, ginkgo nuts, raw	2	1.00	27	124	510	7	0.34	0.274	0.113	0	NA
Nuts, hazelnuts or filberts	114	4.70	163	290	680	0	2.45	1.725	6.175	2.4	NA
Nuts, macadamia nuts, dry roasted, without salt added	70	2.65	118	198	363	4	1.29	0.570	3.036	11.7	NA
Nuts, macadamia nuts, raw	85	3.69	130	188	368	5	1.30	0.756	4.131	3.6	NA
Nuts, mixed nuts with peanuts, dry roasted, with salt added	70	3.70	225	435	597	669	3.80	1.279	1.937	7.5	0
Nuts, mixed nuts with peanuts, dry roasted, without salt added	70	3.70	225	435	597	669	3.80	1.279	1.937	0	0
Nuts, mixed nuts with peanuts, oil roasted, with salt added	108	3.21	235	464	581	419	5.08	1.661	1.892	140.2	NA
Nuts, pecans	70	2.53	121	277	410	0	4.53	1.200	4.500	3.8	NA
Nuts, pine nuts, dried	16	5.53	251	575	597	2	6.45	1.324	8.802	0.7	NA
Nuts, pistachio nuts, raw	107	4.15	121	490	1025	1	2.20	1.300	1.200	7.0	NA
Nuts, walnuts, English	98	2.91	158	346	441	2	3.09	1.586	3.414	4.9	NA
Seeds, breadfruit seeds, raw	36	3.67	54	175	941	25	0.90	1.148	0.142	0	NA
Seeds, breadnut tree seeds, dried	94	4.60	115	178	2011	53	1.91	2.455	0.303	1.9	NA
Seeds, breadnut tree seeds, raw	98	2.09	68	67	1183	31	1.13	1.444	0.178	0	NA

Seeds, flaxseed	255	5.73	392	642	813	30	4.34	1.220	2.482	25.4	NA
Seeds, lotus seeds, dried	163	3.53	210	626	1368	5	1.05	0.350	2.318	0	NA
Seeds, pumpkin & squash seed kernels, dried	43	14.97	535	1174	807	18	7.46	1.387	3.021	5.6	7
Seeds, sesame seeds, whole, dried	975	14.55	351	629	468	11	7.75	4.082	2.460	5.7	NA
Seeds, sunflower kernels, dried	78	5.25	325	660	645	9	5.00	1.800	1.950	53.0	7
Seeds, watermelon seed kernels, dried	54	7.28	515	755	648	99	10.24	0.686	1.641	0	NA
Fish and Shellfish											
Fish, anchovy, European, raw	147	3.25	41	174	383	104	1.72	0.211	0.070	36.5	NA
Fish, bass, striped, raw	15	0.84	40	198	256	69	0.40	0.031	0.015	36.5	0
Fish, bluefish, raw	7	0.48	33	227	372	60	0.81	0.053	0.021	36.5	NA
Fish, butterfish, raw	22	0.50	25	240	375	89	0.77	0.054	0.015	36.5	NA
Fish, catfish, channel, farmed, raw	9	0.50	23	202	299	53	0.74	0.101	0.018	12.6	0
Fish, catfish, channel, wild, raw	14	0.30	23	209	358	43	0.51	0.034	0.025	12.6	0
Fish, cod, Atlantic, raw	16	0.38	32	203	413	54	0.45	0.028	0.015	33.1	7
Fish, cod, Pacific, raw	7	0.26	24	174	403	71	0.40	0.026	0.012	36.5	7
Crustaceans, crab, Alaska king, raw	46	0.59	49	219	204	836	5.95	0.922	0.035	36.4	0
Crustaceans, crab, blue, raw	89	0.74	34	229	329	293	3.54	0.669	0.150	37.4	0

Crustaceans, crab, queen, raw	26	2.50	49	133	173	539	2.80	0.570	0.030	34.6	0
Fish, drum, freshwater, raw	60	0.90	30	180	275	75	0.66	0.232	0.700	12.6	NA
Fish, haddock, raw	33	1.05	39	188	311	68	0.37	0.026	0.025	30.2	5
Fish, halibut, Atlantic & Pacific, raw	47	0.84	83	222	450	54	0.42	0.027	0.015	36.5	1
Fish, halibut, Greenland, raw	3	0.66	26	164	268	80	0.40	0.030	0.012	36.5	1
Fish, herring, Atlantic, raw	57	1.10	32	236	327	90	0.99	0.092	0.035	36.5	NA
Fish, herring, Pacific, raw	83	1.12	32	228	423	74	0.53	0.078	0.045	36.5	0
Crustaceans, lobster, northern, raw	48	0.30	27	144	275	296	3.02	1.663	0.055	41.4	2
Fish, mackerel, Atlantic, raw	12	1.63	76	217	314	90	0.63	0.073	0.015	44.1	4
Fish, mackerel, king, raw	31	1.78	32	248	435	158	0.56	0.026	0.005	36.5	NA
Fish, mackerel, Spanish, raw	11	0.44	33	205	446	59	0.49	0.055	0.014	36.5	NA
Fish, monkfish, raw	8	0.32	21	200	400	18	0.41	0.028	0.024	36.5	NA
Fish, mullet, striped, raw	41	1.02	29	221	357	65	0.52	0.051	0.016	36.5	NA
Fish, ocean perch, Atlantic, raw	107	0.92	30	216	273	75	0.48	0.026	0.015	43.3	0
Fish, pike, walleye, raw	110	1.30	30	210	389	51	0.62	0.178	0.800	12.6	NA
Fish, pollock, Atlantic, raw	60	0.46	67	221	356	86	0.47	0.050	0.015	36.5	NA
Fish, pollock, walleye, raw	5	0.23	57	376	326	99	0.44	0.043	0.015	21.9	NA

Fish, roe, mixed species, raw	22	0.60	20	402	221	91	1.00	0.100	0.010	40.3	NA
Fish, sablefish, raw	35	1.28	55	168	358	56	0.32	0.022	0.015	36.5	NA
Fish, salmon, Atlantic, farmed, raw	12	0.36	28	233	362	59	0.40	0.049	0.015	36.5	1
Fish, salmon, Atlantic, wild, raw	12	0.80	29	200	490	44	0.64	0.250	0.016	36.5	1
Fish, salmon, chinook, raw	26	0.25	95	289	394	47	0.44	0.041	0.015	36.5	NA
Fish, salmon, coho, wild, raw	36	0.56	31	262	423	46	0.41	0.051	0.014	36.5	NA
Fish, salmon, pink, raw	13	0.77	26	230	323	67	0.55	0.077	0.015	44.6	NA
Fish, sardine, Pacific, canned in tomato sauce, drained solids with bone	240	2.30	34	366	341	414	1.40	0.272	0.206	40.6	NA
Fish, shad, America, raw	47	0.97	30	272	384	51	0.37	0.064	0.042	36.5	NA
Fish, shark, mixed species, raw	34	0.84	49	210	160	79	0.43	0.033	0.015	36.5	0
Crustaceans, shrimp, mixed species, raw	52	2.41	37	205	185	148	1.11	0.264	0.050	38.0	12
Fish, swordfish, raw	4	0.81	27	263	288	90	1.15	0.126	0.019	48.1	0
Fish, tuna, fresh, bluefin, raw	8	1.02	50	254	252	39	0.60	0.086	0.015	36.5	5
Fish, wolffish, Atlantic, raw	6	0.09	30	200	300	85	0.78	0.029	0.015	36.5	NA

Meat and Poultry

Beef, bottom sirloin, tri-tip, separable lean only, trimmed to 0" fat, select, raw	22	1.55	23	204	344	54	3.85	0.074	0.011	29.7	7
Beef, brisket, flat half, separable lean and fat, trimmed to 1/8" fat, all grades, raw	16	1.59	18	165	276	59	4.32	0.077	0.011	19.4	NA
Beef, brisket, point half, separable lean and fat, trimmed to 1/4" fat, all grades, raw	7	1.54	16	150	231	65	3.71	0.065	0.011	15.1	NA
Beef, chuck, clod steak, separable lean only, trimmed to 1/4" fat, all grades, raw	6	2.45	22	201	370	67	4.83	0.093	0	30.0	NA
Beef, flank, separable lean only, trimmed to 0" fat, all grades, raw	24	1.57	23	202	340	55	3.94	0.073	0.013	26.4	NA
Beef, ground, 70% lean meat / 30% fat, raw	24	1.64	14	132	218	67	3.57	0.050	0.011	13.5	NA
Beef, rib, shortribs, separable lean only, choice, raw	8	2.16	22	190	357	65	4.78	0.069	0.014	14.4	NA
Beef, round, bottom round, separable lean only, trimmed to 1/2" fat, prime, raw	4	2.38	25	214	371	59	3.51	0.083	0.014	20.8	NA

Beef, tenderloin, separable lean only, trimmed to 1/4" fat, prime, raw	6	2.77	24	211	367	54	3.59	0.109	0.014	17.8	NA
Beef, brain, raw	43	2.55	13	362	274	126	1.02	0.287	0.026	21.3	NA
Beef, heart, raw	7	4.31	21	212	287	98	1.70	0.396	0.035	21.8	NA
Beef, kidneys, raw	13	4.60	17	257	262	182	1.92	0.426	0.142	141.0	NA
Beef, liver, raw	5	4.90	18	387	313	69	4.00	9.755	0.310	39.7	NA
Beef, lung, raw	10	7.95	14	224	340	198	1.61	0.260	0.019	44.3	NA
Beef, spleen, raw	9	44.55	22	296	429	85	2.11	0.169	0.073	62.2	NA
Pork, boneless loin, fresh	4	0.60	21	310	358	1.60	0	0.100	0	0	NA
Pork, center cut chops, fresh	14	0.60	21	0	307	378	1.50	0.100	0	0	NA
Pork, cured, bacon, raw	6	0.48	12	188	208	833	1.17	0.070	0.020	20.2	NA
Pork, cured, patties, grilled	9	1.61	10	101	244	1063	1.90	0.100	0.022	21.1	NA
Pork, fresh, backfat, raw	2	0.18	2	38	65	11	0.37	0.018	0.002	8.0	NA
Pork, fresh, backribs, separable lean and fat, raw	32	0.91	16	143	233	75	2.31	0.062	0.007	24.0	NA
Pork, fresh, belly, raw	5	0.52	4	108	185	32	1.02	0.052	0.006	8.0	NA
Pork, fresh, loin, tenderloin, separable lean only, raw	5	0.98	27	247	399	53	1.89	0.090	0.015	30.8	NA
Pork, fresh, ground, raw	14	0.88	19	175	287	56	2.20	0.045	0.010	24.6	NA

Pork, fresh, leg(ham), whole, separable lean and fat, raw	5	0.85	20	199	315	47	1.93	0.065	0.023	29.4	NA
Pork, flesh, loin, country-style ribs, separable lean only, raw	21	0.90	23	204	338	67	3.00	0.083	0.012	34.8	9
Pork, flesh, separable fat, raw	36	0.39	7	84	125	23	0.67	0.037	0	8.6	NA
Pork, flesh, shoulder, arm picnic, separable lean only, raw	6	1.19	21	218	341	82	2.86	0.097	0.013	30.2	NA
Pork, flesh, brain , raw	10	1.60	14	282	258	120	1.27	0.240	0.094	15.9	NA
Pork, flesh, feet, raw	70	0.58	6	75	63	132	0.76	0.070	0	23.3	NA
Pork, flesh, heart, raw	5	4.68	19	169	294	56	2.80	0.408	0.063	10.4	NA
Pork, flesh, kidneys, raw	9	4.87	17	204	229	121	2.75	0.622	0.123	190.0	NA
Pork, flesh, liver, raw	9	23.30	18	288	273	87	5.76	0.677	0.344	52.7	NA
Pork, flesh, lung, raw	7	18.90	14	196	303	153	2.03	0.083	0.017	17.8	NA
Pork, fresh, spleen, raw	10	22.32	13	260	396	98	2.54	0.131	0.072	32.8	NA
Pork, fresh, stomach, raw	11	1.01	11	130	140	75	1.85	0.169	0.038	31.1	NA
Chicken breast tender, raw	19	1.11	23	211	214	451	0.78	0.205	0.229	24.7	NA
Chicken patty, frozen, raw	20	0.93	25	196	248	518	0.94	0.207	0.254	21.4	NA
Chicken, broiler or fryer, back, meat only, raw	17	1.04	22	151	204	82	1.85	0.060	0.021	13.5	NA

Chicken, broiler or fryer, breast, meat & skin, raw	11	0.74	25	174	220	63	0.80	0.039	0.018	16.6	NA
Chicken, broiler or fryer, leg, meat & skin, raw	10	1.01	21	149	198	79	1.77	0.058	0.020	13.1	NA
Chicken, broiler or fryer, leg, meat only, raw	11	1.02	23	167	229	86	2.06	0.064	0.021	13.5	NA
Chicken, broiler or fryer, light meat, meat & skin, raw	11	0.79	23	163	204	65	0.93	0.040	0.018	16.4	11
Chicken, heart, all classes, raw	12	5.96	15	177	176	74	6.59	0.346	0.089	4.3	NA
Chicken, liver, all classes, raw	8	8.99	19	297	230	71	2.67	0.492	0.255	54.6	NA
Chicken, roasting, meat & skin, raw	10	1.01	19	166	196	68	1.07	0.046	0.018	15.3	NA
Chicken, roasting, meat only, raw		1.03	23	198	238	75	1.19	0.050	0.018	16.9	NA
Chicken, wing, frozen, glazed, barbecue flavored	28	2.41	20	205	190	615	1.14	0.039	0	33.2	NA
Lamb, domestic, shoulder, arm, separable lean & fat, trimmed to 1/4" fat, choice, raw	14	1.56	21	159	238	60	3.43	0.102	0.019	19.3	8
Lamb, ground, raw	16	1.55	21	157	222	59	3.41	0.101	0.019	18.8	NA
Lamb, New Zealand, frozen, shoulder, whole, separable lean & fat, trimmed to 1/8" fat, raw	17	1.36	15	168	137	42	2.91	0.083	0.019	2.7	NA

Lamb, brain, raw	9	1.75	12	270	296	112	1.17	0.240	0.044	9.0	NA
Lamb, heart, raw	6	4.60	17	175	316	89	1.87	0.397	0.046	32.0	NA
Lamb, kidneys, raw	13	6.38	17	246	277	156	2.24	0.446	0.118	126.9	NA
Lamb, liver, raw	7	7.37	19	364	313	70	4.66	6.979	0.184	82.4	NA
Lamb, lungs, raw	10	6.40	14	219	238	157	1.80	0.254	0.019	17.7	NA
Lamb, spleen, raw	9	41.89	21	280	358	84	2.84	0.121	0.051	32.4	NA
Turkey, dark meat, raw	17	1.75	22	184	286	77	3.22	0.147	0.022	28.6	11
Turkey, leg, meat & skin, raw	17	1.72	21	177	273	74	3.09	0.142	0.022	26.4	NA
Turkey, light meat, raw	12	1.19	27	204	305	63	1.62	0.075	0.019	24.4	11
Turkey, meat & skin, raw	15	1.43	22	178	266	65	2.20	0.103	0.020	24.4	NA
Turkey, wing, meat & skin, raw	14	1.26	21	165	240	55	1.54	0.077	0.017	22.4	NA
Oil											
Avocado oil	0	0	0	0	0	0	0	0	0	0	0
Canola oil	0	0	0	0	0	0	0	0	0	0	0
Coconut oil	0	0.04	0	0	0	0	0	0	0	0	NA
Corn oil	0	0	0	0	0	0	0	0	0	0	47
Cottonseed oil	0	0	0	0	0	0	0	0	0	0	NA
Flaxseed oil	0	0	0	0	0	0	0	0	0	0	NA
Grapeseed oil	0	0	0	0	0	0	0	0	0	0	0

Oil											
Olive oil	1	0.56	0	0	1	0	2	0	0	0	0
Palm oil	0	0.01	0	0	0	0	0	0	0	0	0
Palm kernel oil	0	0	0	0	0	0	0	0	0	0	0
Peanut oil	0	0.03	0	0	0	0	0	0.01	0	0	NA
Safflower oil, linoleic (>70%)	0	0	0	0	0	0	0	0	0	0	0
Safflower oil, oleic (>70%)	0	0	0	0	0	0	0	0	0	0	0
Sesame oil	0	0	0	0	0	0	0	0	0	0	0
Sunflower oil, high oleic (>70%)	0	0	0	0	0	0	0	0	0	0	7
Sunflower oil, linoleic (~65%)	0	0	0	0	0	0	0	0	0	0	7

Note: (1) Ca = Calcium, Fe = Iron, Mg = Magnesium, P = Phosphorus, K = Potassium, Na = Sodium, Zn = Zinc, Cu = Copper, Mn = Manganese, Se = Selenium, Cr = Chromium.

(2) *Cr data are taken from The 120 Year Diet (author: Roy L. Walford) published by Simon and Schuster Press in 1986.

(3) Other data are taken from SR Search 20 database – 2008 published by the U.S. department of Agriculture.

(4) NA: not available.

Table A-3 Nutrition values per 100 grams of selected foods: vitamins

Food category and name	A (µg)	C (mg)	D (µg)	E (mg)	K (µg)	B₁ (mg)	B₂ (mg)	B₃ (mg)	B₅ (mg)	B₆ (mg)	*B₇ (µg)	B₉ (µg)	B₁₂ (µg)	Choline (mg)
Vegetables														
Artichoke, raw	1	11.7	0	0.19	14.8	0.072	0.066	1.046	0.338	0.116	4.1	68	0	34.4
Asparagus, raw	38	5.6	0	1.13	41.6	0.143	0.141	0.978	0.274	0.091	1.7	52	0	16.0
Beets, raw	2	4.9	0	0.04	0.2	0.031	0.040	0.334	0.155	0.067	2.7	109	0	6.0
Broccoli, raw	31	89.2	0	0.78	101.6	0.071	0.117	0.639	0.573	0.175	0.5	63	0	18.7
Broccoli, cooked, boiled, drained, without salt	77	64.9	0	1.45	141.1	0.063	0.123	0.553	0.616	0.200	NA	108	0	40.1
Broccoli raab, raw	131	20.2	0	1.62	224.0	0.162	0.129	1.221	0.332	0.171	NA	83	0	18.3
Broccoli raab, cooked	227	37.0	0	2.53	256	0.169	0.140	2.015	0.448	0.220	NA	77	0	33.6
Broccoli, frozen, spears, unprepared	57	68.3	0	1.35	101.4	0.072	0.114	0.462	0.242	0.175	NA	94	0	0
Brussels sprouts, raw	38	85	0	0.88	177.0	0.139	0.090	0.745	0.309	0.219	0.4	61	0	19.1
Cabbage, raw	5	36.6	0	0.15	76.0	0061	0.040	0.234	0.212	0.124	2.4	43	0	10.7
Cabbage, Chinese(pe-tsai), raw	16	27.0	0	0.12	42.9	0.040	0.050	0.400	0.105	0.232	0	79	0	7.6
Cabbage, red, raw	56	57	0	0.11	38.2	0.064	0.069	0.418	0.147	0.209	0.1	18	0	17.1
Carrots, baby, raw	690	2.6	0	0	9.4	0.030	0.036	0.556	0.401	0.105	NA	27	0	7.5

Carrots, raw	835	5.9	0	0.66	13.2	0.066	0.058	0.983	0.273	0.138	2.5	19	0	8.8
Cauliflower, raw	1	46.4	0	0.08	16.0	0.057	0.063	0.526	0.652	0.222	17	57	0	45.2
Celery, raw	22	3.1	0	0.27	29.3	0.021	0.057	0.320	0.246	0.076	0.1	36	0	6.1
Chard, Swiss, raw	306	30	0	1.89	830.0	0.040	0.090	0.400	0.172	0.400	0	14	0	18.0
Corn, sweet, yellow, raw	9	6.8	0	0.07	0.3	0.200	0.060	1.700	0.760	0.055	6.0	46	0	23.0
Cucumber, peeled, raw	4	3.2	0	0.03	7.2	0.031	0.025	0.037	0.340	0.051	0.4	14	0	5.7
Cucumber, with peel, raw	5	2.8	0	0.03	16.4	0.027	0.033	0.098	0.259	0.040	0.4	7	0	6.0
Eggplant, raw	1	2.2	0	0.30	3.5	0.039	0.037	0.649	0.281	0.081	0	22	0	6.9
Garlic, raw	0	31.2	0	0.08	1.7	0.200	0.110	0.700	0.596	1.235	0	3	0	23.2
Kale, raw	769	120.0	0	0	817.0	0.110	0.130	1.000	0.091	0.271	0.5	29	0	0
Leeks (bulb & lower leaf-portion), raw	83	12.0	0	0.92	47.0	0.060	0.030	0.400	0.140	0.233	1.4	64	0	9.5
Lettuce, butterhead (includes boston & bibb types), raw	166	3.7	0	0.18	102.3	0.057	0.062	0.357	0.150	0.086	NA	73	0	8.4
Lettuce, cos or romaine, raw	290	24.0	0	0.13	102.5	0.072	0.067	0.313	0.148	0.076	0.7	136	0	9.9
Lettuce, green leaf, raw	370	18.0	0	0.29	173.6	0.070	0.080	0.375	0.134	0.090	NA	38	0	13.4
Lettuce, iceberg (includes crisphead types), raw	25	2.8	0	0.18	24.1	0.041	0.025	0.123	0.091	0.042	3.0	29	0	6.7
Lettuce, red leaf, raw	375	3.7	0	0.15	140.3	0.064	0.077	0.321	0.144	0.100	NA	36	0	11.8

Mushrooms, brown, Italian or Crimini, raw	0	0	0	0.01	0	0.095	0.490	3.800	1.500	0.110	NA	14	0.10	22.1
Mushrooms, enoki, raw	0	0	0	0.01	0	0.179	0.162	5.903	1.067	0.081	NA	52	0	47.7
Mushrooms, Maitake, raw	0	0	0	0.01	0	0.146	0.242	6.585	0.270	0.056	NA	29	0	0
Mushrooms, portabella, raw	0	0	0	0.02	0	0.077	0.480	4.500	1.500	0.100	NA	22	0.05	21.2
Mushrooms, Shiitake, dried	0	3.5	0	0	0	0.300	1.270	14.10	21.879	0.965	0	163	0	201.7
Mushrooms, white, raw	0	2.1	0.45	0.01	0	0.081	0.402	3.609	1.497	0.104	16.0	16	0.04	17.3
Onions, raw	0	7.4	0	0.02	0.4	0.046	0.027	0.116	0.123	0.120	3.5	19	0	6.1
Onions, sweet, raw	0	4.8	0	0.02	0.3	0.041	0.020	0.133	0.098	0.130	3.5	23	0	5.5
Parsley, raw	421	133.0	0	0.75	1640	0.086	0.098	1.313	0.400	0.090	0.4	152	0	12.8
Peppers, sweet, green, raw	18	80.4	0	0.37	7.4	0.057	0.028	0.480	0.099	0.224	0	10	0	5.5
Peppers, sweet, red, raw	157	127.7	0	1.58	4.9	0.054	0.085	0.979	0.317	0.291	0	46	0	5.6
Peppers, sweet, yellow, raw	10	183.5	0	0	0	0.028	0.025	0.890	0.168	0.168	0	26	0	0
Potatoes, red, flesh & skin, raw	0	8.6	0	0.01	2.9	0.081	0.031	1.149	0.279	0.170	NA	18	0	16.4
Potatoes, white, flesh & skin, raw	0	19.7	0	0.02	1.6	0.071	0.034	1.066	0.281	0.203	0.4	18	0	11.0
Radishes, raw	0	14.8	0	0	1.3	0.012	0.039	0.254	0.165	0.071	0	25	0	6.5
Spinach, raw	469	28.1	0	2.03	482.9	0.078	0.189	0.724	0.065	0.195	7	194	0	18.0

Squash, summer, zucchini, includes skin, raw	10	17.0	0	0.12	4.3	0.048	0.142	0.487	0.155	0.218	0	29	0	9.5
Squash, winter, butternut, raw	532	21.0	0	1.44	1.1	0.100	0.020	1.200	0.400	0.154	0	27	0	0
Soybean, mature seeds, sprouted, raw	1	15.3	0	0	0	0.340	0.118	1.148	0.929	0.176	NA	172	0	0
Tomato, red, ripe, raw, year round average	42	12.7	0	0.54	7.9	0.037	0.019	0.594	0.089	0.080	4	15	0	6.7
Turnip greens, raw	579	60.0	0	2.86	251.0	0.070	0.100	0.600	0.380	0.263	0.4	194	0	0
Waterchestnut, Chinese, (matai), raw	0	4.0	0	1.30	0.3	0.140	0.200	1.000	0.479	0.328	0	16	0	36.2
Fruits														
Apples, raw, with skin	3	4.6	0	0.18	2.2	0.017	0.026	0.091	0.061	0.041	0.9	3	0	3.4
Apples, raw, without skin	2	4.0	0	0.05	0.6	0.019	0.028	0.091	0.071	0.037	0.9	0	0	3.4
Applesauce, canned, unsweetened, without added ascorbic acid	1	1.2	0	0.21	0.6	0.013	0.025	0.188	0.095	0.026	0.3	1	0	3.4
Apricots, raw	96	10.0	0	0.89	3.3	0.030	0.040	0.600	0.240	0.054	0	9	0	2.8
Avocados, raw, all commercial varieties	7	10.0	0	2.07	21.0	0.069	0.130	1.738	1.389	0.257	5.5	81	0	14.2
Avocados, raw, California	7	8.8	0	1.97	21.0	0.075	0.143	1.912	1.463	0.287	5.5	89	0	14.2

Food	n													
Avocados, raw, Florida	7	17.4	0	2.66	0	0.021	0.053	0.672	0.931	0.078	5.5	35	0	0
Bananas, raw	3	8.7	0	0.10	0.5	0.031	0.073	0.665	0.334	0.367	4.4	20	0	9.8
Bananas, dehydrated, banana powder	12	7.0	0	0.39	2.0	0.180	0.240	2.800		0.440	NA	14	0	19.6
Blackberries, raw	11	21.0	0	1.17	19.8	0.020	0.026	0.646	0.276	0.030	NA	25	0	8.5
Blueberries, raw	3	9.7	0	0.57	19.3	0.037	0.041	0.418	0.124	0.052	0	6	0	6.0
Cranberries, raw	3	13.3	0	1.20	5.1	0.012	0.020	0.101	0.295	0.056	0	1	0	5.5
Elderberries, raw	30	36.0	0	0	0	0.070	0.060	0.500	0.140	0.230	NA	6	0	0
Figs, raw	7	2.0	0	0.11	4.7	0.060	0.050	0.400	0.300	0.113	0.3	6	0	4.7
Grapefruit, raw, pink & red, all areas	58	31.2	0	0.13	0	0.043	0.031	0.204	0.262	0.053	3	13	0	7.7
Grapes, American style (slip skin), raw	5	4.0	0	0.19	14.6	0.092	0.057	0.300	0.024	0.110	1.6	4	0	5.6
Grapes, red & green, seedless, raw	3	10.8	0	0.19	14.6	0.069	0.070	0.188	0.050	0.086	1.6	2	0	5.6
Honeydew melons, raw	3	18.0	0	0.02	2.9	0.038	0.012	0.418	0.155	0.088	NA	19	0	7.6
Lemon, raw, with peel	2	77.0	0	0	0	0.050	0.040	0.200	0.232	0.109	0	0	0	0
Limes, raw	2	29.1	0	0.22	0.6	0.030	0.020	0.200	0.217	0.043	0	8	0	5.1
Kiwi fruit (Chinese gooseberries), fresh, raw	4	92.5	0	1.46	40.3	0.027	0.025	0.341	0.183	0.063	NA	25	0	7.8

Mangos, raw	38	27.7	0	1.12	4.2	0.058	0.057	0.584	0.160	0.134	NA	14	0	7.6
Nectarine, raw	17	5.4	0	0.77	2.2	0.034	0.027	1.125	0.185	0.025	0	5	0	6.2
Oranges, raw, navels	12	59.1	0	0.15	0	0.068	0.051	0.425	0.261	0.079	1.9	34	0	8.4
Oranges, mandarin, tangerines, raw	34	26.7	0	0.20	0	0.058	0.036	0.376	0.216	0.078	1.9	16	0	10.2
Peaches, raw	16	6.6	0	0.73	2.6	0.024	0.031	0.806	0.153	0.025	1.7	4	0	6.1
Pears, raw	1	4.2	0	0.12	4.5	0.012	0.025	0.157	0.048	0.028	0.1	7	0	5.1
Persimmon, native, raw	0	66.0	0	0	0	0	0	0	0	0	0	0	0	0
Pineapple, raw, all varieties	3	47.8	0	0.02	0.7	0.079	0.032	0.500	0.213	0.112	0	18	0	5.5
Plums, raw	17	9.5	0	0.26	6.4	0.028	0.026	0.417	0.135	0.029	0.1	5	0	1.9
Raisins, seedless	0	2.3	0	0.12	3.5	0.106	0.125	0.766	0.095	0.174	NA	5	0	11.1
Raspberries, raw	2	26.2	0	0.87	7.8	0.032	0.038	0.598	0.329	0.055	1.9	21	0	12.3
Strawberries, raw	1	58.8	0	0.29	2.2	0.024	0.022	0.386	0.125	0.047	4.0	24	0	5.7
Watermelon, raw	28	8.1	0	0.05	0.1	0.033	0.021	0.178	0.221	0.045	3.6	3	0	4.1
Apple juice, canned or bottled	1	0.9	0	0.01	0	0.021	0.017	0.100	0.063	0.030	NA	0	0	1.8
Cranberry juice, cocktail, bottled	0	42.3	0	0.22	1.0	0	0	0.041	0.052	0	NA	0	0	1.1
Grape juice drink, canned	0	26.5	0	0	0.2	0.225	0.354	0.142	0.023	0.035	NA	1	0	0.3
Grapefruit juice, pink, raw	22	38.0	0	0	0	0.040	0.020	0.200	0.189	0.044	NA	10	0	0

Grapefruit juice, white, raw	1	38.0	0	1.22	0	0.040	0.020	0.200	0.189	0.044	NA	10	0	7.7
Lemon juice, raw	1	46.0	0	0.15	0	0.030	0.010	0.100	0.103	0.051	NA	13	0	5.1
Lime juice, raw	2	30.0	0	0.22	0.6	0.025	0.015	0.142	0.123	0.038	NA	10	0	5.1
Orange juice, raw	10	50.0	0	0.04	0.1	0.090	0.030	0.400	0.190	0.040	0.8	30	0	6.2
Prune juice, canned	0	4.1	0	0.12	3.4	0.016	0.070	0.785	0.107	0.218	NA	0	0	2.7
Legumes														
Beans, black, mature seeds, raw	0	0	0	0.21	5.6	0.900	0.193	1.955	0.899	0.286	NA	444	0	66.4
Beans, kidney, red mature seeds, raw	0	4.5	0	0.21	5.6	0.608	0.215	2.110	0.780	0.397	NA	394	0	65.9
Beans, navy, mature seeds, raw	0	0	0	0.02	2.5	0.775	0.164	2.188	0.744	0.428	NA	364	0	87.4
Beans, pink, mature seeds, raw	0	0	0	0.21	5.7	0.772	0.192	1.892	0.997	0.527	NA	463	0	67.2
Beans, pinto, mature seeds, raw	0	6.3	0	0.21	5.6	0.713	0.212	1.174	0.785	0.474	0	525	0	66.2
Beans, pinto, mature seeds, cooked, boiled, with salt	0	0.8	0	0.94	3.5	0.193	0.062	0.318	0.210	0.229	0	172	0	0
Beans, snap, green, raw	35	16.3	0	0.41	14.4	0.084	0.105	0.752	0.094	0.074	0.4	37	0	15.3
Chickpeas (garbanzo beans), mature seeds, raw	3	4.0	0	0.82	9.0	0.477	0.212	1.541	1.588	0.535	NA	557	0	95.2

Cowpeas, common, mature seeds, raw	3	1.5	0	0.39	5.0	0.853	0.226	2.075	1.496	0.357	21.0	633	0	94.7
Lentils, raw	2	4.4	0	0.49	5.0	0.873	0.211	2.605	2.140	0.540	0	479	0	96.4
Peas, split, mature seeds, raw	7	1.8	0	0.09	14.5	0.726	0.215	2.889	1.758	0.174	9.0	274	0	95.5
Soybeans, mature seeds, raw	1	6.0	0	0.85	47.0	0.874	0.870	1.623	0.793	0.377	60.0	375	0	115.9
Tofu, silken, firm (MURI-NU)	0	0	0	0	0	0.101	0.041	0.247	0	0.011	0	0	0	0
Tofu, silken, soft (MURI-NU)	0	0	0	0	0	0.100	0.040	0.300	0	0.011	0	0	0	0
Tofu, yogurt	2	2.5	0	0.31	3.5	0.060	0.020	0.024	0	0.020	NA	6	0	48.4
Tofu, dried-frozen (koyatofu)	26	0.7	0	0	0	0.494	0.317	1.189	0.415	0.286	NA	92	0	0
Tofu, dried-frozen (koyatofu), prepared with calcium sulfate	0	0.7	0	0	0	0.494	0.317	1.189	0.415	0.286	NA	92	0	0
Tofu, fried	1	0	0	0	0	0.170	0.050	0.100	0.140	0.099	NA	27	0	0
Tofu, fried, prepared with calcium sulfate	0	0	0	0	0	0.170	0.050	0.100	0.140	0.099	NA	27	0	0
Tofu, hard, prepared with nigari	0	0.3	0	0	0	0.042	0.077	0.639	0.037	0.039	NA	22	0	0
Tofu, regular, prepared with calcium sulfate	4	0.1	0	0	0	0.081	0.052	0.195	0.068	0.047	NA	15	0	0

Tofu, salted and fermented (fuyu), prepared with calcium sulfate	0	0.2	0	0	0	0	0.157	0.101	0.379	0.132	0.091	NA	29	0	0
Cereal															
Buckwheat	0	0	0	0	0	0	0.101	0.425	7.020	1.233	0.210	0	30	0	0
Buckwheat flour, whole-groat	0	0	0	0.32	7.0	0.417	0.190	6.150	0.440	0.528	NA	54	0	54.2	
Cereals ready-to-eat, granola, homemade	1	1.2	0	11.1	8.7	0.735	0.292	2.143	1.563	0.294	NA	82	0	49.1	
Cereals ready-to-eat, bran flakes, single brand	751	0	3.33	0.85	1.4	1.250	1.420	16.67	0.868	1.670	NA	333	0	27.6	
Cereals ready-to-eat, bran, malted flour, single brand	776	0	0	2.32	1.6	1.290	1.470	17.24	1.930	1.730	NA	345	0	29.0	
Cereals ready-to-eat, corn & oat flour, puffed presweetened, single brand	748	0	3.45	0.19	0.7	1.290	1.470	17.24	0.198	1.730	NA	345	0	14.4	
Cereals ready-to-eat, GERNERAL MILLS, CHEERIOS	867	24.4	3.33	0.68	3.2	1.932	1.608	19.10	1.073	1.775	NA	975	0	26.2	
Cereals ready-to-eat, GERNERAL MILLS, Cinnamon Grahams	501	20.0	3.33	0.31	0.8	1.250	1.420	16.70	0	1.670	NA	333	0	14.0	

Cereals ready-to-eat, GERNERAL MILLS, FIBER ONE	2	20.0	0	0.91	0.8	1.250	1.420	16.70	0.816	1.667	NA	333	5.00	24.0
Cereals ready-to-eat, GERNERAL MILLS, HARMONY	273	55.0	1.83	24.54	0.5	2.730	1.550	18.20	0	1.820	NA	727	7.60	9.6
Cereals ready-to-eat, Malt-O-Meal, High Fiber Bran Flakes	1771	57.1	6.20	26.64	1.6	1.560	2.030	30.30	1.357	9.680	NA	1290	28.30	0
Cereal, oats, instant, fortified, plain, dry	1072	0	0	0.47	1.9	2.050	1.200	16.55	1.100	1.600	NA	286	0	40.6
Cereals ready-to-eat, KELLOGG, KELLOGG'S Complete Wheat Bran Flakes	1294	207.0	3.45	11.93	1.6	5.400	5.900	69.00	34.900	7.000	NA	1390	20.70	27.6
Cereals, Whole wheat hot, natural cereal, dry	0	0	0	1.31	2.4	0.400	0.300	4.900	0.915	0.391	0	78	0	23.1
Grain														
Barley, pearled, raw	1	0	0	0.02	2.2	0.191	0.114	4.604	0.282	0.260	31.0	23	0	37.8
Barley, pearled, cooked	0	0	0	0.01	0.8	0.083	0.062	2.063	0.135	0.115	31.0	16	0	13.4
Barley malt flour	1	0.6	0	0.57	2.2	0.309	0.308	5.636	0.577	0.655	NA	38	0	0
Cocoa, dry powder, unsweetened	0	0	0	0.10	2.5	0.078	0.241	2.185	0.254	0.118	NA	32	0	12.0

Cornmeal, whole-grain, white	0	0	0	0.42	0.3	0.385	0.201	3.632	0.428	0.304	6.6	25	0	21.6
Cornmeal, whole-grain, yellow	11	0	0	0.42	0.3	0.385	0.201	3.632	0.425	0.304	6.6	25	0	21.6
Cornmeal, white (Navajo)	0	0	0	0.37	0.4	0.310	0.137	2.800	2.490	0.583	6.6	36	0	0
Cornmeal, yellow (Navajo)	0	0	0	0.37	0.2	0.300	0.093	2.470	2.490	0.595	6.6	39	0	0
Corn flour, whole-grain, white	0	0	0	0.42	0.3	0.246	0.080	1.900	0.658	0.370	NA	25	0	21.6
Corn flour, whole-grain, yellow	11	0	0	0.42	0.3	0.246	0.080	1.900	0.658	0.370	NA	25	0	21.6
Corn, sweet, yellow, raw	9	6.8	0	0.07	0.3	0.200	0.060	1.700	0.760	0.055	NA	46	0	23.0
Oat flour, partially debranned	0	0	0	0.70	3.2	0.692	0.125	1.474	0.201	0.125	NA	32	0	29.9
Peanut flour, defatted	0	0	0	0.05	0	0.700	0.480	27.00	2.744	0.504	NA	248	0	108.7
Peanut flour, low fat	0	0	0	0	0	0.457	0.172	11.50	1.543	0.304	NA	133	0	0
Popcorn, air-popped	10	0	0	0.29	1.2	0.104	0.083	2.308	0.510	0.157	0	31	0	21.2
Potato flour	0	3.8	0	0.25	0	0.228	0.051	3.507	0.474	0.769	NA	25	0	39.5
Rice bran, crude	0	0	0	4.92	1.9	2.753	0.284	33.99	7.390	4.070	NA	63	0	32.2
Rice flour, brown	0	0	0	1.20	0	0.443	0.080	6.340	1.591	0.736	0	16	0	0
Rice flour, white	0	0	0	0.11	0	0.138	0.021	2.590	0.819	0.436	0	4	0	5.8

Rice noodles, cooked	0	0	0	0	0.018	0.004	0.072	0.011	0.006	0	3	0	0
Rice noodles, dry	0	0	0	0	0.031	0.017	0.221	0.051	0.015	0	3	0	0
Rice, brown, long-grain, cooked	0	0	0.03	0.6	0.096	0.025	1.528	0.285	0.145	0	4	0	9.2
Rice, brown, long-grain, raw	0	0	1.2	1.9	0.401	0.093	5.091	1.493	0.509	0	20	0	30.7
Rice, brown, medium-grain, cooked	0	0	0	0	0.102	0.012	1.330	0.392	0.149	0	4	0	0
Rice, brown, medium-grain, raw	0	0	0	0	0.413	0.043	4.308	1.493	0.509	0	20	0	0
Rice, white, long-grain, regular, cooked	0	0.077	0.04	0	0.163	0.013	1.476	0.390	0.093	0	58	0	2.1
Rice, white, long-grain, regular, raw, unenriched	0	0	0.11	0.1	0.070	0.049	1.600	1.014	0.164	0	8	0	5.8
Rice, white, medium-grain, cooked	0	0	0	0	0.167	0.016	1.835	0.411	0.050	0	58	0	0
Rice, white, medium-grain, raw	0	0	0	0	0.070	0.048	1.600	1.342	0.145	0	9	0	0
Rice, white, short-grain, cooked	0	0	0	0	0.164	0.016	1.493	0.397	0.059	0	59	0	0
Rice, white, short-grain, raw	0	0	0	0	0.565	0.048	4.113	1.287	0.171	0	231	0	0
Rye flour, dark	1	0	1.41	5.9	0.316	0.251	4.270	1.456	0.443	6	60	0	30.4

Rye flour, light	0	0	0	0.43	5.9	0.331	0.090	0.800	0.665	0.234	6	22	0	10.8
Rye flour, medium	0	0	0	0.79	5.9	0.287	0.114	1.727	0.492	0.268	6	19	0	20.6
Seeds, cottonseed flour, low fat (glandless)	22	2.4	0	0	0	2.089	0.396	4.039	0.445	0.764	NA	228	0	0
Seeds, sesame flour, high fat	3	0	0	0	0	2.684	0.286	13.37	2.928	0.152	NA	31	0	0
Seeds, sesame flour, low fat	3	0	0	0	0	2.516	0.269	12.53	2.745	0.142	NA	29	0	0
Seeds, sunflower flour, partially defatted	2	1.3	0	0	0	3.187	0.266	7.313	6.595	0.753	NA	222	0	
Soy flour, full-fat, raw	6	0	0	1.95	70.0	0.581	1.160	4.320	1.590	0.461	NA	345	0	190.6
Wheat flour, white, all-purpose, enriched bleached	0	0	0	0.06	0.3	0.785	0.494	5.904	0.438	0.044	1.0	183	0	10.4
Wheat flour, white, all-purpose, enriched unbleached	0	0	0	0.23	0.3	0.785	0.494	5.904	0.438	0.044	1.0	183	0	0
Wheat flour, white, all-purpose, self-rising, enriched	0	0	0	0.05	0.3	0.674	0.414	5.832	0.438	0.050	1.0	196	0	10.4
Wheat flour, whole-grain	0	0	0	0.82	1.9	0.447	0.215	6.365	1.008	0.341	9.0	44	0	31.2
Bread														
Bread, cracked-wheat	0	0	0	0	0	0.385	0.240	3.671	0.512	0.304	NA	61	0	0
Bread, egg	63	0	0.40	0.26	0.9	0.438	0.436	4.848	0.282	0.064	NA	105	0	84.0
Bread, French or Vienna (includes sourdough)	0	0.2	0	0.18	0.6	0.433	0.287	4.760	0.334	0.100	NA	148	0	14.8

Bread, Italian	0	0	0	0.29	1.2	0.473	0.292	4.381	0.378	0.04	NA	191	0	14.8
Bread, oat bran	2	0	0	0.44	1.2	0.504	0.346	4.831	0.581	0.073	NA	81	0	14.6
Bread, oatmeal	5	0	0	0.48	1.5	0.399	0.240	3.136	0.341	0.068	NA	62	0	14.6
Bread, pumpernickel	0	0	0	0.42	0.8	0.327	0.305	3.091	0.404	0.126	0	93	0	14.6
Bread, raisin,	0	0.1	0	0	0	0.177	0.173	1.495	0.387	0.069	NA	34	0	0
Bread, rye	0	0.4	0	0.33	1.2	0.434	0.335	3.805	0.440	0.075	0	110	0	14.6
Bread, wheat	0	0.2	0	0.19	4.9	0.373	0.311	5.190	0.820	0.119	2	85	0	18.7
Bread, white, commercially prepared (includes soft bread crumbs)	0	0	0	0.22	3.1	0.455	0.331	4.385	0.203	0.084	NA	111	0	14.6
Dairy														
Milk, buttermilk, dried	49	5.7	0	0.10	0.4	0.392	1.579	0.876	3.170	0.338	NA	47	3.82	118.7
Milk, buttermilk, fluid, cultured, low fat	7	1.0	0	0.05	0.1	0.034	0.154	0.058	0.275	0.034	NA	5	0	16.0
Milk, chocolate, fluid, reduced fat	64	0	1.00	0.04	0.2	0.045	0.183	0.164	0.539	0.024	NA	2	0.33	17.1
Milk, chocolate, fluid, whole	26	0.9	1.00	0.06	0.2	0.037	0.162	0.125	0.295	0.040	NA	5	0.33	17.0
Milk, dry, whole	257	8.6	7.80	0.48	1.8	0.283	1.205	0.646	2.271	0.302	NA	37	3.25	119.3
Milk, goat, fluid	57	1.3	0.30	0.07	0.3	0.048	0.138	0.277	0.310	0.046	NA	1	0.07	16.0
Milk, human, mature, fluid	61	5.0	0.10	0.08	0.3	0.014	0.036	0.177	0.223	0.011	NA	5	0.05	16.0

Milk, fluid, 1% milkfat, with added vitamin A	58	0	1.30	0.01	0.1	0.020	0.185	0.093	0.361	0.037	NA	5	0.44	17.7
Milk, fluid, nonfat (fat free or skim)	2	1.0	0	0.04	0	0.036	0.140	0.088	0.329	0.040	1.5	5	0.38	0
Milk, producer, fluid, 3.7% milkfat	33	1.5	0	0	0	0.038	0.161	0.084	0.313	0.042	NA	5	0.36	0
Milk, fluid, 2% milkfat, with added vitamin A	55	0.2	1.08	0.03	0.2	0.039	0.185	0.092	0.356	0.038	0	5	0.46	16.4
Milk, sheep, fluid	44	4.2	0	0	0	0.065	0.355	0.417	0.407	0.060	NA	7	0.71	0
Milk, whole, 3.25% milkfat	28	0	1.00	0.06	0.2	0.044	0.183	0.107	0.362	0.036	NA	5	0.44	14.3
Egg														
Egg, duck, whole, fresh, raw	194	0	0	1.34	0.4	0.156	0.404	0.200	1.862	0.250	NA	80	5.40	263.4
Egg, goose, whole, fresh, raw	187	0	0	1.29	0.4	0.147	0.382	0.189	1.759	0.236	NA	76	5.10	263.4
Egg, quail, whole, fresh, raw	156	0	0	1.08	0.3	0.130	0.790	0.150	1.761	0.150	NA	66	1.58	263.4
Egg, turkey, whole, fresh, raw	166	0	0	0	0	0.110	0.470	0.024	1.889	0.131	NA	71	1.69	0
Egg, white, raw, fresh	0	0	0	0	0	0.004	0.439	0.105	0.190	0.005	7.0	4	0.09	1.1
Egg, whole, cooked, fried	198	0	0.93	1.22	5.6	0.075	0.518	0.077	1.558	0.155	23.0	51	1.39	272.6
Egg, whole, cooked, hard-boiled	169	0	0	1.03	0.3	0.066	0.513	0.064	1.398	0.121	23.0	44	1.11	225.3
Egg, whole, cooked, omelet	155	0	0.73	1.22	4.5	0.058	0.404	0.060	1.210	0.121	23.0	39	1.09	211.7

Egg, whole, cooked, poached	139	0	0.85	0.96	0.3	0.055	0.405	0.059	1.433	0.121	23.0	35	1.28	200.1
Egg, whole, cooked, scrambled	143	0.2	0.85	1.09	4.0	0.052	0.437	0.079	1.007	0.118	23.0	30	0.77	189.5
Egg, whole, raw, fresh	140	0	0.88	0.97	0.3	0.069	0.478	0.070	1.438	0.143	23.0	47	1.29	251.1
Egg, yolk, raw, fresh	381	0	2.68	2.58	0.7	0.176	0.528	0.024	2.990	0.350	52.0	146	1.95	682.3
Cheese														
Cheese, America cheddar, imitation	114	0	0	0.27	2.7	0.050	0.430	0.130	0	0.120	NA	7	0.40	0
Cheese, blue	198	0	0	0.25	2.4	0.029	0.382	1.016	1.729	0.166	NA	36	1.22	15.4
Cheese, brick	292	0	0	0.26	2.5	0.014	0.351	0.118	0.288	0.065	NA	20	1.26	15.4
Cheese, brie	174	0	0	0.24	2.3	0.070	0.520	0.380	0.690	0.235	NA	65	1.65	15.4
Cheese, camembert	241	0	0.30	0.21	2.0	0.028	0.488	0.630	1.364	0.227	NA	62	1.30	15.4
Cheese, caraway	271	0	0	0	0	0.031	0.450	0.180	0.190	0.074	NA	18	0.27	0
Cheese, cheddar	265	0	0.30	0.29	2.8	0.027	0.375	0.080	0.413	0.074	3.6	18	0.83	16.5
Cheese, cheshire	233	0	0	0	0	0.046	0.293	0.080	0.413	0.074	NA	18	0.83	0
Cheese, Colby	264	0	0	0.28	2.7	0.015	0.375	0.093	0.210	0.079	NA	18	0.83	15.4
Cheese, cottage, 1% milkfat	11	0	0	0.01	0.1	0.021	0.165	0.128	0.215	0.068	0	12	0.63	17.5
Cheese, cottage, 2% milkfat	21	0	0	0.02	0.2	0.024	0.185	0.144	0.242	0.076	NA	13	0.71	16.3
Cheese, cream, fat free	279	0	0	0.01	0.1	0.050	0.172	0.160	0.194	0.050	NA	37	0.55	27.2

Cheese, edam	242	0	0.90	0.24	2.3	0.037	0.389	0.082	0.281	0.076	NA	16	1.54	15.4
Cheese, feta	125	0	0	0.18	1.8	0.154	0.844	0.991	0.967	0.424	0	32	1.69	15.4
Cheese, Mexican, blend, reduced fat	155	0	0	0.17	1.6	0.030	0.300	0.060	0	0.084	NA	20	1.66	13.5
Cheese, Mexican, queso anejo	54	0	0	0.26	2.5	0.020	0.209	0.032	0.252	0.047	NA	1	1.38	15.4
Cheese, Monterey	198	0	0	0.26	2.5	0.015	0.390	0.093	0.210	0.079	0	18	0.83	15.4
Cheese, Monterey, low fat	142	0	0	0.19	1.8	0.020	0.360	0.090	0	0.080	0	18	0.83	15.4
Cheese, Mozzarella, part skim	127	0	0	0.14	1.6	0.018	0.303	0.105	0.079	0.070	0	9	0.82	15.4
Cheese, muenster	298	0	0	0.26	2.5	0.013	0.320	0.103	0.190	0.056	NA	12	1.47	15.4
Cheese, parmesan, hard	108	0	0.70	0.23	1.7	0.039	0.332	0.271	0.453	0.091	NA	7	1.20	15.4
Cheese, provolone, reduced fat	141	0	0	0.15	1.5	0.019	0.321	0.156	0.476	0.073	NA	10	1.46	12.9
Cheese, Ricotta, part skim	107	0	0	0.07	0.7	0.021	0.185	0.078	0.242	0.020	0	13	0.29	17.5
Cheese, Swiss	220	0	1.10	0.38	2.5	0.063	0.296	0.092	0.429	0.083	0	6	3.34	15.5
Cheese, tilsit	249	0	0	0	0	0.061	0.359	0.205	0.346	0.065	NA	20	2.10	0
Nuts and Seeds														
Nuts, acorns, raw	2	0	0	0	0	0.112	0.118	1.827	0.715	0.528	NA	87	0	0
Nuts, almonds	0	0	0	26.22	0	0.211	1.014	3.385	0.469	0.143	18	50	0	52.1

Nuts, cashew nuts, raw	0	0	0.5	0	0.90	34.1	0.423	0.058	1.062	0.864	0.417	0	25	0	0
Nuts, chestnuts, Chinese, raw	10	0	36.0	0	0	0	0.160	0.180	0.800	0.555	0.410	1.5	68	0	0
Nuts, chestnuts, European, raw	1	0	43.0	0	0	0	0.238	0.168	1.179	0.509	0.376	1.5	62	0	0
Nuts, chestnuts, Japanese, raw	2	0	26.3	0	0	0	0.344	0.163	1.500	0.206	0.283	1.5	47	0	0
Nuts, coconut meat, raw	0	0	3.3	0	0.24	0.2	0.066	0.020	0.540	0.300	0.054	NA	26	0	12.1
Nuts, ginkgo nuts, raw	28	0	15.0	0	0	0	0.220	0.090	6.000	0.160	0.328	NA	54	0	0
Nuts, hazelnuts or filberts	1	0	6.3	0	15.03	14.2	0.643	0.113	1.800	0.918	0.563	NA	113	0	45.6
Nuts, macadamia nuts, dry roasted, without salt added	0	0	0.7	0	0.57	0	0.710	0.087	2.274	0.603	0.359	NA	10	0	44.6
Nuts, macadamia nuts, raw	0	0	1.2	0	0.54	0	1.195	0.162	2.473	0.758	0.275	NA	11	0	0
Nuts, mixed nuts /w peanuts, dry roasted, with salt added	0	0	0.4	0	10.94	12.9	0.200	0.200	4.700	1.205	0.296	NA	50	0	54.3
Nuts, mixed nuts /w peanuts, dry roasted, without salt added	1	0	0.4	0	0	0	0.200	0.200	4.700	1.205	0.296	NA	50	0	0
Nuts, mixed nuts /w peanuts, oil roasted, with salt added	1	0	0.5	0	0	0	0.498	0.222	5.061	1.248	0.240	NA	83	0	0

Nuts, pecans	3	1.1	0	1.40	3.5	0.660	0.130	1.167	0.863	0.210	27.0	22	0	40.5
Nuts, pine nuts, dried	1	0.8	0	9.33	53.9	0.364	0.227	4.387	0.313	0.094	NA	34	0	55.8
Nuts, pistachio nuts, raw	28	5.0	0	2.30	0	0.870	0.160	1.300	0.520	1.700	NA	51	0	0
Nuts, walnuts, English	1	1.3	0	0.70	2.7	0.341	0.150	1.125	0.570	0.537	NA	98	0	39.2
Seeds, breadfruit seeds, raw	13	6.6	0	0	0	0.482	0.301	0.438	0.877	0.320	NA	53	0	0
Seeds, breadnut tree seeds, dried	11	46.6	0	0	0	0.030	0.140	2.100	1.875	0.685	NA	113	0	0
Seeds, breadnut tree seeds, raw	12	27.4	0	0	0	0.055	0.055	0.880	1.103	0.403	NA	66	0	0
Seeds, flaxseed	0	0.6	0	0.31	4.3	1.644	0.161	3.080	0.985	0.473	NA	87	0	78.7
Seeds, lotus seeds, dried	3	0	0	0	0	0.640	0.150	1.600	0.851	0.629	NA	104	0	0
Seeds, pumpkin & squash seed kernels, dried	19	1.9	0	0	51.4	0.210	0.320	1.745	0.339	0.224	0	58	0	63.0
Seeds, sesame seeds, whole, dried	0	0	0	0.25	0	0.791	0.247	4.515	0.050	0.790	NA	97	0	25.6
Seeds, sunflower kernels, dried	3	1.4	0	33.23	0	1.480	0.355	8.335	1.130	1.345	0	227	0	55.1
Seeds, watermelon seed kernels, dried	0	0	0	0	0	0.190	0.145	3.550	0.346	0.089	NA	58	0	0
Fish and Shellfish														
Fish, anchovy, European, raw	15	0	0	0.57	0.1	0.055	0.256	14.024	0.645	0.143	NA	9	0.62	0

Fish, bass, striped, raw	27	0	0	0	0	0.100	0.030	2.100	0.750	0.300	0	9	3.82	0
Fish, bluefish, raw	120	0	0	0	0	0.058	0.080	5.950	0.828	0.402	NA	2	5.39	0
Fish, butterfish, raw	30	0	0	0	0	0.120	0.150	4.500	0.750	0.300	NA	15	1.90	0
Fish, catfish, channel, farmed, raw	15	0.6	0	1.20	0.1	0.361	0.075	2.304	0.600	0.188	0	10	2.47	65.0
Fish, catfish, channel, wild, raw	15	0.7	0	0	0	0.210	0.072	1.907	0.765	0.116	0	10	2.23	0
Fish, cod, Atlantic, raw	12	1.0	1.10	0.64	0.1	0.076	0.065	2.063	0.153	0.245	3.0	7	0.91	65.2
Fish, cod, Pacific, raw	8	2.9	0	0.64	0.1	0.022	0.042	2.040	0.140	0.400	3.0	7	0.90	65.0
Crustaceans, crab, Alaska king, raw	7	7.0	0	0	0	0.043	0.043	1.100	0.350	0.150	0	44	9.00	0
Crustaceans, crab, blue, raw	2	3.0	0	0	0	0.080	0.040	2.700	0.350	0.150	0	44	9.00	0
Crustaceans, crab, queen, raw	45	7.0	0	0	0	0.080	0.200	2.500	0.350	0.150	0	44	9.00	0
Fish, drum, freshwater, raw	51	1.0	0	0	0	0.070	0.170	2.350	0.750	0.300	NA	15	2.00	0
Fish, haddock, raw	17	0	0	0.39	0.1	0.035	0.037	3.803	0.127	0.300	5.0	12	1.20	65.0
Fish, halibut, Atlantic & Pacific, raw	47	0	0	0.85	0.1	0.060	0.075	5.848	0.329	0.344	8.0	12	1.18	61.8
Fish, halibut, Greenland, raw	17	0	0	0.85	0.1	0.060	0.080	1.500	0.250	0.420	8.0	1	1.00	61.8
Fish, herring, Atlantic, raw	28	0.7	40.70	1.07	0.1	0.092	0.233	3.217	0.645	0.302	4.5	10	13.67	65.0

Fish, herring, Pacific, raw	32	0	7.88	1.60	0	0.060	0.200	2.200	1.000	0.450	4.5	5	10.00	65.0
Crustaceans, lobster, northern, raw	21	0	0	1.47	0.1	0.006	0.048	1.455	1.630	0.063	5.0	9	0.93	80.9
Fish, mackerel, Atlantic, raw	50	0.4	9.00	1.52	5.0	0.176	0.312	9.080	0.856	0.399	18.0	1	8.71	65.0
Fish, mackerel, king, raw	218	1.6	0	0	0	0.100	0.476	8.590	0.839	0.442	18.0	8	15.60	0
Fish, mackerel, Spanish, raw	30	1.6	0	0.69	0.1	0.130	0.170	2.300	0.750	0.400	18.0	1	2.40	65.0
Fish, monkfish, raw	12	1.0	0	0	0	0.025	0.060	2.100	0.150	0.240	NA	7	0.90	0
Fish, mullet, striped, raw	37	1.2	0	1.00	0.1	0.090	0.080	5.200	0.760	0.425	NA	9	0.22	65.0
Fish, ocean perch, Atlantic, raw	12	0.8	0	1.25	0.1	0.110	0.110	2.000	0.360	0.230	0	9	1.00	65.0
Fish, pike, walleye, raw	21	0	0	0	0	0.270	0.160	2.300	0.750	0.120	NA	15	2.00	0
Fish, pollock, Atlantic, raw	11	0	0	0.23	0.1	0.047	0.185	3.270	0.358	0.287	NA	3	3.19	65.0
Fish, pollock, walleye, raw	20	0	0	0.64	0.1	0.065	0.058	1.290	0.140	0.060	NA	3	3.10	65.0
Fish, roe, mixed species, raw	90	16.0	0	7.00	0.2	0.240	0.740	1.800	1.000	0.160	NA	80	10.00	335.4
Fish, sablefish, raw	93	0	0	0	0	0.100	0.090	4.000	0.750	0.300	NA	15	1.50	0
Fish, salmon, Atlantic, farmed, raw	15	3.9	0	0	0	0.340	0.120	7.505	1.380	0.637	0.9	26	2.80	78.5
Fish, salmon, Atlantic, wild, raw	12	0	0	0	0	0.226	0.380	7.860	1.664	0.818	0.9	25	3.18	0
Fish, salmon, chinook, raw	136	4.0	0	1.22	0	0.054	0.113	8.420	0.750	0.400	0.9	30	1.30	0

Fish, salmon, coho, wild, raw	30	1.0	0	0.65	0.1	0.113	0.140	7.230	0.823	0.549	0.9	9	4.17	94.6
Fish, salmon, pink, raw	35	0	0	0.64	0.4	0.170	0.060	7.000	0.750	0.200	0.9	4	3.00	94.6
Fish, sardine, Pacific, canned in tomato sauce, drained solids with bone	34	1.0	12.00	1.44	0.4	0.044	0.233	4.200	0.730	0.123	5.0	24	9.00	85.0
Fish, shad, America, raw	33	0	0	1.00	0.1	0.150	0.240	8.400	0.750	0.400	NA	15	0.15	65.0
Fish, shark, mixed species, raw	70	0	0	1.00	0.1	0.042	0.062	2.938	0.695	0.400	NA	3	1.49	65.0
Crustaceans, shrimp, mixed species, raw	54	2.0	3.80	1.10	0	0.028	0.034	2.552	0.276	0.104	1.0	3	1.16	80.9
Fish, swordfish, raw	36	1.1	0	0.50	0.1	0.037	0.095	9.680	0.412	0.330	0	2	1.75	65.0
Fish, tuna, fresh, bluefin, raw	655	0	0	1.00	0	0.241	0.251	8.654	1.054	0.455	3.0	2	9.43	65.0
Fish, wolffish, Atlantic, raw	113	0	0	0	0	0.180	0.080	2.133	0.570	0.400	NA	5	2.03	0
Meat and Poultry														
Beef, bottom sirloin, tri-tip, separable lean only, trimmed to 0" fat, select, raw	0	0	0	0.28	1.1	0.072	0.115	6.201	0.627	0.602	0	12	0.90	0
Beef, brisket, flat half, separable lean and fat, trimmed to 1/8" fat, all grades, raw	0	0	0	0.44	1.7	0.065	0.130	4.041	0.516	0.624	NA	10	1.54	0

Beef, brisket, point half, separable lean and fat, trimmed to 1/4" fat, all grades, raw	0	0	0	0	0	0.070	0.130	2.840	0.270	0.330	NA	6	2.11	0
Beef, chuck, clod steak, separable lean only, trimmed to 1/4" fat, all grades, raw	0	0	0	0.13	0	0.129	0.209	3.708	0	0.437	NA	8	3.46	0
Beef, flank, separable lean only, trimmed to 0" fat, all grades, raw	0	0	0	0.30	1.2	0.066	0.108	6.683	0.638	0.604	NA	13	1.06	0
Beef, ground, 70% lean meat / 30% fat, raw	0	0	0	0.49	2.9	0.044	0.139	3.382	0.408	0.278	NA	8	2.07	46.8
Beef, rib, shortribs, separable lean only, choice, raw	0	0	0	0	0	0.094	0.154	3.412	0.320	0.390	NA	6	3.39	0
Beef, round, bottom round, separable lean only, trimmed to 1/2" fat, prime, raw	0	0	0	0	0	0.117	0.196	4.128	0.443	0.570	5.0	10	2.93	0
Beef, tenderloin, separable lean only, trimmed to 1/4" fat, prime, raw	0	0	0	0	0	0.140	0.250	3.410	0.350	0.430	NA	7	2.90	0
Beef, brain, raw	7	10.7	0	0.99	0	0.092	0.199	3.550	2.010	0.226	NA	3	9.51	0
Beef, heart, raw	0	2.0	0	0.22	0	0.238	0.906	7.530	1.790	0.279	NA	3	8.55	0
Beef, kidneys, raw	419	9.4	0.80	0.22	0	0.357	2.840	8.030	3.980	0.665	NA	98	27.50	0

Beef, liver, raw	4968	1.3	0.40	0.38	3.1	0.189	2.755	13.175	7.173	1.083	NA	290	59.30	333.3
Beef, lung, raw	14	38.5	0	0	0	0.047	0.230	4.000	1.000	0.040	NA	11	3.81	0
Beef, spleen, raw	0	45.5	0	0	0	0.050	0.370	8.400	1.081	0.070	NA	4	5.68	0
Pork, boneless loin, fresh	0	1.3	0	0	0	0	0	0	0	0	0	0	0	0
Pork, center cut chops, fresh	0	1.7	0	0	0	0	0	0	0	0	0	0	0	0
Pork, cured, bacon, raw	11	0	0	0.27	0	0.281	0.113	3.828	0.520	0.210	NA	2	0.69	46.6
Pork, cured, patties, grilled	0	0	0	0.46	0	0.350	0.185	3.245	0.262	0.160	NA	3	0.70	52.0
Pork, fresh, backfat, raw	5	0.1	0	0	0	0.084	0.051	0.985	0.115	0.040	NA	1	0.18	15.4
Pork, fresh, backribs, separable lean and fat, raw	3	0.2	0	0	0	0.584	0.258	4.570	0.745	0.395	NA	4	0.82	0
Pork, fresh, belly, raw	3	0.3	0	0.39	0	0.396	0.242	4.647	0.256	0.130	NA	1	0.84	0
Pork, fresh, loin, tenderloin, separable lean only, raw	0	0	0	0.22	0	0.998	0.342	6.684	0.846	0.777	NA	0	0.51	80.8
Pork, fresh, ground, raw	2	0.7	0	0	0	0.732	0.235	4.338	0.668	0.383	NA	5	0.70	0
Pork, fresh, leg(ham), whole, separable lean and fat, raw	2	0.7	0	0	0	0.736	0.200	4.574	0.685	0.401	NA	7	0.63	0
Pork, flesh, loin, country-style ribs, separable lean only, raw	0	0	0	0.25	0	0.349	0.271	3.093	1.737	0.577	NA	0	1.01	87.3
Pork, flesh, separable fat, raw	24	0	0	0.05	0	0.189	0.082	2.937	0.383	0.173	NA	0	0.92	25.2

Pork, flesh, shoulder, arm picnic, separable lean only, raw	2	0.9	0	0.17	0	0.874	0.306	4.628	0.776	0.490	NA	4	0.73	0
Pork, flesh, brain, raw	0	13.5	0	0	0	0.155	0.275	4.275	2.800	0.190	NA	6	2.19	0
Pork, flesh, feet, raw	0	0	0	0.02	0	0.026	0.106	1.130	0.303	0.053	NA	10	0.52	0
Pork, flesh, heart, raw	8	5.3	0	0.63	0	0.613	1.185	6.765	2.515	0.390	NA	4	3.79	0
Pork, flesh, kidneys, raw	59	13.3	0	0	0	0.340	1.697	8.207	3.130	0.440	NA	59	8.49	0
Pork, flesh, liver, raw	6502	25.3	0	0	0	0.283	3.005	15.301	6.650	0.690	NA	212	26.00	NA
Pork, flesh, lung, raw	0	12.3	0	0	0	0.085	0.430	3.345	0.900	0.100	NA	3	2.75	0
Pork, fresh, spleen, raw	0	28.5	0	0	0	0.130	0.300	5.867	1.055	0.060	NA	4	3.26	0
Pork, fresh, stomach, raw	0	0	0	0.04	0	0.051	0.201	2.480	1.220	0.034	NA	3	0.30	194.8
Chicken breast tender, raw	0	0.8	0	0.08	14.7	0.211	0.091	5.710	0.855	0.041	NA	12	0.27	96.4
Chicken patty, frozen, raw	11	0	0	1.18	11.1	0.073	0.054	6.630	1.081	0.155	NA	5	0.23	44.8
Chicken, broiler or fryer, back, meat only, raw	75	1.6	0	0.37	2.4	0.051	0.116	4.835	0.819	0.190	NA	6	0.25	0
Chicken, broiler or fryer, breast, meat & skin, raw	25	0	0	0.31	0	0.063	0.085	9.908	0.804	0.530	NA	4	0.34	67.1
Chicken, broiler or fryer, leg, meat & skin, raw	37	2.5	0	0.44	2.9	0.067	0.164	5.435	1.110	0.290	NA	11	0.32	56.6
Chicken, broiler or fryer, leg, meat only, raw	18	0	0	0.32	2.9	0.079	0.193	6.067	1.178	0.330	NA	10	0.36	61.8

Chicken, broiler or fryer, light meat, meat & skin, raw	30	0	0	0	0.27	2.4	0.059	0.086	8.908	0.794	0.480	11	4	0.34	0
Chicken, heart, all classes, raw	9	0	3.2	0	0	0	0.152	0.728	4.883	2.559	0.360	NA	72	7.29	0
Chicken, liver, all classes, raw	3296	0	17.9	0	0.70	0	0.305	1.778	9.728	6.233	0.853	NA	588	16.58	194.4
Chicken, roasting, meat & skin, raw	38	0	0	0	0.30	2.4	0.058	0.115	6.572	0.885	0.320	NA	6	0.31	0
Chicken, roasting, meat only, raw	13	0	0	0	0.22	2.4	0.069	0.134	7.875	1.032	0.420	NA	7	0.36	0
Chicken, wing, frozen, glazed, barbecue flavored	17	0	0	0	0.36	0	0.074	0.242	5.500	0.545	0.142	NA	10	0.40	0
Lamb, domestic, shoulder, arm, separable lean & fat, trimmed to 1/4" fat, raw	0	0	0	0	0.22	0	0.120	0.230	6.000	0.720	0.150	0	24	2.67	0
Lamb, ground, raw	0	0	0	0	0.20	3.6	0.110	0.210	5.960	0.650	0.130	NA	18	2.31	69.3
Lamb, New Zealand, frozen, shoulder, whole, separable lean & fat, trimmed to 1/8" fat, raw	0	0	0	0	0	0	0.120	0.310	5.460	0.550	0.080	0	1	3.14	0
Lamb, brain, raw	0	0	16.0	0	0	0	0.130	0.300	3.900	0.920	0.290	NA	3	11.30	0
Lamb, heart, raw	0	0	5.0	0	0	0	0.375	0.990	6.140	2.630	0.390	NA	2	10.25	0
Lamb, kidneys, raw	95	0	11.0	0	0	0	0.620	2.240	7.510	4.220	0.220	NA	28	52.41	0

Lamb, liver, raw	7391	4.0	0	0	0	0.340	3.630	16.110	6.130	0.900	NA	230	90.05	NA
Lamb, lungs, raw	27	31.0	0	0	0	0.048	0.237	4.124	0	0.110	NA	12	3.93	0
Lamb, spleen, raw	0	23.0	0	0	0	0.047	0.348	7.895	0	0.110	NA	4	5.34	0
Turkey, dark meat, raw	2	0	0	0	0	0.073	0.202	2.855	1.033	0.320	0	10	0.38	0
Turkey, leg, meat & skin, raw	1	0	0	0	0	0.077	0.211	2.947	1.090	0.340	NA	10	0.39	0
Turkey, light meat, raw	0	0	0	0	0	0.064	0.122	5.844	0.688	0.560	0	8	0.45	0
Turkey, meat & skin, raw	2	0	0	0.35	3.1	0.064	0.155	4.085	0.807	0.410	0	8	0.40	68.0
Turkey, wing, meat & skin, raw	3	0	0	0	0	0.050	0.110	4.425	0.554	0.410	0	7	0.39	0
Oil														
Avocado oil	0	0	0	0	0	0	0	0	0	0	0	0	0	0
Canola oil	0	0	0	17.6	71.3	0	0	0	0	0	0	0	0	0.2
Coconut oil	0	0	0	0.09	0.5	0	0	0	0	0	0	0	0	0.3
Corn oil	0	0	0	14.3	1.9	0	0	0	0	0	0	0	0	0.2
Cottonseed oil	0	0	0	35.3	24.7	0	0	0	0	0	0	0	0	0.2
Flaxseed oil	0	0	0	17.5	0	0	0	0	0	0	0	0	0	0.2
Grapeseed oil	0	0	0	28.8	0	0	0	0	0	0	0	0	0	0.3
Olive oil	0	0	0	14.35	60.2	0	0	0	0	0	0	0	0	0

Palm oil	0	0	15.94	8.0	0	0	0	0	0	0	0	0	0.3
Palm kernel oil	0	0	3.81	24.7	0	0	0	0	0	0	0	0	0.2
Peanut oil	0	0	15.69	0.7	0	0	0	0	0	0	0	0	0.1
Safflower oil, linoleic (>70%)	0	0	34.10	7.1	0	0	0	0	0	0	0	0	0
Safflower oil, oleic (>70%)	0	0	34.1	7.1	0	0	0	0	0	0	0	0	0.2
Sesame oil	0	0	1.40	13.6	0	0	0	0	0	0	0	0	0.2
Sunflower oil, high oleic (>70%)	0	0	41.08	5.4	0	0	0	0	0	0	0	0	0
Sunflower oil, linoleic (~65%)	0	0	41.08	5.4	0	0	0	0	0	0	0	0	0.2

Note: (1) A = vitamin A, C = vitamin C, D = vitamin D, E = vitamin E, K = vitamin K, B_1 = Thiamin, B_2 = Riboflavin, B_3 = Niacin, B_5 = Pantothenic Acid, B_7 = Biotin, B_9 = Folate, B_{12} = Vitamin B_{12}.

(2) *B_7 data are taken from The 120 Year Diet (author: Roy L. Walford) published by Simon and Schuster Press in 1986.

(3) Other data are taken from SR Search 20 database – 2008 published by the U.S. department of Agriculture.

(4) NA: not available.

Table A-4 Nutrition values per 100 grams of selected foods: essential amino acids, EPA, DHA, lutein and zeaxanthin

Food category and name	W (g)	T (g)	I (g)	L (g)	K (g)	M + C (g)	F + Y (g)	V (g)	H (g)	EPA (g)	DHA (g)	Lutein + Zeaxan-thin (µg)
Vegetables												
Artichoke, raw	0	0	0	0	0	0	0	0	0	0	0	464
Asparagus, raw	0.027	0.084	0.075	0.128	0.104	0.062	0.127	0.115	0.049	0	0	710
Beets, raw	0.019	0.047	0.048	0.068	0.058	0.037	0.084	0.056	0.021	0	0	0
Broccoli, raw	0.033	0.088	0.079	0.129	0.135	0.066	0.167	0.125	0.059	0	0	1403
Broccoli, cooked, boiled, drained, without salt	0.034	0.096	0.092	0.147	0.155	0.074	0.176	0.138	0.063	0	0	1080
Broccoli raab, raw	0.043	0.106	0.104	0.170	0.198	0.087	0.203	0.153	0.066	0	0	1121
Broccoli raab, cooked	0.052	0.128	0.125	0.206	0.239	0.105	0.244	0.184	0.080	0	0	1683
Broccoli, frozen, spears, unprepared	0.032	0.099	0.119	0.143	0.154	0.057	0.161	0.140	0.054	0	0	1525
Brussels sprouts, raw	0.037	0.120	0.132	0.152	0.154	0.054	0.098	0.155	0.076	0	0	1590
Cabbage, raw	0.011	0.035	0.030	0.041	0.044	0.023	0.051	0.042	0.022	0	0	30
Cabbage, Chinese(pe-tsai), raw	0.012	0.039	0.068	0.070	0.071	0.020	0.058	0.053	0.021	0	0	48
Cabbage, red, raw	0.012	0.039	0.034	0.046	0.049	0.026	0.058	0.048	0.024	0	0	329
Carrots, baby, raw	0.009	0.031	0.034	0.035	0.033	0.013	0.042	0.036	0.013	0	0	358

Carrots, raw	0.012	0.191	0.077	0.102	0.101	0.103	0.104	0.069	0.040	0	256
Cauliflower, raw	0.026	0.072	0.075	0.116	0.106	0.051	0.114	0.099	0.040	0	33
Celery, raw	0.009	0.020	0.021	0.032	0.027	0.009	0.029	0.027	0.012	0	283
Chard, Swiss, raw	0.017	0.083	0.147	0.130	0.099	0.019	0.110	0.110	0.036	0	11000
Corn, sweet, yellow, raw	0.023	0.129	0.129	0.348	0.137	0.093	0.273	0.185	0.089	0	644
Cucumber, peeled, raw	0.007	0.012	0.012	0.025	0.025	0.019	0.033	0.012	0.002	0	16
Cucumber, with peel, raw	0.005	0.019	0.021	0.029	0.029	0.010	0.030	0.022	0.010	0	23
Eggplant, raw	0.009	0.037	0.045	0.064	0.047	0.017	0.070	0.053	0.023	0	0
Garlic, raw	0.066	0.157	0.217	0.308	0.273	0.141	0.264	0.291	0.113	0	16
Kale, raw	0.040	0.147	0.197	0.231	0.197	0.076	0.286	0.181	0.069	0	39550
Leeks (bulb & lower leaf-portion), raw	0.012	0.063	0.052	0.096	0.078	0.043	0.096	0.056	0.025	0	1900
Lettuce, butterhead (includes boston & bibb types), raw	0.013	0.041	0.039	0.071	0.056	0.023	0.072	0.054	0.017	0	1223
Lettuce, cos or romaine, raw	0.010	0.043	0.045	0.076	0.064	0.021	0.090	0.055	0.021	0	2312
Lettuce, green leaf, raw	0.009	0.059	0.084	0.079	0.084	0.032	0.087	0.070	0.022	0	1730
Lettuce, iceberg (includes crisphead types), raw	0.009	0.025	0.018	0.025	0.024	0.010	0.030	0.024	0.009	0	277
Lettuce, red leaf, raw	0.022	0.048	0.038	0.070	0.045	0.025	0.096	0.048	0.019	0	1724
Mushrooms, brown, Italian or Crimini, raw	0.056	0.113	0.099	0.153	0.252	0.054	0.151	0.115	0.067	0	0

Mushrooms, enoki, raw	0	0	0.070	0.230	0.290	0.050	0.130	0.130	0.090	0.110	0.040
Mushrooms, Maitake, raw	0	0	0	0	0	0	0	0	0	0	0
Mushrooms, portabella, raw	0	0	0.043	0.154	0.098	0.030	0.062	0.080	0.049	0.068	0.031
Mushrooms, Shiitake, dried	0	0	0.159	0.486	0.809	0.375	0.343	0.679	0.405	0.497	0.031
Mushrooms, white, raw	0	0	0.057	0.232	0.129	0.043	0.107	0.120	0.076	0.107	0.035
Onions, raw	4	0	0.014	0.021	0.039	0.006	0.039	0.025	0.014	0.021	0.014
Onions, sweet, raw	6	0	0.011	0.020	0.036	0.018	0.033	0.025	0.014	0.018	0.009
Parsley, raw	5561	0	0.061	0.172	0.207	0.056	0.181	0.204	0.118	0.122	0.045
Peppers, sweet, green, raw	341	0	0.010	0.036	0.104	0.019	0.039	0.036	0.024	0.036	0.012
Peppers, sweet, red, raw	51	0	0.017	0.031	0.059	0.025	0.036	0.036	0.021	0.040	0.012
Peppers, sweet, yellow, raw	0	0	0.020	0.042	0.052	0.031	0.044	0.052	0.032	0.037	0.013
Potatoes, red, flesh & skin, raw	21	0	0.029	0.089	0.195	0.044	0.090	0.090	0.056	0.060	0.017
Potatoes, white, flesh & skin, raw	13	0	0.028	0.084	0.179	0.048	0.085	0.078	0.053	0.055	0.016
Radishes, raw	10	0	0.013	0.035	0.045	0.020	0.033	0.031	0.020	0.023	0.009
Spinach, raw	12198	0	0.064	0.161	0.237	0.088	0.174	0.223	0.147	0.122	0.039
Squash, summer, zucchini, includes skin, raw	2125	0	0.026	0.054	0.075	0.030	0.067	0.071	0.044	0.029	0.010
Squash, winter, butternut, raw		0	0.019	0.043	0.073	0.021	0.037	0.057	0.039	0.030	0.014
Soybean, mature seeds, sprouted, raw	0	0	0.348	0.620	1.118	0.295	0.752	0.938	0.580	0.503	0.159

Tomato, red, ripe, raw, year round average	0.006	0.027	0.018	0.025	0.027	0.015	0.081	0.018	0.014	0	123
Turnip greens, raw	0.026	0.082	0.078	0.137	0.098	0.051	0.150	0.102	0.036	0	12825
Waterchestnut, Chinese, (matai), raw	0	0	0	0	0	0	0	0	0	0	0
Fruits											
Apples, raw, with skin	0.001	0.006	0.006	0.013	0.012	0.002	0.007	0.012	0.005	0	29
Apples, raw, without skin	0.001	0.006	0.006	0.014	0.013	0.002	0.008	0.012	0.005	0	18
Applesauce, canned, unsweetened, without added ascorbic acid	0.002	0.006	0.006	0.010	0.010	0.004	0.008	0.008	0.003	0	18
Apricots, raw	0.015	0.047	0.041	0.077	0.097	0.009	0.081	0.047	0.027	0	89
Avocados, raw, all commercial varieties	0.025	0.073	0.084	0.143	0.132	0.065	0.281	0.107	0.049	0	271
Avocados, raw, California	0.025	0.072	0.083	0.141	0.129	0.064	0.276	0.105	0.048	0	271
Avocados, raw, Florida	0.028	0.082	0.094	0.160	0.147	0.073	0.314	0.120	0.055	0	0
Bananas, raw	0.009	0.028	0.028	0.068	0.050	0.017	0.058	0.047	0.077	0	22
Bananas, dehydrated, banana powder	0	0.171	0.167	0.359	0.162	0.137	0.322	0.282	0.333	0	84
Blackberries, raw	0	0	0	0	0	0	0	0	0	0	118
Blueberries, raw	0.003	0.020	0.023	0.044	0.013	0.020	0.035	0.031	0.011	0	80
Cranberries, raw	0.003	0.028	0.033	0.053	0.039	0.006	0.068	0.045	0.018	0	91
Elderberries, raw	0.013	0.027	0.027	0.060	0.026	0.029	0.091	0.033	0.015	0	0

Figs, raw	0.006	0.024	0.023	0.033	0.030	0.018	0.050	0.028	0.011	0	9
Grapefruit, raw, pink & red, all areas	0.008	0.013	0.008	0.015	0.019	0.015	0.054	0.015	0.008	0	5
Grapes, American style (slip skin), raw	0.003	0.017	0.005	0.013	0.014	0.031	0.024	0.017	0.023	0	72
Grapes, red & green, seedless, raw	0.011	0.022	0.011	0.022	0.027	0.019	0.020	0.022	0.022	0	72
Honeydew melons, raw	0.005	0.013	0.013	0.016	0.018	0.010	0.025	0.018	0.005	0	27
Lemon, raw, with peel	0	0	0	0	0	0	0	0	0	0	0
Limes, raw	0.003	0	0	0	0.014	0.002	0	0	0	0	0
Kiwi fruit (Chinese gooseberries), fresh, raw	0.015	0.047	0.051	0.066	0.061	0.055	0.078	0.057	0.027	0	122
Mangos, raw	0.008	0.019	0.018	0.031	0.041	0.005	0.027	0.026	0.012	0	0
Nectarine, raw	0.005	0.009	0.009	0.014	0.016	0.011	0.018	0.013	0.008	0	130
Oranges, raw, navels	0.009	0.018	0.017	0.028	0.038	0.019	0.066	0.026	0.013	0	129
Oranges, mandarin, tangerines, raw	0.002	0.016	0.017	0.028	0.032	0.004	0.033	0.021	0.011	0	138
Peaches, raw	0.010	0.016	0.017	0.027	0.030	0.022	0.033	0.022	0.013	0	91
Pears, raw	0.002	0.011	0.011	0.019	0.017	0.004	0.013	0.017	0.002	0	45
Persimmon, native, raw	0.014	0.041	0.035	0.058	0.045	0.025	0.059	0.042	0.016	0	0
Pineapple, raw, all varieties	0.005	0.019	0.019	0.024	0.026	0.026	0.040	0.024	0.010	0	0
Plums, raw	0.009	0.010	0.014	0.015	0.016	0.010	0.022	0.016	0.009	0	73
Raisins, seedless	0.050	0.077	0.057	0.096	0.084	0.040	0.152	0.083	0.072	0	0

Raspberries, raw	0	0	0	0	0	0	0	0	0	0	136
Strawberries, raw	0.008	0.020	0.016	0.034	0.026	0.008	0.041	0.019	0.012	0	26
Watermelon, raw	0.007	0.027	0.019	0.018	0.062	0.008	0.027	0.016	0.006	0	8
Apple juice, canned or bottled	0	0	0	0	0	0	0	0	0	0	16
Cranberry juice, cocktail, bottled	0	0	0	0	0	0	0	0	0	0	13
Grape juice drink, canned	0	0	0	0	0	0	0	0	0	0	19
Grapefruit juice, pink, raw	0	0	0	0	0	0	0	0	0	0	0
Grapefruit juice, white, raw	0	0	0	0	0	0	0	0	0	0	10
Lemon juice, raw	0	0	0	0	0	0	0	0	0	0	9
Lime juice, raw	0.002	0.002	0.002	0.016	0.016	0.014	0.013	0.011	0.002	0	0
Orange juice, raw	0.002	0.008	0.008	0.013	0.009	0.008	0.013	0.011	0.003	0	115
Prune juice, canned	0	0	0	0	0	0	0	0	0	0	40
Legumes											
Beans, black, mature seeds, raw	0.256	0.909	0.954	1.725	1.483	0.560	1.776	1.130	0.601	0	0
Beans, kidney, red mature seeds, raw	0.267	0.948	0.995	1.799	1.547	0.584	1.842	1.179	0.627	0	0
Beans, navy, mature seeds, raw	0.247	0.711	0.952	1.723	1.280	0.460	1.642	1.241	1.020	0	0
Beans, pink, mature seeds, raw	0.248	0.882	0.925	1.673	1.438	0.543	1.723	1.096	0.583	0	0
Beans, pinto, mature seeds, raw	0.237	0.810	0.871	1.558	1.356	0.446	1.522	0.998	0.556	0	0

Beans, pinto, mature seeds, cooked, boiled, with salt	0.098	0.350	0.368	0.664	0.571	0.216	0.684	0.435	0.232	0	0	0
Beans, snap, green, raw	0.019	0.079	0.066	0.112	0.088	0.040	0.109	0.090	0.034	0	0	640
Chickpeas (garbanzo beans), mature seeds, raw	0.185	0.716	0.828	1.374	1.291	0.512	1.513	0.809	0.531	0	0	0
Cowpeas, common, mature seeds, raw	0.290	0.895	0.956	1.820	1.591	0.595	2.133	1.121	0.730	0	0	0
Lentils, raw	0	0	0	0	0	0	0	0	0	0	0	0
Peas, split, mature seeds, raw	0.275	0.872	1.014	1.760	1.772	0.624	1.843	1.159	0.597	0	0	0
Soybeans, mature seeds, raw	0.591	1.766	1.971	3.309	2.706	1.202	3.661	2.029	1.097	0	0	0
Tofu, silken, firm (MURI-NU)	0.085	0.286	0.349	0.586	0.459	0.206	0.693	0.385	0.169	0	0	0
Tofu, silken, soft (MURI-NU)	0.068	0.215	0.233	0.279	0.341	0.146	0.496	0.295	0.117	0	0	0
Tofu, yogurt	0	0	0	0	0	0	0	0	0	0	0	0
Tofu, dried-frozen (koyatofu)	0.747	1.956	2.376	3.644	3.157	1.276	3.938	2.418	1.394	0	0	0
Tofu, dried-frozen (koyatofu), prepared with calcium sulfate	0.747	1.956	2.376	3.644	3.157	1.276	3.938	2.418	1.394	0	0	0
Tofu, fried	0.268	0.701	0.852	1.306	1.131	0.458	1.412	0.867	0.499	0	0	0
Tofu, fried, prepared with calcium sulfate	0.268	0.701	0.852	1.306	1.131	0.458	1.412	0.867	0.499	0	0	0
Tofu, hard, prepared with nigari	0.198	0.517	0.628	0.963	0.835	0.337	0.841	0.640	0.369	0	0	0

Tofu, regular, prepared with calcium sulfate	0.126	0.330	0.400	0.614	0.532	0.215	0.663	0.408	0.235	0	0
Tofu, salted and fermented (fuyu), prepared with calcium sulfate	0.127	0.332	0.404	0.619	0.537	0.217	0.670	0.411	0.237	0	
Cereal											
Buckwheat	0.192	0.506	0.498	0.832	0.672	0.401	0.761	0.678	0.309	0	0
Buckwheat flour, whole-groat	0.183	0.482	0.474	0.792	0.640	0.382	0.725	0.646	0.294	0	220
Cereals ready-to-eat, granola, home-made	0.196	0.540	0.586	1.050	0.643	0.545	1.173	0.753	0.390	0	137
Cereals ready-to-eat, bran flakes, single brand	0	0	0	0	0	0	0	0	0	0	0
Cereals ready-to-eat, bran, malted flour, single brand	0	0	0	0	0	0	0	0	0	0	0
Cereals ready-to-eat, corn & oat flour, puffed presweetened, single brand	0	0	0	0	0	0	0	0	0	0	721
Cereals ready-to-eat, GERNERAL MILLS, CHEERIOS	0.157	0.392	0.402	0.852	0.343	0.363	0.931	0.549	0.245	0	176
Cereals ready-to-eat, GERNERAL MILLS, Cinnamon Grahams	0	0	0	0	0	0	0	0	0	0	0
Cereals ready-to-eat, GERNERAL MILLS, FIBER ONE	0	0	0	0	0	0	0	0	0	0	782

Cereals ready-to-eat, GERNERAL MILLS, HARMONY	0	0	0	0	0	0	0	0	0	0	0	0
Cereals ready-to-eat, Malt-O-Meal, High Fiber Bran Flakes	0	0	0	0	0	0	0	0	0	0	0	0
Cereal, oats, instant, fortified, plain, dry	0.180	0.366	0.495	0.960	0.675	0.651	1.040	0.705	0.285	0	0	0
Cereals ready-to-eat, KELLOGG, KELLOGG'S Complete Wheat Bran Flakes	0	0	0	0	0	0	0	0	0	0	0	0
Cereals, Whole wheat hot, natural cereal, dry	0	0	0	0	0	0	0	0	0	0	0	227
Grain												
Barley, pearled, raw	0.165	0.337	0.362	0.673	0.369	0.409	0.840	0.486	0.223	0	0	160
Barley, pearled, cooked	0.038	0.077	0.083	0.154	0.084	0.093	0.192	0.111	0.051	0	0	56
Barley malt flour	0.132	0.407	0.361	0.746	0.535	0.451	0.566	0.503	0.275	0	0	160
Cocoa, dry powder, unsweetened	0.293	0.776	0.760	1.189	0.983	0.441	1.676	1.177	0.339	0	0	38
Cornmeal, whole-grain, white	0.057	0.305	0.291	0.996	0.228	0.316	0.729	0.411	0.248	0	0	5
Cornmeal, whole-grain, yellow	0.057	0.305	0.291	0.996	0.228	0.316	0.729	0.411	0.248	0	0	1355
Cornmeal, white (Navajo)	0.070	0.345	0.404	1.375	0.319	0.475	0.955	0.554	0.292	0	0	0
Cornmeal, yellow (Navajo)	0.050	0.307	0.370	1.275	0.301	0.414	0.793	0.494	0.265	0	0	0
Corn flour, whole-grain, white	0.049	0.261	0.248	0.850	0.195	0.270	0.622	0.351	0.211	0	0	5

Corn flour, whole-grain, yellow	0.049	0.261	0.248	0.850	0.195	0.270	0.622	0.351	0.211	0	0	1355
Corn, sweet, yellow, raw	0.023	0.129	0.129	0.348	0.137	0.093	0.273	0.185	0.089	0	0	644
Oat flour, partially debranned	0	0	0	0	0	0	0	0	0	0	0	180
Peanut flour, defatted	0.507	1.788	1.836	3.384	1.874	1.301	4.827	2.189	1.319	0	0	0
Peanut flour, low fat	0.328	1.158	1.188	2.191	1.213	0.848	3.126	1.418	0.854	0	0	0
Popcorn, air-popped	0.085	0.452	0.431	1.473	0.338	0.469	1.078	0.607	0.367	0	0	1450
Potato flour	0.115	0.280	0.299	0.425	0.413	0.177	0.540	0.356	0.166	0	0	0
Rice bran, crude	0.108	0.555	0.568	1.022	0.650	0.623	1.046	0.881	0.355	0	0	220
Rice flour, brown	0.092	0.265	0.306	0.598	0.276	0.251	0.644	0.424	0.184	0	0	0
Rice flour, white	0.072	0.210	0.244	0.488	0.207	0.251	0.631	0.348	0.149	0	0	0
Rice noodles, cooked	0.011	0.033	0.039	0.075	0.033	0.040	0.079	0.056	0.021	0	0	0
Rice noodles, dry	0.040	0.123	0.149	0.284	0.124	0.152	0.299	0.210	0.081	0	0	0
Rice, brown, long-grain, cooked	0.033	0.095	0.109	0.214	0.099	0.089	0.230	0.11	0.066	0	0	0
Rice, brown, long-grain, raw	0.101	0.291	0.336	0.657	0.303	0.275	0.708	0.466	0.202	0	0	0
Rice, brown, medium-grain, cooked	0.030	0.085	0.098	0.191	0.088	0.080	0.206	0.136	0.059	0	0	0
Rice, brown, medium-grain, raw	0.096	0.275	0.318	0.620	0.286	0.230	0.668	0.440	0.190	0	0	0
Rice, white, long-grain, regular, cooked	0.031	0.096	0.116	0.222	0.097	0.118	0.234	0.164	0.063	0	0	0
Rice, white, long-grain, regular, raw, unenriched	0.083	0.255	0.308	0.589	0.258	0.314	0.619	0.435	0.168	0	0	0

Rice, white, medium-grain, cooked	0.028	0.085	0.103	0.197	0.086	0.105	0.207	0.145	0	0.056	0	0
Rice, white, medium-grain, raw	0.077	0.236	0.285	0.546	0.239	0.290	0.574	0.403	0	0.155	0	0
Rice, white, short-grain, cooked	0.027	0.084	0.102	0.195	0.085	0.104	0.185	0.144	0	0.056	0	0
Rice, white, short-grain, raw	0.075	0.233	0.281	0.538	0.235	0.286	0.565	0.397	0	0.153	0	0
Rye flour, dark	0.159	0.486	0.541	0.970	0.486	0.486	0.987	0.703	0	0.313	0	210
Rye flour, light	0.095	0.291	0.324	0.580	0.291	0.290	0.589	0.420	0	0.187	0	210
Rye flour, medium	0.106	0.325	0.362	0.649	0.325	0.325	0.660	0.470	0	0.209	0	210
Seeds, cottonseed flour, low fat (glandless)	0.752	1.843	1.796	3.404	2.529	2.116	4.899	2.557	0	1.570	0	0
Seeds, sesame flour, high fat	0.674	1.278	1.342	2.358	0.987	1.637	2.921	1.719	0	0.906	0	0
Seeds, sesame flour, low fat	1.097	2.081	2.157	3.841	1.608	2.668	4.758	2.800	0	1.476	0	0
Seeds, sunflower flour, partially defatted	0.735	1.959	2.403	3.500	1.977	1.995	3.872	2.775	0	1.333	0	0
Soy flour, full-fat, raw	0.502	1.500	1.675	2.812	2.298	1.022	3.108	1.724	0	0.931	0	0
Wheat flour, white, all-purpose, enriched bleached	0.127	0.281	0.357	0.710	0.228	0.402	0.832	0.415	0	0.230	0	18
Wheat flour, white, all-purpose, enriched unbleached	0.127	0.281	0.357	0.710	0.228	0.402	0.832	0.415	0	0.230	0	79
Wheat flour, white, all-purpose, self-rising, enriched	0.121	0.269	0.342	0.680	0.219	0.385	0.796	0.397	0	0.220	0	18
Wheat flour, whole-grain	0.212	0.395	0.508	0.926	0.378	0.529	1.046	0.618	0	0.317	0	220

Bread

Bread, cracked-wheat	0.112	0.261	0.338	0.606	0.244	0.338	0.672	0.387	0.193	0	0	0
Bread, egg	0.112	0.306	0.394	0.692	0.311	0.397	0.767	0.443	0.210	0.001	0.012	45
Bread, French or Vienna (includes sour-dough)	0.121	0.284	0.374	0.686	0.295	0.387	0.677	0.428	0.211	0	0	12
Bread, Italian	0.103	0.245	0.333	0.614	0.197	0.349	0.681	0.376	0.188	0	0	48
Bread, oat bran	0.131	0.299	0.399	0.733	0.297	0.413	0.842	0.461	0.225	0	0	46
Bread, oatmeal	0.116	0.247	0.325	0.608	0.270	0.360	0.677	0.393	0.186	0	0	72
Bread, pumpernickel	0.097	0.267	0.334	0.602	0.248	0.345	0.660	0.396	0.196	0	0	46
Bread, raisin	0.083	0.222	0.287	0.516	0.200	0.280	0.565	0.329	0.167	0	0	0
Bread, rye	0.096	0.255	0.319	0.579	0.233	0.312	0.624	0.379	0.182	0	0	54
Bread, wheat	0.078	0.172	0.217	0.388	0.181	0.208	0.403	0.260	0.126	0	0	44
Bread, white, commercially prepared (includes soft bread crumbs)	0.089	0.225	0.298	0.533	0.203	0.297	0.593	0.335	0.165	0	0	44

Dairy

Milk, buttermilk, dried	0.484	1.548	2.075	3.360	2.720	1.177	3.302	2.296	0.930	0	0	0
Milk, buttermilk, fluid, cultured, low fat	0.036	0.158	0.204	0.329	0.277	0.112	0.313	0.243	0.095	0	0	0
Milk, chocolate, fluid, reduced fat	0.045	0.140	0.140	0.275	0.230	0.100	0.260	0.180	0.080	0	0	0
Milk, chocolate, fluid, whole	0.045	0.143	0.192	0.311	0.251	0.108	0.306	0.212	0.086	0	0	0

Milk, dry, whole	0.371	1.188	1.592	2.578	2.087	0.903	2.541	1.762	0.714	0	0	0
Milk, goat, fluid	0.044	0.163	0.207	0.314	0.290	0.126	0.334	0.240	0.089	0	0	0
Milk, human, mature, fluid	0.017	0.046	0.056	0.095	0.068	0.040	0.099	0.063	0.023	0	0	0
Milk, fluid, 1% milkfat, with added vitamin A	0.040	0.089	0.187	0.375	0.287	0.199	0.309	0.217	0.084	0	0	0
Milk, fluid, nonfat (fat free or skim)	0.048	0.154	0.206	0.334	0.270	0.118	0.330	0.228	0.092	0	0	0
Milk, producer, fluid, 3.7% milkfat	0.046	0.148	0.198	0.321	0.260	0.112	0.316	0.220	0.089	0	0	0
Milk, fluid, 2% milkfat, with added vitamin A	0.040	0.103	0.183	0.331	0.233	0.190	0.315	0.218	0.073	0	0	0
Milk, sheep, fluid	0.084	0.268	0.338	0.587	0.513	0.190	0.565	0.448	0.167	0	0	0
Milk, whole, 3.25% milkfat	0.075	0.143	0.165	0.265	0.140	0.092	0.299	0.192	0.075	0	0	0
Egg												
Egg, duck, whole, fresh, raw	0.260	0.735	0.598	1.097	0.951	0.861	1.453	0.885	0.320	0	0	459
Egg, goose, whole, fresh, raw	0.282	0.797	0.647	1.188	1.030	0.933	1.574	0.958	0.346	0	0	442
Egg, quail, whole, fresh, raw	0.209	0.641	0.816	1.146	0.881	0.732	1.280	0.940	0.315	0	0	369
Egg, turkey, whole, fresh, raw	0.219	0.672	0.855	1.201	0.924	0.768	1.342	0.985	0.330	0	0	0
Egg, white, raw, fresh	0.125	0.449	0.661	1.016	0.806	0.686	1.143	0.809	0.290	0	0	0
Egg, whole, cooked, fried	0.180	0.601	0.726	1.174	0.986	0.704	1.274	0.928	0.334	0.004	0.040	358
Egg, whole, cooked, hard-boiled	0.153	0.604	0.686	1.075	0.904	0.684	1.181	0.767	0.298	0.005	0.038	353

Egg, whole, cooked, omelet	0.140	0.468	0.565	0.915	0.768	0.549	0.992	0.723	0.260	0.003	0.031	279
Egg, whole, cooked, poached	0.166	0.554	0.670	1.083	0.910	0.650	1.176	0.856	0.308	0.004	0.037	330
Egg, whole, cooked, scrambled	0.136	0.528	0.608	0.854	0.800	0.585	1.060	0.678	0.264	0.003	0.030	245
Egg, whole, raw, fresh	0.167	0.556	0.672	1.088	0.914	0.652	1.181	0.859	0.309	0.004	0.037	331
Egg, yolk, raw, fresh	0.177	0.687	0.866	1.399	1.217	0.642	1.259	0.949	0.416	0.011	0.114	1094
Cheese												
Cheese, America cheddar, imitation	0	0	0	0	0	0	0	0	0	0	0	0
Cheese, blue	0.312	0.785	1.124	1.919	1.852	0.691	2.382	1.556	0.758	0	0	0
Cheese, brick	0.324	0.882	1.137	2.244	2.124	0.696	2.346	1.472	0.823	0	0	0
Cheese, brie	0.322	0.751	1.015	1.929	1.851	0.706	2.358	1.340	0.716	0	0	0
Cheese, camembert	0.307	0.717	0.968	1.840	1.766	0.675	2.250	1.279	0.683	0	0	0
Cheese, caraway	0.324	0.896	1.563	2.412	2.095	0.785	2.542	1.682	0.884	0	0	0
Cheese, cheddar	0.320	0.886	1.546	2.385	2.072	0.777	2.513	1.663	0.874	0	0	0
Cheese, cheshire	0.300	0.832	1.451	2.238	1.945	0.729	2.359	1.560	0.821	0	0	0
Cheese, Colby	0.305	0.845	1.475	2.275	1.978	0.741	2.398	1.586	0.834	0	0	0
Cheese, cottage, 1% milkfat	0.138	0.550	0.728	1.274	1.002	0.488	1.328	0.767	0.412	0	0	0
Cheese, cottage, 2% milkfat	0.153	0.609	0.808	1.413	1.111	0.540	1.473	0.851	0.457	0	0	0
Cheese, cream, fat free	0	0	0	0	0	0	0	0	0	0	0	0
Cheese, edam	0.352	0.932	1.308	2.570	2.660	0.976	2.891	1.810	1.034	0	0	0

Cheese, feta	0.200	0.637	0.803	1.395	1.219	0.451	1.343	1.065	0.397	0	0
Cheese, Mexican, blend, reduced fat	0	0	0	0	0	0	0	0	0	0	0
Cheese, Mexican, queso anejo	0.215	0.731	1.054	2.017	1.452	0.625	2.309	1.338	0.679	0	0
Cheese, Monterey	0.315	0.871	1.519	2.344	2.037	0.763	2.471	1.635	0.859	0	0
Cheese, Monterey, low fat	0	0	0	0	0	0	0	0	0	0	0
Cheese, Mozzarella, part skim	0.339	0.924	1.164	2.365	2.464	0.821	2.669	1.517	0.913	0	0
Cheese, muenster	0.327	0.888	1.145	2.260	2.139	0.681	2.363	1.482	0.829	0	0
Cheese, parmesan, hard	0.482	1.317	1.894	3.452	3.306	1.193	3.917	2.454	1.384	0	0
Cheese, provolone, reduced fat	0.345	0.982	1.091	2.297	2.646	0.802	2.807	1.640	1.115	0	0
Cheese, Ricotta, part skim	0.127	0.523	0.596	1.235	1.353	0.384	1.152	0.700	0.464	0	0
Cheese, Swiss	0.401	1.038	1.537	2.959	2.585	0.874	3.355	2.139	1.065	0	0
Cheese, tilsit	0.352	0.899	1.484	2.548	2.039	0.892	2.816	1.752	0.704	0	0
Nuts and Seeds											
Nuts, acorns, raw	0.074	0.236	0.285	0.489	0.384	0.212	0.456	0.345	0.170	0	0
Nuts, almonds	0.214	0.598	0.702	1.488	0.580	0.340	1.572	0.817	0.557	0	1
Nuts, cashew nuts, raw	0.287	0.688	0.789	1.472	0.928	0.755	1.459	1.094	0.456	0	22
Nuts, chestnuts, Chinese, raw	0.049	0.167	0.157	0.259	0.228	0.211	0.315	0.220	0.121	0	0
Nuts, chestnuts, European, raw	0.027	0.086	0.095	0.143	0.143	0.134	0.169	0.135	0.067	0	0
Nuts, chestnuts, Japanese, raw	0.032	0.090	0.111	0.139	0.147	0.119	0.153	0.134	0.056	0	0

Nuts, coconut meat, raw	0.039	0.121	0.131	0.247	0.147	0.128	0.272	0.202	0.077	0	0	0
Nuts, ginkgo nuts, raw	0.071	0.268	0.209	0.316	0.206	0.078	0.232	0.283	0.102	0	0	0
Nuts, hazelnuts or filberts	0.193	0.497	0.545	1.063	0.420	0.498	1.025	0.701	0.432	0	0	92
Nuts, macadamia nuts, dry roasted, without salt added	0.066	0.364	0.309	0.592	0.018	0.028	1.154	0.357	0.192	0	0	0
Nuts, macadamia nuts, raw	0.067	0.370	0.314	0.602	0.018	0.029	1.176	0.363	0.195	0	0	0
Nuts, mixed nuts /w peanuts, dry roasted, with salt added	0.264	0.597	0.744	1.371	0.712	0.515	1.629	0.934	0.480	0	0	21
Nuts, mixed nuts /w peanuts, dry roasted, without salt added	0.264	0.597	0.744	1.371	0.712	0.515	1.629	0.934	0.480	0	0	0
Nuts, mixed nuts /w peanuts, oil roasted, with salt added	0.247	0.569	0.724	1.344	0.658	0.632	1.575	0.936	0.471	0	0	10
Nuts, pecans	0.093	0.306	0.336	0.598	0.287	0.335	0.641	0.411	0.262	0	0	17
Nuts, pine nuts, dried	0.107	0.370	0.542	0.991	0.540	0.548	1.033	0.687	0.341	0	0	9
Nuts, pistachio nuts, raw	0.273	0.673	0.900	1.554	1.151	0.695	1.477	1.239	0.507	0	0	0
Nuts, walnuts, English	0.170	0.596	0.625	1.170	0.424	0.444	1.117	0.753	0.391	0	0	9
Seeds, breadfruit seeds, raw	0.123	0.385	0.443	0.563	0.570	0.212	1.341	0.535	0.207	0	0	0
Seeds, breadnuttree seeds, dried	0.234	0.335	0.488	0.935	0.376	0.185	1.041	0.834	0.132	0	0	0
Seeds, breadnuttree seeds, raw	0.162	0.232	0.338	0.647	0.260	0.128	0.721	0.578	0.091	0	0	0
Seeds, flaxseed	0.297	0.766	0.896	1.235	0.862	0.710	1.450	1.072	0.472	0	0	651

Seeds, lotus seeds, dried	0.221	0.747	0.765	1.215	0.985	0.468	1.142	0.991	0.430	0	0	0
Seeds, pumpkin & squash seed kernels, dried	0.431	0.903	1.246	2.079	1.833	0.852	2.241	1.972	0.681	0	0	0
Seeds, sesame seeds, whole, dried	0.388	0.736	0.763	1.358	0.569	0.944	1.683	0.990	0.522	0	0	0
Seeds, sunflower kernels, dried	0.348	0.928	1.139	1.659	0.937	0.945	1.835	1.315	0.632	0	0	0
Seeds, watermelon seed kernels, dried	0.390	1.112	1.342	2.149	0.887	1.272	3.047	1.556	0.775	0	0	0
Fish and Shellfish												
Fish, anchovy, European, raw	0.228	0.892	0.938	1.654	1.869	0.820	1.481	1.048	0.599	0.538	0.911	0
Fish, bass, striped, raw	0.199	0.777	0.817	1.441	1.628	0.715	1.291	0.914	0.522	0.169	0.585	0
Fish, bluefish, raw	0.224	0.878	0.923	1.629	1.840	0.608	1.458	1.032	0.590	0.252	0.519	0
Fish, butterfish, raw	0.194	0.758	0.796	1.405	1.587	0.697	1.258	0.890	0.509	0	0	0
Fish, catfish, channel, farmed, raw	0.174	0.682	0.717	1.264	1.429	0.627	1.132	0.801	0.458	0.067	0.207	0
Fish, catfish, channel, wild, raw	0.183	0.718	0.755	1.331	1.504	0.661	1.192	0.844	0.482	0.130	0.234	0
Fish, cod, Atlantic, raw	0.199	0.781	0.821	1.447	1.635	0.718	1.296	0.917	0.524	0.064	0.120	0
Fish, cod, Pacific, raw	0.200	0.785	0.825	1.455	1.644	0.722	1.303	0.922	0.527	0.080	0.135	0
Crustaceans, crab, Alaska king, raw	0.255	0.741	0.887	1.452	1.592	0.720	1.382	0.861	0.372	0	0	0
Crustaceans, crab, blue, raw	0.251	0.731	0.875	1.433	1.572	0.710	1.364	0.849	0.367	0.170	0.150	0
Crustaceans, crab, queen, raw	0.258	0.749	0.897	1.468	1.610	0.728	1.387	0.870	0.376	0.259	0.113	0
Fish, drum, freshwater, raw	0.196	0.769	0.808	1.425	1.611	0.707	1.277	0.904	0.516	0.230	0.287	0

Fish, haddock, raw	0.212	0.829	0.871	1.537	1.736	0.763	1.376	0.974	0.557	0.059	0.126	0
Fish, halibut, Atlantic & Pacific, raw	0.233	0.912	0.959	1.692	1.911	0.839	1.516	1.072	0.613	0.071	0.292	0
Fish, halibut, Greenland, raw	0.161	0.630	0.662	1.168	1.320	0.579	1.046	0.740	0.423	0.526	0.393	0
Fish, herring, Atlantic, raw	0.201	0.787	0.828	1.460	1.650	0.725	1.307	0.925	0.529	0.709	0.862	0
Fish, herring, Pacific, raw	0.184	0.719	0.755	1.332	1.506	0.671	1.193	0.845	0.483	0.969	0.689	0
Crustaceans, lobster, northern, raw	0.262	0.761	0.911	1.492	1.636	0.740	1.420	0.884	0.382	0	0	0
Fish, mackerel, Atlantic, raw	0.208	0.815	0.857	1.512	1.708	0.750	1.354	0.958	0.548	0.898	1.401	0
Fish, mackerel, king, raw	0.227	0.889	0.935	1.648	1.863	0.817	1.477	1.045	0.597	0.136	0.177	0
Fish, mackerel, Spanish, raw	0.216	0.846	0.889	1.568	1.771	0.778	1.404	0.994	0.568	0.329	1.012	0
Fish, monkfish, raw	0.162	0.635	0.667	1.177	1.330	0.584	1.054	0.746	0.426	0	0	0
Fish, mullet, striped, raw	0.217	0.848	0.892	1.573	1.777	0.780	1.408	0.997	0.570	0.217	0.108	0
Fish, ocean perch, Atlantic, raw	0.209	0.817	0.858	1.514	1.711	0.751	1.356	0.960	0.548	0.080	0.211	0
Fish, pike, walleye, raw	0.214	0.839	0.882	1.555	1.758	0.771	1.393	0.986	0.563	0.086	0.225	0
Fish, pollock, Atlantic, raw	0.218	0.852	0.896	1.580	1.786	0.784	1.415	1.002	0.572	0.071	0.350	0
Fish, pollock, walleye, raw	0.192	0.753	0.792	1.396	1.578	0.693	1.251	0.885	0.506	0.150	0.222	0
Fish, roe, mixed species, raw	0.293	1.017	1.142	1.956	1.699	0.952	2.213	1.307	0.607	0.983	1.363	0
Fish, sablefish, raw	0.150	0.588	0.618	1.090	1.232	0.541	0.977	0.691	0.395	0.677	0.718	0
Fish, salmon, Atlantic, farmed, raw	0.223	0.872	0.917	1.617	1.828	0.802	1.449	1.025	0.586	0.618	1.293	0
Fish, salmon, Atlantic, wild, raw	0.222	0.870	0.914	1.613	1.822	0.800	1.445	1.022	0.584	0.321	1.115	0

Fish, salmon, chinook, raw	0.225	0.879	0.924	1.630	1.842	0.809	1.460	1.033	0.590	1.008	0.944	0
Fish, salmon, coho, wild, raw	0.242	0.948	0.996	1.757	1.985	0.872	1.574	1.114	0.636	0.429	0.656	0
Fish, salmon, pink, raw	0.223	0.874	0.919	1.621	1.831	0.804	1.451	1.027	0.587	0.419	0.586	0
Fish, sardine, Pacific, canned in tomato sauce, drained solids with bone	0.157	0.795	0.795	1.358	1.400	0.615	1.418	0.926	0.680	0.532	0.865	0
Fish, shad, America, raw	0.190	0.742	0.780	1.376	1.555	0.683	1.233	0.872	0.498	1.086	1.321	0
Fish, shark, mixed species, raw	0.235	0.920	0.967	1.705	1.926	0.846	1.527	1.081	0.618	0.316	0.527	0
Crustaceans, shrimp, mixed species, raw	0.283	0.822	0.985	1.612	1.768	0.800	1.534	0.956	0.413	0.258	0.222	0
Fish, swordfish, raw	0.222	0.868	0.912	1.609	1.818	0.798	1.441	1.020	0.583	0.108	0.531	0
Fish, tuna, fresh, bluefin, raw	0.261	1.023	1.075	1.896	2.142	0.940	1.698	1.202	0.687	0.283	0.890	0
Fish, wolffish, Atlantic, raw	0.196	0.767	0.806	1.422	1.607	0.706	1.274	0.902	0.515	0.307	0.316	0
Meat and Poultry												
Beef, bottom sirloin, tri-tip, separable lean only, trimmed to 0" fat, select, raw	0.140	0.853	0.971	1.698	1.804	0.831	1.523	1.059	0.681	0	0	0
Beef, brisket, flat half, separable lean and fat, trimmed to 1/8" fat, all grades, raw	0.127	0.769	0.876	1.531	1.627	0.749	1.373	0.955	0.614	0	0	0
Beef, brisket, point half, separable lean and fat, trimmed to 1/4" fat, all grades, raw	0.181	0.704	0.725	1.274	1.341	0.594	1.171	0.784	0.552	0	0	0

Beef, chuck, clod steak, separable lean only, trimmed to 1/4" fat, all grades, raw	0.228	0.977	1.091	1.868	1.983	1.826	1.691	1.143	0.681	0	0	0
Beef, flank, separable lean only, trimmed to 0" fat, all grades, raw	0.142	0.862	0.982	1.716	1.823	0.840	1.539	1.070	0.689	0	0	0
Beef, ground, 70% lean meat / 30% fat, raw	0.049	0.533	0.645	1.119	1.174	0.491	0.999	0.709	0.442	0	0	0
Beef, rib, shortribs, separable lean only, choice, raw	0.213	0.832	0.856	1.506	1.585	0.701	1.384	0.927	0.652	0	0	0
Beef, round, bottom round, separable lean only, trimmed to 1/2" fat, prime, raw	0.245	0.955	0.983	1.729	1.819	0.805	1.589	1.064	0.749	0	0	0
Beef, tenderloin, separable lean only, trimmed to 1/4" fat, prime, raw	0.233	0.908	0.934	1.643	1.729	0.765	1.509	1.011	0.712	0	0	0
Beef, brain, raw	0	0	0	0	0	0	0	0	0	0	0.851	0
Beef, heart, raw	0	0	0	0	0	0	0	0	0	0	0	0
Beef, kidneys, raw	0	0	0	0	0	0	0	0	0	0	0	0
Beef, liver, raw	0.263	0.869	0.967	1.910	1.607	0.919	1.891	1.260	0.629	0	0	0
Beef, lung, raw	0.148	0.604	0.772	1.190	1.148	0.573	1.023	0.798	0.492	0	0	0
Beef, spleen, raw	0.190	0.720	0.706	1.616	1.323	0.867	1.256	1.101	0.656	0	0	0
Pork, boneless loin, fresh	0	0	0	0	0	0	0	0	0	0	0	0

Pork, center cut chops, fresh	0	0	0	0	0	0	0	0	0	0	0	0	0	0
Pork, cured, bacon, raw	0.097	0.454	0.544	0.903	0.962	0.387	0.823	0.617	0	0	0	0	0	0
Pork, cured, patties, grilled	0.155	0.592	0.581	1.051	1.130	0.530	1.000	0.579	0.485	0	0	0	0	0
Pork, fresh, backfat, raw	0.037	0.133	0.137	0.234	0.263	0.114	0.219	0.158	0.117	0	0	0	0	0
Pork, fresh, backribs, separable lean and fat, raw	0.205	0.736	0.755	1.293	1.450	0.633	1.205	0.875	0.644	0	0	0	0	0
Pork, fresh, belly, raw	0	0	0	0	0	0	0	0	0	0	0	0	0	0
Pork, fresh, loin, tenderloin, separable lean only, raw	0.220	0.940	1.031	1.784	1.943	0.819	1.678	1.095	0.905	0	0	0	0	0
Pork, fresh, ground, raw	0.214	0.771	0.790	1.354	1.518	0.662	1.262	0.916	0.674	0	0	0	0	0
Pork, fresh, leg(ham), whole, separable lean and fat, raw	0.208	0.776	0.787	1.376	1.550	0.660	1.272	0.931	0.659	0	0	0	0	0
Pork, flesh, loin, country-style ribs, separable lean only, raw	0.204	0.868	0.952	1.648	1.794	0.756	1.549	1.011	0.836	0	0	0	0	0
Pork, flesh, separable fat, raw	0.061	0.261	0.286	0.496	0.540	0.227	0.466	0.304	0.251	0	0	0	0	0
Pork, flesh, shoulder, arm picnic, separable lean only, raw	0.251	0.902	0.925	1.585	1.776	0.775	1.456	1.071	0.789	0	0	0	0	0
Pork, flesh, brain , raw	0.132	0.480	0.475	0.896	0.204	0.523	0.586	0.586	0.276	0.220	0.450	0	0	0
Pork, flesh, feet, raw	0	0	0	0	0	0	0	0	0	0	0	0	0	0
Pork, flesh, heart, raw	0.199	0.757	0.831	1.558	1.428	0.751	1.353	0.914	0.439	0	0	0	0	0

Pork, flesh, kidneys, raw	0.213	0.682	0.879	1.477	1.185	0.714	1.369	0.948	0.395	0	0	0
Pork, flesh, liver, raw	0.301	0.910	1.085	1.906	1.649	0.934	1.776	1.321	0.582	0	0.020	0
Pork, flesh, lung, raw	0.124	0.496	0.563	1.093	1.027	0.449	0.984	0.838	0.356	0.010	0.010	0
Pork, fresh, spleen, raw	0.183	0.714	0.797	1.460	1.334	0.560	1.263	0.971	0.426	0	0	0
Pork, fresh, stomach, raw	0	0	0	0	0	0	0	0	0	0	0	0
Chicken breast tender, raw	0.184	0.557	0.603	1.019	0.988	0.467	0.856	0.659	0.435	0	0	0
Chicken patty, frozen, raw	0.178	0.542	0.586	0.991	0.961	0.454	0.832	0.641	0.423	0	0	0
Chicken, broiler or fryer, back, meat only, raw	0.228	0.826	1.033	1.467	1.661	0.791	1.436	0.970	0.607	0.020	0.060	0
Chicken, broiler or fryer, breast, meat & skin, raw	0.237	0.869	1.063	1.537	1.725	0.837	1.500	1.020	0.625	0.010	0.020	0
Chicken, broiler or fryer, leg, meat & skin, raw	0.204	0.752	0.911	1.325	1.484	0.726	1.295	0.883	0.536	0.010	0.030	0
Chicken, broiler or fryer, leg, meat only, raw	0.235	0.850	1.063	1.511	1.710	0.815	1.479	0.999	0.625	0.010	0.040	0
Chicken, broiler or fryer, light meat, meat & skin, raw	0.227	0.839	1.015	1.477	1.654	0.811	1.443	0.985	0.597	0.010	0.020	0
Chicken, heart, all classes, raw	0.199	0.704	0.833	1.355	1.303	0.587	1.253	0.880	0.408	0	0	0
Chicken, liver, all classes, raw	0.176	0.725	0.813	1.512	1.332	0.704	1.477	0.998	0.507	0	0	0
Chicken, roasting, meat & skin, raw	0.190	0.706	0.851	1.244	1.390	0.684	1.215	0.831	0.501	0.010	0.030	0

Chicken, roasting, meat only, raw	0.237	0.859	1.073	1.526	1.727	0.823	1.493	1.008	0.631	0.010	0.030	0
Chicken, wing, frozen, glazed, barbecue flavored	0.180	0.743	0.745	1.278	1.352	0.598	1.219	0.809	0.462	0	0.010	0
Lamb, domestic, shoulder, arm, separable lean & fat, trimmed to 1/4" fat, raw	0.196	0.719	0.810	1.306	1.483	0.631	1.247	0.906	0.532	0	0	0
Lamb, ground, raw	0.193	0.709	0.799	1.288	1.462	0.623	1.230	0.893	0.524	0	0	0
Lamb, New Zealand, frozen, shoulder, whole, separable lean & fat, trimmed to 1/8" fat, raw	0.201	0.736	0.829	1.337	1.518	0.646	1.278	0.927	0.544	0	0	0
Lamb, brain, raw	0.107	0.466	0.414	0.813	0.667	0.315	0.881	0.495	0.276	0	0.490	0
Lamb, heart, raw	0.178	0.777	0.714	1.401	1.240	0.499	1.225	0.819	0.377	0.040	0.030	0
Lamb, kidneys, raw	0.212	0.741	0.626	1.181	1.020	0.498	1.284	0.923	0.396	0.050	0.030	0
Lamb, liver, raw	0.236	0.882	0.878	1.665	1.102	0.656	1.637	1.122	0.479	0	0	0
Lamb, lungs, raw	0.171	0.614	0.527	1.337	1.080	0.563	1.159	0.920	0.420	0	0	0
Lamb, spleen, raw	0.190	0.702	1.090	1.530	1.332	0.557	1.283	1.123	0.572	0	0	0
Turkey, dark meat, raw	0.228	0.893	1.044	1.600	1.892	0.790	1.589	1.067	0.626	0	0.030	0
Turkey, leg, meat & skin, raw	0.219	0.861	0.998	1.537	1.809	0.766	1.526	1.028	0.598	0	0.030	0
Turkey, light meat, raw	0.268	1.048	1.225	1.877	2.220	0.927	1.866	1.251	0.735	0	0.020	0
Turkey, meat & skin, raw	0.226	0.891	1.024	1.587	1.857	0.798	1.574	1.063	0.614	0	0.020	0
Turkey, wing, meat & skin, raw	0.217	0.866	0.975	1.531	1.773	0.785	1.514	1.031	0.585	0	0.010	0

Oil													
Avocado oil	0	0	0	0	0	0	0	0	0	0	0	0	0
Canola oil	0	0	0	0	0	0	0	0	0	0	0	0	0
Coconut oil	0	0	0	0	0	0	0	0	0	0	0	0	0
Corn oil	0	0	0	0	0	0	0	0	0	0	0	0	0
Cottonseed oil	0	0	0	0	0	0	0	0	0	0	0	0	0
Flaxseed oil	0	0	0	0	0	0	0	0	0	0	0	0	0
Grapeseed oil	0	0	0	0	0	0	0	0	0	0	0	0	0
Olive oil	0	0	0	0	0	0	0	0	0	0	0	0	0
Palm oil	0	0	0	0	0	0	0	0	0	0	0	0	0
Palm kernel oil	0	0	0	0	0	0	0	0	0	0	0	0	0
Peanut oil	0	0	0	0	0	0	0	0	0	0	0	0	0
Safflower oil, linoleic (>70%)	0	0	0	0	0	0	0	0	0	0	0	0	0
Safflower oil, oleic (>70%)	0	0	0	0	0	0	0	0	0	0	0	0	0
Sesame oil	0	0	0	0	0	0	0	0	0	0	0	0	0
Sunflower oil, high oleic (>70%)	0	0	0	0	0	0	0	0	0	0	0	0	0
Sunflower oil, linoleic (~65%)	0	0	0	0	0	0	0	0	0	0	0	0	0

Note: *(1) W = Tryptophan, T = Threonine, I = Isoleucine, L = Leucine, K = Lysine, M = Methionie, C = Cysteine, F = Phenylalanine, Y = Tyrosine, V = Valine, H = Histidine, EPA = Eicosapentaenoic acid, DHA = Docosahexaenoic acid. (2) All data are taken from SR Search 20 database – 2008 published by the U.S. department of Agriculture.*

References

Introduction

Pizzorno, J. *Total wellness: improving your health by understanding the body's healing systems.* Rocklin, California: Prima Publishing, 1996.

Chapter One

Allen L.H. 2002. Iron supplements: scientific issues concerning efficacy and implications for research and programs. *J. Nutr.* 32: 813S–839S.

Anderson J.B. 1996. Calcium, phosphorus, and human bone development. *J. Nutr.* 126: 1153–1157.

Anderson R.A., Kozlovsky A.S. 1985. Chromium intake, absorption, and exretion of subjects consuming self-selected diets. *Am., J., Clin. Nutr.* 41: 1177–1183.

Bhaskaram P. 2001. Immunobiology of mild micronutrient deficiencies. *Br. J. Nutr.* 85: S75–80.

Bible, NIV—New International Version. Grand Rapids, Michigan: Zondervan Publishing, 2007.

Bogden J., Louria D. 1999. Aging and the immune system: role of micronutrient nutrition. *Nutrition* 15: 593–562.

Brody T. *Nutritional Biochemistry*, San Diego: Academic Press, 1999.

Brown R.O., et al. 1986. Chromium deficiency after long-term total parenteral nutrition. *Dig. Dis. Sci.* 31: 661–664.

Casey C.E., Neville M.C. 1987. Studies in human lactation 3: molybdenum and nickel in human milk during the first month of lactation. *Am. J. Clin. Nutr.* 45: 921–926.

Cordano A. 1998. Clinical manifestations of nutritional copper deficiency in infants and children. *Am. J. Clin. Nutr.* 67(suppl.): 1012S–1016S.

Cotzias G.C., Miller S.T., et al. 1976. Interaction between manganese and brain dopamine. *Med. Clin. N. Am.* 60: 729–738.

Emsley J. *The elements*, 3rd ed. Oxford: Clarendon Press, 1998.

Forbes R.M. 1945. The composition of the adult human body as determined by chemical analysis. *J. Biol. Chem.* 166: 359–366.

Grant A.M., et al. 2005. Oral vitamin D_3 and calcium for secondary prevention of low-trauma fractures in elderly people (randomized evaluation of calcium or vitamin D, RECORD): a randomized placebo-controlled trial, *Lancet* 365(9471): 1621–1628.

Greenwood N.N., Earnshaw A. *Chemistry of the elements*, 2nd Edition. Oxford: Butterworth-Heinemann, 1997.

Haas J.D., Brownlie T. 2001. 4th iron deficiency and reduced work capacity: a critical review of the research to determine a causal relationship. *J. Nutr.* 131: 691S–696S.

Institute of Medicine, Food and Nutrition Board. *Dietary reference intakes for vitamin A, vitamin K, arsenic, boron, chromium, copper, iodine, iron, manganese, molybdenum, nickel, silicon, vanadium and zinc.* Washington, DC: National Academy Press, 2001.

Jackson R.D.,et al. 2006. Calcium plus vitamin D supplementation and the risk of fractures. *N. Engl. J. Med.* 354(7): 669–683.

Keshan Disease Research Group. 1979. Epidemiologic studies on the etiologic relationship of selenium and Keshan disease. *China Med. J.* 92: 477–482.

Keshan Disease Research Group. 1979. Observation on effect of sodium selenite in prevention of Keshan disease. *China Med. J.* 92: 471–476.

Lappe J.M., Travers-Gustafson D., et al. 2007. Vitamin D and calcium supplementation reduces cancer risk: results of a randomized trial. *Am. J. Clin. Nutr.* 85(6): 1586–1591.

Lee K., Bradley R., et al. 1999. Too much versus too little: the implications of current iodine intake in the United States. *Nutr. Rev.* 57: 177–182.

Lee N., Reasner C. 1994. Beneficial effect of chromium supplementation on serum triglyceride levels in NIDDM. *Diabetes Care* 17: 1449–1453.

Liberman S., Bruning N. *The real vitamin & mineral book*, Garden City Park, New York: Pavery Publishing Group Inc., 1990.

Lin J., Manson J.E., et al. 2007. Intakes of calcium and vitamin d and breast cancer risk in women, *Arch. Intern. Med.* 167(10): 1050–1059.

Mahan L.K., Escott-Stump S. *Krause's food, nutrition, & diet therapy*, 11th Edition. Philadelphia, Pennsylvania: Saunders, 2004.

Maheshwari U.R., McDonald J.T., et al. 1981. Fluoride balance studies in ambulatory healthy men with and without fluoride supplements. *Am. J. Clin. Nutr.* 34: 2679–2684.

Neve J. 2000. New approaches to assess selenium status and requirement. *Nutr. Rev.* 58: 363–369.

Palmer C., Anderson J.B. 2000. Position of the American Dietetic Association: the impact of fluoride on health. *J. Am. Diet. Assoc.* 200: 1208–1213.

Patrick L. 2008. Iodine: deficiency and therapeutic considerations. *Altern. Med. Rev.* 13(2): 116–127.

Pennington J.A.T., Schoen S.A. 1996. Total diet study: estimated dietary intakes of nutritional elements. *Int. J. Vitam. Nutr. Res.* 66: 350–362.

Porthouse J., et al. 2005. Randomized controlled trial of calcium and supplementation with cholecalciferol (vitamin D₃) for prevention of fractures in primary care. *BMJ* 330(7498): 1003–1006.

Prince R.L., et al. 2006. Effects of calcium supplementation on clinical fracture and bone structure: results of a 5-year, double-blind, placebo-controlled trial in elderly women. *Arch. Intern. Med.* 166(8): 869–875.

Rajagopalan K.V. 1988. Molybdenum: an essential trace element in human nutrition. *Annu. Rev. Nutr.* 8: 401–427.

Rucker R.B. 1998. Copper, lysyl oxidase, and extracellular matrix cross-linking. *Am. J. Clin. Nutr.* 67(suppl.): 996S–1002S.

Rude R.K. 1998. Magnesium deficiency: a cause of heterogeneous disease in humans. *J. Bone Miner. Res.* 13: 749–758.

Saltman P.D., Strause L.G. 1993. The role of trace minerals in osteoporosis. *J. Am. Coll. Nutr.* 12(4): 384–389.

Shaw J.C.L. 1980. Trace elements in the fetus and young infant II: copper manganese, selenium, and chromium. *Am. J. Dis. Child* 134: 74–81.

Spencer H.D., Lender M. 1981. Studies of fluoride metabolism in man: a review and report of original data. *Sci. Total Environ.* 17: 1–12.

Tang Y.-L., Wang S.-W., et al. 2008. Both inorganic and organic selenium supplements decrease brain monoamine oxidase B enzyme activity in adult rats. *Br. J. Nutr.* 100: 660–665.

The role of elements in life processes. Retrieved on 5-10-08 from http://www.mii.org/periodic/LifeElement.html.

Underwood E.J. 1981. The incidence of trace element deficiency disease. *Phil. Trans. R. Sco. Lond. B* 294: 3–8.

Wactawski-Wende J., Kotchen J.M., et al. 2006. Calcium plus vitamin D supplementation and the risk of colorectal cancer. *N. Engl. J. Med* 354(7): 684–696.

Wood R.J., Zheng J.J. 1997. High dietary calcium intakes reduce zinc absorption and balance in humans. *Am. J. Clin. Nutr.* 65(6): 1803–1809.

Chapter Two

Carbohydrate from http://en.wikipedia.org/wiki/Carbohydrate.

Cunnane S.C. 2005. Essential Fatty Acids: Time for a New Paradigm? *PUFA Newsletter.* Retrieved on 2008-3-14.

Crowe F.L., Skeaff C.M., et al. 2007. Serum phospholipid n-3 long-chain polyunsaturated fatty acids and physical and mental health in a population-based survey of New Zealand adolescents and adults. *Am. J.Clin.Nutr.* 86(5): 1278–1285.

Dekkers J.C. 1996. The role of antioxidant vitamins and enzymes in the prevention of exercise-induced muscle damage. *Sports Med.* 21: 213–238.

Dietary fiber from http://en.wikipedia.org/wiki/Dietary_fiber.

Drozdowski L.A., Dixon W.T., et al. 2002. Short-chain fatty acids and total parenteral nutrition affect intestinal gene expression. *J. Parenter. Enteral. Nutr.* 26(3): 145–150.

Fatty acid from http://en.wikipedia.org/wiki/Fatty_acid.

Mozaffarian D., Katan M.B., et al. 2006. Trans Fatty Acids and Cardiovascular Disease. *New Eng. J. Med.* 354(15): 1601–1613.

National Institute of Health. Omega-3 fatty acids, fish oil, alpha-linolenic acid, 2005-08-01. Retrieved on 2008-3-26.

OH R. 2005. Practical applications of fish oil (n-3 fatty acids) in primary care. *J. Am. Board Family Prac.* 18(1): 28–36.

Oxygen and your health (http://www.inspiredliving.com/health/oxygen.htm). Retrieved on 12-12-2007.

Protein from http://en.wikipedia.org/wiki/Protein.

Ravnskov U. *The cholesterol myths: exposing the fallacy that saturated fat and cholesterol cause heart disease.* Winona Lake, IN: New Trends Pub. Inc., 2002.

Roy C.C., Kien C.L., et al. 2006. Short-chain fatty acids: ready for prime time? *Nutr. Clin. Pract.* 21(4): 351–366.

Scholz-Ahrens K.E., Ade P., et al. 2007. Prebiotics, probiotics, and synbiotics affect mineral absorption, bone mineral content, and bone structure. *J. Nutr.* 137(3): 838S–846S.

Sears B. *The Zone: A Dietary Road Map.* New York: ReganBooks, 1995.

Simopoulos A. 2000. Evolutionary aspects of diet and essential fatty acids. *World Rev. Nutr. Diet* 88: 18–27.

Singh M. 2005. Essential fatty acids, DHA and the human brain. *Indian J. Pediatrics* 72(3): 239–242.

Sjodin T. 1990. Biochemical mechanisms for oxygen free radical formation during exercise. *Sports Med.* 10: 236–254.

Stacewicz-Sapuntzakis M., Bowen P.E., et al. 2001. Chemical composition and potential health effects of prunes: a functional food? *Crit. Rev. Food Sci. Nutr.* 41(4): 251–286.

Subcommittee on the Tenth Edition of the RDAs, Food and Nutrition Board Commission on Life Sciences, National Research Council. *Recommended Dietary Allowances*, 10th Edition. Washington DC: National Academy Press, 1989.

Trans fat: Avoid this cholesterol double whammy, Mayo Foundation for Medical Education and Research (MFMER) (http://www.mayoclinic.com/health/trans-fat/CL00032). Retrieved on 12-10-2008.

Trans fat from http://en.wikipedia.org/wiki/Trans_fat.

Watkim D.M. *Handbook of nutrition, health, and age.* Noyes Publications, Park Ridge, New Jersey: Noyes Publications, 1983.

Warburg O. 1931. The oxygen-transferring ferment of respiration. *Nobel Lecture.* (http://nobelprize.org/nobel_prizes/medicine/laureates/1931/warburg-lecture.pdf). Retrieved on 12-10-2007.

WHO (World Health Organization). Energy and protein requirements. Report of a joint FAO/WHO/UNU expert consultation. Technical report series 724. Geneva: WHO press, 1985.

Wong J.M., de Souza R., et al., Colonic health: fermentation and short chain fatty acids. *J. Clin. Gastroenterol.* 40(3): 235–243.

Chapter Three

Bauernfeind J.C. 1972. Carotenoid vitamin A precursors and analogs in foods and feeds. *J. Agric. Food. Chem.* 20: 456–473.

Brody T. *Nutritional Biochemistry*, San Diego: Academic Press, 1999.

Campbell R.K. 2006. A critical review of chromium picolinate and biotin. *U.S. Pharmacist* 31: 11–15.

Can C., et al. 2002. Vascular endothelial dysfunction associated with elevated serum homocysteine levels in rat adjuvant arthritis: effect of vitamin E administration. *Life Sci.* 71(4): 401–410.

Canty D.J., Zeisel S.J. 1994. Lecithin and choline in human health and disease. *Nutr. Rev.* 52: 327–331.

Carethers M. 1988. Diagnosing vitamin B_{12} deficiency, a common geriatric disorder. *Geriatrics* 43: 89–93.

Combs G.F. 2008. *The vitamins: Fundamental Aspects in Nutrition and Health*, 3rd Edition. Ithaca, New York: Elsevier Academic Press, 2008.

Dam H. 1935. The antihaenorrhagic vitamin of the chick: occurrence and chemical nature. *Nature* 135: 652–653.

Delmas P.D. 2002. Treatment of postmenopausal osteoporosis. *Lancet* 359(9322): 2018–2026.

Dunn W.A., Rettura G., et al. 1984. Effect of ascorbate deficiency on the in situ activity of gamma-butyrobetaine hydroxylase. *J. Biol. Chem.* 259(17): 10764–10770.

Durga J., van Boxtel M.P.J., et al. 2007. Effect of 3-year folic acid supplementation on cognitive function in older adults in the FACIT trial: a randomized, double blind, controlled trial. *Lancet* 369: 208–216.

Eipper B.A., et al. 1992. The biosynthesis of neuropeptides: peptide alpha-amidatio. *Annu. Rev. Neurosci.* 15: 57–85.

Eipper B.A., Milgram S.L., et al. 1993. Peptidylglycine alpha-amidating monooxygenase, a multifunctional protein with catalytic, processing, and routing domains. *Protein Sci.* 2: 489–497.

England S., Seifter S. 1986. The biochemical functions of ascorbic acid. *Annu. Rev. Nutr.* 6: 365–406.

Ericson U., Sonestedt E., et al. 2007. High folate intake is associated with lower breast cancer incidence in postmenopausal women in the Malmö Diet and Cancer cohort. *Am. J. Clin. Nutr.* 86(2): 434–443.

Gale C.R., Hall N.F. 2003. Lutein and zeaxanthin status and risk of age-related macular degeneration. *Invest. Ophthalmol. Vis. Sci.* 44(6): 2461–2465.

Huang J., Agus D.B., et al. 2001. Dehydroascorbic acid, a blood-brain barrier transportable form of vitamin C, mediates potent cerebroprotection in experimental stroke. *Proceedings of the National Academy of Sciences* 98(20): 11720–11724.

Fairfield K.M., Fletcher R.H. 2002. Vitamins for chronic disease prevention in adults, *JAMA* 287: 3116–3126.

Ferland G. 1998. The vitamin K-dependent proteins: an update, *Nutr. Rev.* 56(8): 223–230.

Jaconello P. 1992. Niacin versus niacinamide. *CMAJ* 147(7): 990–994.

Kallner A. 1977. On the absorption of ascorbic acid in man. Int. *J. Vitam. Nutr. Res.* 47: 383–388.

Kaufman S. 1974. Dopamine-beta-hydroxylase. *J. Psychiatr. Res.* 11: 303–316.

Knip M. 2000. Safety of high-dose nicotinamide: a review. *Diabetologia* 43(11): 1337–1345.

Krinsky N.I., Landrum J.T., et al. 2003. Biologic mechanisms of the protective role of lutein and zeaxanthin in the eye, *Annu. Rev. Nutr.*, 2003, 23:171–201.

Larsson S.C., Håkansson N., et al.2006. Folate intake and pancreatic cancer incidence: a prospective study of Swedish women and men. *J. Natl. Cancer Inst.* 98(6): 407–413.

Lewis C.J., Crane N.T., et al. 1999. Estimated folate intakes: data updated to reflect food fortification, increased bioavailability, and dietary supplement use. *Am. J. Clin. Nutr.* 70: 198–207.

Levine M., Dhariwal K.R. 1992. Ascorbic acid and reaction kinetics in situ: a new approach to vitamin requirements. *J. Nutr. Sci. Vitaminol. (Tokyo)* Spec No: 169–172.

Levine M., Rumsey S.C., et al. Vitamin C. In Stipanuk M.H. (ed.): *Biochemical and Physiological Aspects of Human Nutrition*, Philadelphia: W B Saunders, 2000.

Liberman S., Bruning N. *The real vitamin & mineral book*, Garden City Park, New York: Pavery Publishing Group Inc., 1990.

Lindblad B., et al. 1970.The mechanism of enzymic formation of homogentisate from p-hydroxyphenylpyruvate. *J. Am. Chem. Soc.* 92: 7446–7449.

Mahan L.K. Escott-Stump S. *Krause's food, nutrition, & diet therapy*, 11th Edition. Philadelphia, Pennsylvania: Saunders, 2004.

Malmberg K.J., et al. 2002. A short term dietary supplementation of high does of vitamin E increases T helper 1 cytokine production in patients with advanced colorectal cancer. *Clin. Cancer Res.* 8: 1772–1778.

Meister A. 1994. Glutathione-ascorbic acid antioxidant system in animals. *J. Biol. Chem.* 269(13): 9397–9400.

Morris M.C. 2002. Dietary intake of antioxidant nutrients and the risk of incident Alzeimer disease in biracial community study. *JAMA* 287: 3261–3263.

Olson J.A. 1972. The prevention of childhood blindness by the administration of massive doses of vitamin A. *Isr. J. Med. Sci.* 8: 1199–1206.

Packer L., Fuchs J., eds., *Vitamin C in health and disease*. New York: Marcel Dekker, 1997.

Rao C.N., Rao B.S.N. 1970. Absorption of dietary carotenes in human subjects. *Am. J. Clin. Nutr.* 23: 105–109.

Rebouche C.J. 1991. Ascorbic acid and carnitine biosynthesis. *Am. J. Clin. Nutr.* 54 (6 Suppl): 1147S–1152S.

Reddy V., Sivakumar B. 1972. Studies on vitamin A absorption. *Indian Pediatr.* 9: 307–310.

Sanjoaquin M.A., Allen N., et al. 2005. Folate intake and colorectal cancer risk: a meta-analytical approach. *Int. J. Cancer* 113(5): 825–828.

Shawn M. Choline, *a guide to understanding dietary supplements*. New York: Haworth Press, Inc., 2002.

Stevenson N.R. 1974. Active transport of L-ascorbic acid in human ileum. *Gastroenterology* 67: 952–956.

Thomas M.K. 1998. Hypovitaminosis D in medical patients. *N. Engl. J. Med.* 338(12): 777–783.

Vermeer C. 1996. Effects of vitamin K on bone mass and bone metabolism. *J. Nutr.* 126: 1228–1232.

Zeisel S.H., Blusztajn J.K. 1994.Choline and human nutrition. *Annu. Rev. Nutr.* 14: 269–274.

Chapter Four

Allen L.H. 2002. Iron supplements: scientific issues concerning efficacy and implications for research and programs. *J. Nutr.* 32: 813S–839S.

Anderson J.B. 1996. Calcium, phosphorus, and human bone development. *J. Nutr.* 126: 1153–1157.

Anderson R.A., Kozlovsky A.S. 1985. Chromium intake, absorption, and exretion of subjects consuming self-selected diets. *Am., J., Clin. Nutr.* 41: 1177–1183.

Baron J.A., Beach M., et al. 1999. Calcium supplements for the prevention of colorectal adenomas. *N. Engl. J. Med.* 340(2): 101–107.

Bhaskaram P. 2001. Immunobiology of mild micronutrient deficiencies. *Br. J. Nutr.* 85: S75–80.

Bogden J., Louria D. 1999. Aging and the immune system: role of micronutrient nutrition. *Nutrition* 15: 593–562.

Bonithon-Kopp C., Kronborg O., et al. 2000. Calcium and fiber supplementation in prevention of colorectal adenoma recurrence: a randomized intervention trial. European Cancer Prevention Organization Study Group. *Lancet* 356(9238): 1300–1306.

Brody T. *Nutritional Biochemistry*, San Diego: Academic Press, 1999.

Brown R.O., et al. 1986. Chromium deficiency after long-term total parenteral nutrition. *Dig. Dis. Sci.* 31: 661–664.

Casey C.E., Neville M.C. 1987. Studies in human lactation 3: molybdenum and nickel in human milk during the first month of lactation. *Am. J. Clin. Nutr.* 45: 921–926.

Cordano A. 1998. Clinical manifestations of nutritional copper deficiency in infants and children. *Am. J. Clin. Nutr.* 67(suppl.): 1012S–1016S.

Cotzias G.C., Miller S.T., et al. 1976. Interaction between manganese and brain dopamine. *Med. Clin. N. Am.* 60: 729–738.

Grant A.M., et al. 2005. Oral vitamin D_3 and calcium for secondary prevention of low-trauma fractures in elderly people (randomized evaluation of calcium or vitamin D, RECORD): a randomized placebo-controlled trial, *Lancet* 365(9471): 1621–1628.

Haas J.D., Brownlie T. 2001. 4th iron deficiency and reduced work capacity: a critical review of the research to determine a causal relationship. *J. Nutr.* 131: 691S–696S.

Institute of Medicine, Food and Nutrition Board. *Dietary reference intakes for vitamin A, vitamin K, arsenic, boron, chromium, copper, iodine, iron, manganese, molybdenum, nickel, silicon, vanadium and zinc*. Washington, DC: National Academy Press, 2001.

Jackson R.D.,et al. 2006. Calcium plus vitamin D supplementation and the risk of fractures. *N. Engl. J. Med.* 354(7): 669–683.

Keshan Disease Research Group. 1979. Epidemiologic studies on the etiologic relationship of selenium and Keshan disease. *China Med. J.* 92: 477–482.

Keshan Disease Research Group. 1979. Observation on effect of sodium selenite in prevention of Keshan disease. *China Med. J.* 92: 471–476.

Lappe J.M., Travers-Gustafson D., et al. 2007. Vitamin D and calcium supplementation reduces cancer risk: results of a randomized trial. *Am. J. Clin. Nutr.* 85(6): 1586–1591.

Lee K., Bradley R., et al. 1999. Too much versus too little: the implications of current iodine intake in the United States. *Nutr. Rev.* 57: 177–182.

Lee N., Reasner C. 1994. Beneficial effect of chromium supplementation on serum triglyceride levels in NIDDM. *Diabetes Care* 17: 1449–1453.

Liberman S., Bruning N. *The real vitamin & mineral book*, Garden City Park, New York: Pavery Publishing Group Inc., 1990.

Lin J., Manson J.E., et al. 2007. Intakes of calcium and vitamin d and breast cancer risk in women, *Arch. Intern. Med.* 167(10): 1050–1059.

Mahan L.K., Escott-Stump S. *Krause's food, nutrition, & diet therapy*, 11th Edition. Philadelphia, Pennsylvania: Saunders, 2004.

Maheshwari U.R., McDonald J.T., et al. 1981. Fluoride balance studies in ambulatory healthy men with and without fluoride supplements. *Am. J. Clin. Nutr.* 34: 2679–2684.

Neve J. 2000. New approaches to assess selenium status and requirement. *Nutr. Rev.* 58: 363–369.

Palmer C., Anderson J.B. 2000. Position of the American Dietetic Association: the impact of fluoride on health. *J. Am. Diet. Assoc.* 200: 1208–1213.

Patrick L. 2008. Iodine: deficiency and therapeutic considerations. *Altern. Med. Rev.* 13(2): 116–127.

Pennington J.A.T., Schoen S.A. 1996. Total diet study: estimated dietary intakes of nutritional elements. *Int. J. Vitam. Nutr. Res.* 66: 350–362.

Porthouse J., et al. 2005. Randomized controlled trial of calcium and supplementation with cholecalciferol (vitamin D_3) for prevention of fractures in primary care. *BMJ* 330(7498): 1003–1006.

Prince R.L., et al. 2006. Effects of calcium supplementation on clinical fracture and bone structure: results of a 5-year, double-blind, placebo-controlled trial in elderly women. *Arch. Intern. Med.* 166(8): 869–875.

Rajagopalan K.V. 1988. Molybdenum: an essential trace element in human nutrition. *Annu. Rev. Nutr.* 8: 401–427.

Rucker R.B. 1998. Copper, lysyl oxidase, and extracellular matrix cross-linking. *Am. J. Clin. Nutr.* 67(suppl.): 996S–1002S.

Rude R.K. 1998. Magnesium deficiency: a cause of heterogeneous disease in humans. *J. Bone Miner. Res.* 13: 749–758.

Saltman P.D., Strause L.G. 1993. The role of trace minerals in osteoporosis. *J. Am. Coll. Nutr.* 12(4): 384–389.

Shaw J.C.L. 1980. Trace elements in the fetus and young infant II: copper manganese, selenium, and chromium. *Am. J., Dis., Child* 134: 74–81.

Spencer H.D., Lender M. 1981. Studies of fluoride metabolism in man: a review and report of original data. *Sci. Total Environ.* 17: 1–12.

Tang Y.-L., Wang S.-W., et al. 2008. Both inorganic and organic selenium supplements decrease brain monoamine oxidase B enzyme activity in adult rats. *Br. J. Nutr.* 100: 660–665.

Underwood E.J. 1981. The incidence of trace element deficiency disease. *Phil. Trans. R. Sco. Lond. B* 294: 3–8.

Wactawski-Wende J., Kotchen J.M., et al. 2006. Calcium plus vitamin D supplementation and the risk of colorectal cancer. *N. Engl. J. Med* 354(7): 684–696.

Weingarten M.A. 2005. Dietary calcium supplementation for preventing colorectal cancer, adenomatous polyps and calcium metabolisism disorder. *Cochrane database of systematic reviews (Online)* (3): CD003548.

William G.H., Dluhy R.G. Hypertensive states: associated fluid and electrolyte disturbances. In Narins R.G. eds: *Maxwell and Kleeman's clinical disorders of fluid and electrolyte metabolism*, 5th Edition. New York: McGraw-Hill, 1994.

Wood R.J., Zheng J.J. 1997. High dietary calcium intakes reduce zinc absorption and balance in humans. *Am. J. Clin. Nutr.* 65(6): 1803–1809.

Chapter Five

Cao G. 1993. Oxygen-radical absorbance capacity assay for antioxidants. *Free Radic. Biol. Med.* 14(3): 303–311.

Dekkers J.C. 1996. The role of antioxidant vitamins and enzymes in the prevention of exercise-induced muscle damage. *Sports Med.* 21: 213–238.

Harman D. 1956. Aging: a theory based on free radical and radiation chemistry. J. *Gerontology* 11(3): 298–300.

Harman D. 1972. A biologic clock: the mitochondria? *J. Am. Geriatrics Soc.* 20(4): 145–147.

Ishii N. 2000. Oxidative stress and aging in caenorhabditis elegans. *Free Radical Res.* 33(6): 857–864.

Ou B. 2001. Development and validation of an improved oxygen radical absorbance capacity assay using fluorescein as the fluorescent probe. *J. Agric. Food Chem.* 49(10): 4619–4626.

Oxygen Radical Absorbance Capacity of Selected Foods—2007. Nutrient Data Laboratory, Agricultural Research Service, United States Department of Agriculture. November 2007.

Schriner S.E., Linford N.J., et al. 2005. Extension of murine life span by overexpression of catalase targeted to mitochondria. *Science* 308(5730): 1909–1911.

Sjodin T. 1990. Biochemical mechanisms for oxygen free radical formation during exercise. *Sports Med.* 10: 236–254.

Chapter Six

Anthea M., Hopkins J., et al. *Human biology and health.* Englewood Cliffs, New Jersey: Prentice Hall, 1993.

Bible, NIV—New International Version. Grand Rapids, Michigan: Zondervan Publishing, 2007.

Bruce A. *Leukocyte functions and percentage breakdown, Molecular biology of the cell,* NCBI Bookshelf, 2005.

Kim B. Essential details on acid and alkaline-forming effects of food and how your body maintains a healthy pH from www.DrBenKim.com. Retrieved on 9-20-08.

Kim B. The truth about saturated fats and cholesterol from www.DrBenKim.com. Retrieved on 9-20-08.

Oxygen content of blood from http://www.frca.co.uk/article.aspx?articleid=100175. Retrieved on 8-10-08.

Shmukler M. 2004. Density of Blood. *The physics fact book.* From http://hypertextbook.com/facts/2004/MichaelShmukler.shtml. Retrieved on 1-25-09.

The acidification theory of aging from
http://www.anti-aging-today.org/aging/theory/acidification.htm. Retrieved on 6-7-09.

Trudnowski R.J., Rico R.C. 1974. Specific gravity of blood and plasma at 4°C and 37°C, *Clin. Chem.* 20: 615–616.

Tunsky G. What in the cell is going on? —The battle over pH (http://www.itshealthywater.com/documents/What in the Cell is Goingon.pdf). Retrieved on 5-9-09.

Chapter Seven

Bahr R., Ingnes I., et al. 1987. Effect of duration of exercise on excess postexercise O_2 consumption. *J. Appl. Physiol.* 62: 485–490.

FAO/WHO/UNU. *Protein and amino acid requirements in human nutrition.* Technical Report Series 935. Geneva: WHO Press, 2007.

Gaesser G.A., Brooks G.A. 1984. Metabolic bases of excess post-exercise oxygen consumption: A review. *Med. Sci. Sports Exerc.* 16: 29–43.

Institute of Medicine, Food and Nutrition Board. *Dietary reference intakes for energy, carbohydrate, fiber, fat, fatty acids, protein, amino acids.* Washington DC: The National Academies Press, 2002/2005.

Kuczmarski R.J., Ogden C.L., et al. 2000. CDC growth charts: United States. *Adv. Data* 314:1–28.

Nelson K.M., Weinsier R.L., et al. 1992. Prediction of resting energy expenditure from fat-free mass and fat mass. *Am. J. Clin. Nutr.* 56: 848–856.

NHLBI/NIDDK (National Heart, Lung, and Blood Institute/National Institute of Diabetes and Digestive and Kidney Diseases). *Clinical Guidelines on the Identification, Evaluation, and Treatment of Overweight and Obesity in Adults*, The Evidence Report. NIH Publication No. 98-4083. Bethesda, MD: National Institutes of Health, 1998.

Owen O.E., Holup J.L. 1987. A reappraisal of the caloric requirements of men. *Am. J. Clin. Nutr.* 46: 875–885.

Owen O.E., Kavle E., et al. 1986. A reappraisal of caloric requirements in healthy women. *Am. J. Clin. Nutr.* 44: 1–19.

Poehlman E.T. 1993. Regulation of energy expenditure in aging humans. *Geriatr. Biosci.* 41: 552-559.

Poehlman E.T., Horton E.S. Energy needs: assessment and requirements in humans. In Bloch A.S., Shils M.E. eds: *Modern nutrition in health and disease.* Baltimore: Williams & Wilkins, 1998.

Ravussin E., Harper I.T., et al. 1991. Energy expenditure by doubly labeled water: validation in lean and obese subjects. *Am. J. Physiol.* 261: E402–E409.

Ravussin E., Lillioja S., et al. 1986. Determinants of 24-hour energy expenditure in man: Methods and results using a respiratory chamber. *J. Clin. Invest.* 78:1568–1578.

Ravussin E., Lillioja S., et al. 1988. Reduced rate of energy expenditure as a risk factor for body-weight gain. *N. Engl. J. Med.* 318: 467–472.

Webb P. 1986. 24-hour energy expenditure and the menstrual cycle. *Am. J. Clin. Nutr.* 44: 614–619.

WHO (World Health Organization). *Energy and protein requirement, Report of a Joint Food and Agriculture Organization/World Health Organization/United Nations University (FAO/WHO/UNU) Expert Consultation.* Technical Report Series 724. Geneva: WHO Press, 1985.

WHO (World Health Organization). Principles for the Safety Assessment of Food Additives and Contaminants in Food. *Environmental Health Criteria 70.* Geneva: WHO Press, 1987.

WHO (World Health Organization). *Trace Elements in Human Nutrition and Health*, Geneva: WHO Press, 1996.

Chapter Eight

SR 20 Search Database, USDA, 2008.

Walford R.L. *The 120-year diet.* New York: Simon and Schuster, 1986.

Chapter Nine

Centre for Affordable Water and Sanitation Technology, Household water treatment guide, March 2008.

Lide D.R. Editor-in-Chief, *CRC Handbook of Chemistry and Physics*, 1997 Edition. Boston: CRC press, 1997.

Popkin B.M., et al. 2006. Recommended intakes of beverages. *Am. J. Clin. Nutr.* 83: 529-542.

Research on health and air quality from http://www.hc-sc.gc.ca/ewh-semt/air/out-ext/research-recherche-eng.php. Retrieved on 8-19-08.

The acidification theory of aging from http://www.anti-aging-today.org/aging/theory/acidification.htm. Retrieved on 6-7-09.

U.S. Centers for Disease Control and Prevention, Safe water system: a low-cost technology for safe drinking water, Fact Sheet, World Water Forum 4 Update, Atlanta, GA, March 2006.

Walford R.L. *Maximum life span*. New York: W.W. Norton & Company, 1983.

Walford R.L. *The 120 year diet*, New York: Simon and Schuster, 1986.

WHO's guidelines for drinking water quality. Geneva: WHO Press, 2008.

Chapter Ten

Dietary Supplement Health and Education Act of 1994, Food and Drug Administration web site: fda.gov/opacom/laws/dshea.html. Retrieved on 5-11-09.

Dietary supplements: overview. U.S. Food and Drug Administration, Center for Food Safety and Applied Nutrition web site: cfsan.fda.gov/~dms/supplmnt.html. Retrieved on 5-20-09.

Institute of Medicine, Food and Nutrition Board. *Dietary reference intakes for energy, carbohydrate, fiber, fat, fatty acids, protein, amino acids*. Washington DC: The National Academies Press, 2002/2005.

Pizzorno J. *Total wellness: improving your health by understanding the body's healing systems*. California: Prima Publishing, 1996.

Chapter Eleven

Adams M. High cholesterol, high blood pressure raises risk of Alzheimer's by 600%. Accessed at: http://www.newstarget.com/001422.htm.

Alafuzoff I., Helisalmi S. 2000. Selegiline treatment and the extent of degenerative changes in brain tissue of patients with Alzheimer's disease. *Eur. J. Clin. Pharmocol.* 55: 815–819.

Benedetti S.M., Dostert P. 1989. Monoamine oxidase, brain aging and degenerative diseases. *Biochem. Pharmacol.* 38: 555–561.

Bible, NIV—New International Version. Grand Rapids, Michigan: Zondervan Publishing, 2007.

Buettner D. *The blue zone: lessons for living longer from the people who've lived the longest*. Whashinton DC: National Geographic, 2008.

Courmot M., Marquie J.C. et al., 2006. Relation between body mass index and congnitive function in healthy middle-aged men and women. *Neurology* 67: 1208–1214.

Cournil A., Kirkwood T.B. 2001. If you would live long, choose your parents well. *Trends in Genetics* 17(5): 233–235.

Early S. February 06, 2007. The relationship between exercise and human longevity. Retrieved 7-16-2009, from http://today.reuters.com/news/newsarticle.aspx?type=healthNews&storyid=2006-11-14T190915Z_01_N10395594_RTRUKOC_0_US-AGE.xml.

Ferr C.P., et al. 2005.Global prevalence of dementia: a delphi consensus study. *Lancet* 366(9503): 2112-2117.

Finch C.E., Tanzi R.E. 1997. *Science* 278: 407–410.

Lai M.-H., Huang C.-L., et al. 2000. Correlation between blood chromium (III) level, blood glucose and lipid concentrations in diabetes. *J. Nutr. Sci.* 25(3): 140–147.

Lean M.E. 2000. Pathophysiology of obesity. *Proceedings of the Nutrition Society* 59(3): 331–336.

Robine J.M., Allard M. 1998. The oldest human. *Science* 279(5358): 1834–1835.

Whitmer R.A., Gunderson E.P., et al. 2005.Obesity in middle age and future risk of dementia: a 27-year longitudinal population-based study. *BMJ* 330(7504): 1360–1365.

Ruston D., et al. *National diet and nutrition survey: adults aged 19 to 64 years. Volume 4, Nutritional status (anthropometry and blood analytes), blood pressure and physical activity*. London: TSO, 2004.

Saura J., Luque J.M., et al. 1994. Increased monoamine oxidase B activity in plaque-associated astrocytes of Alzheimer brains revealed by quantitative enzyme radioautography. *Neuroscience* 62: 15–30.

Tang Y.-L., Wang S.-W., et al. 2008. Both inorganic and organic selenium supplements decrease brain monoamine oxidase B enzyme activity in adult rats. *Br. J. Nutr.*100: 660–665.

Walford R.L. *The 120 year diet*. New York: Simon and Schuster, 1986.

WHO (World Heath Organization). *Obesity: preventing and managing the global epidemic*. WHO Technical Report Series 894. Geneva: WHO Press, 2000.

Summary

Finkelstein E.A., et al.2003. National medical spending attributable to overweight and obesity: How much, and who's paying? *Health Affairs* W3: 219–226.

Katzmarzyk P., Janssen I. 2004. The economic costs associated with physical inactivity and obesity in Canada: An update. *Can. J. Appl. Physiol.* 29(1): 90–115.

Wolf A.M., Colditz G.A. 1998. Current estimates of the economic cost of obesity in the United States. *Obesity Research* 6(2): 97–106.

Glossary

Acidemia: a state in which the pH of arterial blood decreases below the normal range of 7.35 to 7.45 because of an increase in circulating acids or a reduction in bicarbonate levels

Acidosis: a physiologic process or disease state that if left untreated results in acidemia

Acetylcholine: a white crystalline derivative of choline that is released at the ends of nerve fibers in the somatic and parasympathetic nervous systems and is involved in the transmission of nerve impulses in the body

Acetyl coenzyme A (acetyl CoA): a molecule produced by fatty acid oxidation

Active transport: the movement of particles via a carrier protein across cell membranes and epithelial layers; requires expenditure of energy

Adenosine triphosphate (ATP): an adenosine-derived nucleotide that supplies large amounts of energy to cells for various biochemical processes, including muscle contraction and sugar metabolism, through its hydrolysis to adenosine diphosphate (ADP)

Albumin: a class of simple, water-soluble proteins that can be coagulated by heat and precipitated by strong acids and are found in egg white, blood serum, milk, and many other animal and plant juices and tissues; also called albumen

Aldosterone: a steroid hormone secreted by the adrenal cortex that regulates the salt and water balance in the body

Alkalemia: a state in which the pH of arterial blood exceeds the normal range of 7.35 to 7.45 because of an increase in bicarbonate levels or a reduction in circulating acids

Alkalosis: a physiologic process or disease state that if left untreated results in alkalemia

Alzheimer's disease (AD): one form of dementia, is a progressive, degenerative brain disease; it affects memory, thinking, and behavior

Amino acid: an organic compound containing an amino (NH_2) group and a carboxyl (COOH) group; links with other amino acids to form proteins

Amylase: an enzyme that is secreted in saliva and from the pancreas and catalyzes the hydrolysis of starch

Amylopectin: a form of starch made up of highly branched glucose polymers

Anemia: a decrease in normal number of red blood cells (RBCs) or less than the normal quantity of hemoglobin in the blood

Anorexia: loss of appetite, especially as a result of disease

Antagonist: a chemical substance that interferes with the physiological action of another, especially by combining with and blocking its nerve receptor

Antioxidant: a substance that can inhibit reactions of free radicals such as reactive species of oxygen

Asbestos: either of two incombustible, chemical-resistant, fibrous mineral forms of impure magnesium silicate, used for fireproofing, electrical insulation, building materials, brake linings, and chemical filters

Atherosclerosis: a form of arteriosclerosis characterized by the deposition of atheromatous plaques containing cholesterol and lipids on the innermost layer of the walls of large and medium-sized arteries

Basal energy expenditure (BEE): the measurement of the basal metabolic rate; usually expressed as kilocalories per 24 hours (kcal/24 hr)

Basal metabolic rate (BMR): the energy needed to sustain the metabolic activities of cells and tissues and to maintain circulatory, respiratory, gastrointestinal, and renal processes

Beriberi: a neuropathy caused by thiamin deficiency

Buffer: a proton donor and acceptor system that helps preserve homeostasis of the hydrogen ion concentration

Butyrate: a salt or ester of butyric acid

Calcitonin: a 32-amino acid linear polypeptide hormone that is produced in humans primarily by the parafollicular cells (also known as C-cells) of the thyroid, and in many other animals in the ultimobranchial body

Calorie: the amount of energy required to raise the temperature of 1 ml of water at 15°C by 1°C

Candida albicans: a diploid fungus (a form of yeast) and a causal agent of opportunistic oral and genital infections in humans

Catabolism: the metabolic breakdown of complex molecules into simpler ones, often resulting in a release of energy

Catalase: an enzyme that decomposes hydrogen peroxide into oxygen and water

Cataract: a clouding of the natural lens, the part of the eye responsible for focusing light and producing clear, sharp images

Catecholamine: any of a group of amines derived from catechol that have important physiological effects as neurotransmitters and hormones and include epinephrine, norepinephrine, and dopamine

Cellulose: a carbohydrate made of long, straight glucose polymers in βlinkage that resists hydrolysis in the human digestive tract; a dietary fiber

Ceruloplasmin: a serum glycoprotein involved in the storage and transport of copper and iron

Cheilosis: a disorder of the lips often due to riboflavin deficiency and other B-complex vitamin deficiencies and characterized by fissures, especially in the corners of the mouth

Chelate: a chemical compound in the form of a heterocyclic ring, containing a metal ion attached by coordinate bonds to at least two nonmetal ions

Cholecystokinin (CCK): a hormone that is secreted by the proximal small bowel and stimulates the pancreas to secrete enzymes (and to a lesser extent, bicarbonate and water), stimulates gallbladder contraction, slow gastric emptying, stimulates colonic activity, and may regulate appetite

Cholesterol: a sterol found in cell membranes of all animal tissues that is also necessary for production of bile and steroid hormones

Choline: a natural amine, $C_5H_{15}NO_2$, often classed in the vitamin B complex and a constituent of many other biologically important molecules, such as acetylcholine and lecithin

Chylomicron: a large plasma lipoprotein particle, occurring as a droplet consisting primarily of triglycerides and functioning in the transport of neutral lipids from the intestine to the tissues by way of the lymph

Cocarboxylase: a coenzyme $C_{12}H_{19}ClN_4O_7P_2S \cdot H_2O$ that is important in metabolic reactions (as decarboxylation in the Krebs cycle) called also thiaminepyrophosphate

Colonic salvage: the process of fermenting and absorbing end products of dietary carbohydrates, fiber, and amino acids from the large intestine

Conjunctivitis: inflammation of the conjunctiva, characterized by redness and often accompanied by a discharge

Corrin: the cyclic system of four pyrrole rings forming the central structure of the vitamin B_{12} and related compounds

Creatine: an amino acid, $C_4H_9N_3O_2$, which is a constituent of the muscles of vertebrates and is phosphorylated to store energy used for muscular contraction

Creatinine: a creatine anhydride, $C_4H_7N_3O$, formed by the metabolism of creatine, which is found in muscle tissue and blood and normally excreted in the urine as a metabolic waste

Cretinism: a congenital disease due to absence or deficiency of normal thyroid secretion, characterized by physical deformity, dwarfism, and mental retardation, and often by goiter

Cryptosporidium: an intestinal parasite in humans and other vertebrates and sometimes causes diarrhea that is especially severe in immunocompromised individuals

Cytochrome: any of a class of iron-containing proteins important in cell respiration as catalysts of oxidation-reduction reactions

Cytosol: the water-soluble components of cell cytoplasm, constituting the fluid portion that remains after removal of the organelles and other intracellular structures

Dehydration: excessive loss of body water

Delusion: a false belief strongly held in spite of invalidating evidence, especially as a symptom of mental illness

Dementia: deterioration of intellectual faculties, such as memory, concentration, and judgment, resulting from an organic disease or a disorder of the brain, and often accompanied by emotional disturbance and personality changes

Diabetes: any of several metabolic disorders marked by excessive discharge of urine and persistent thirst, especially one of the two types of diabetes mellitus

Diacylglycerols (diglycerides): lipids with only two fatty acids attached to the glycerol molecule

Dietary fiber: the amount of plant material remaining after treatment with digestive enzymes and reduction of acid and alkali; may be soluble or insoluble

Dietary reference intakes (DRIs): a set of nutrient reference values; they are used to help people select healthful diets, set national nutrition policy, and establish safe upper limits of intake

Disaccharides: sugars capable of being hydrolyzed into two monosacchacharide molecules

Doubly labeled water (DLW): used to measure total energy expenditure in free-living people using two stable isotopes of water (deuterium [^2H_2O] and oxygen-18 [$H_2^{18}O$]); the difference in the turnover rates of the two isotopes measures the carbon dioxide production rate, from which total energy expenditure can be calculated

Dopamine: a catecholamine neurotransmitter in the central nervous system, retina, and sympathetic ganglia, acting within the brain to help regulate movement and emotion: its depletion may cause Parkinson's disease

Edema: an accumulation of an excessive amount of watery fluid in cells, tissues, or serous cavities

Eicosanoid: any of a class of compounds (as prostaglandins, leukotrienes, and thromboxanes) derived from polyunsaturated fatty acids (as arachidonic acid) and involved in cellular activity

Energy expended in physical activity (EEPA): the energy expended during voluntary exercise and involuntary activities such as shivering and fidgeting; the most variable component of total energy expenditure

Ergometer: a device designed to measure muscle power

Erythropoeisis: the formation or production of red blood cells

Estimated energy requirement (EER): the average dietary energy intake that is predicted to maintain energy balance in a healthy adult of a defined age, gender, weight, height, and level of physical activity consistent with good health. In children and pregnant and lactating women, the EER is taken to include the energy needs associated with the deposition of tissues or the secretion of milk at rates consistent with good health

Ethanolamine: a colorless liquid ($NH_2(CH_2)_2OH$) used in the purification of petroleum, as a solvent in dry cleaning, and as an ingredient in paints and pharmaceuticals

Extracellular fluid: the water and dissolved substances in the spaces outside cells

Facilitated diffusion: the movement of particles across a membrane via a carrier protein

Facultative thermogenesis: a portion of the thermic effect of food; "excess" energy expended in addition to the obligatory thermogenesis, thought to be partially mediated by sympathetic nervous system activity

Ferritin: an iron-containing protein complex, found principally in the intestinal mucosa, spleen, and liver, that functions as the primary form of iron storage in the body

Fibrosis: the formation of fibrous tissue as a reparative or reactive process

Fluoroapatite: a crystalline mineral, $Ca_5(PO_4)_3F$, formed from hydroxyapatite in the presence of fluoride, that has a hardening effect on bones and teeth

Fructose: a monosaccharide in fruit, honey, and some vegetables; the sweetest of the monosaccharides

Gamma-aminobutyric acid (GABA): an amino acid, $C_4H_9NO_2$, which is not found in proteins, but occurs in the central nervous system and is associated with the transmission of nerve impulses

Gastric inhibitory polypeptide (GIP): a hormone that is released from the intestine mucosa in the presence of fat and glucose and inhibits gastric acid secretion and stimulates insulin release

Gastrin: a hormone that is produced by the antral mucosa of the stomach and stimulates gastric secretions and motility

Glossitis: inflammation of the tongue

Glucagon: a hormone secreted by the pancreas that acts in opposition to insulin in the regulation of blood glucose levels

Gluconeogenesis: glucose formation in animals from a noncarbohydrate source, as from proteins or fats

Glucose: the main monosaccharide in blood and an important source of energy for living organisms; usually found as a disaccharide linked to fructose (sucrose), galatose (lactose), or glucose (maltose)

Glutamine synthetase: is an enzyme that plays an essential role in the metabolism of nitrogen by catalyzing the condensation of glutamate and ammonia to form glutamine

Glutathione peroxidase (GPX): an enzyme in the body that is a powerful scavenger of free radicals

Glycogen: a branched-chain glucose polymer used for glucose storage in animals

Glycolipids: membrane lipids with one or more sugar molecules attached to the polar head group; high concentration in the brain

Glycoprotein: any of a group of conjugated proteins that contain a carbohydrate as the nonprotein component

Goiter: a chronic enlargement of the thyroid gland, visible as a swelling at the front of the neck; commonly associated with iodine deficiency

Gum: any of numerous colloidal polysaccharide substances of plant origin that are gelatinous when moist but harden on drying and are salts of complex organic acids.

Homeostasis: the maintenance of relatively stable internal physiological conditions (as body temperature or the pH of blood) in higher animals under fluctuating environmental conditions; the process of maintaining a stable psychological state in the individual under varying psychological pressures or stable social conditions in a group under varying social, environmental, or political factors

Hemicellulose: any of several polysaccharides that are more complex than a sugar and less complex than cellulose, found in plant cell walls and produced commercially from corn grain hulls, and that hydrolyze to monosaccharides more readily than cellulose

Hemoglobin: a conjugated protein containing four heme groups and globin, with the property of reversible oxygenation

Hemorrhage: a profuse discharge of blood, as from a ruptured blood vessel; bleeding

Hemosiderin: an insoluble protein that contains iron and that is produced by phagocytic digestion of hematin and found as granules in most tissues, especially in the liver

High-Density Lipoprotein (HDL): a lipoprotein of blood plasma that is composed of a high proportion of protein with little triglyceride and cholesterol and that is associated with decreased probability of developing athero-sclerosis called also good cholesterol

Humerus: the long bone of the arm or forelimb, extending from the shoulder to the elbow

Huntington's disease: an incurable neurodegenerative genetic disorder that affects muscle coordination and some cognitive functions, typically becoming noticeable in middle age

Homocysteine: an amino acid that is a homologue of cysteine, is produced by the demethylation of methionine, and forms a complex with serine that metabolizes to produce cysteine and homoserine

Hydrogenation: the process of adding hydrogen across the unsaturated fatty acid double bond; commercial hydrogenation of oils increases saturation and makes the oil more solid at room temperature

Hydroxyapatite: the principal bone salt, $Ca_5(PO_4)_3OH$, which provides the compression strength of vertebrate bone

Hypercholesterolemia: an abnormally high concentration of cholesterol in the blood

Hyperglycaemia: an abnormally high level of glucose in the blood

Hypertension: persistent high blood pressure; arterial disease in which chronic high blood pressure is the primary symptom

Hyperthyroidism: pathologically excessive production of thyroid hormones; the condition resulting from excessive activity of the thyroid gland, character-ized by increased basal metabolism

Hypoprothrombinemia: deficiency of prothrombin in the blood usually due to vitamin K deficiency or liver disease (especially obstructive jaundice) and resulting in delayed clotting of blood or spontaneous bleeding (as from the nose or into the skin) called also prothrombinopenia

Hypocalcemia: abnormally low levels of calcium in blood

Hypochromia: an anemic condition in which the percentage of hemoglobin in red blood cells is abnormally low

Hypoglycemia: an abnormally low level of glucose in the blood

Hypokalemia: an abnormally low concentration of potassium ions in the blood; also called hypopotassemia

Infertility: the inability of a couple to conceive and reproduce

Insomnia: chronic inability to fall asleep or remain asleep for an adequate length of time

Intelligence quotient (IQ): the ratio of tested mental age to chronological age, usually expressed as a quotient multiplied by 100

Intracellular fluid: the water and dissolved substances contained within cells

Isoxazole: a liquid heterocyclic compound (C_3H_3NO), isomeric with oxazole and having a penetrating odor like that of pyridine

Kilocalorie (kcal): 1000 calories; sometimes written as Calorie

Lactase: an intestinal enzyme that hydrolyzes lactose into glucose and galactose

Lactose: the principal sugar in mammalian milk; a disaccharide composed of glucose and galactose

Lecithin (phosphatidylcholine): a phospholipid containing choline; found in the membranes of biologic organisms; is part of bile, where it emulsifies fats, and is part of lipoproteins, where it transports triglyceride and cholesterol

Lethargy: a state of sluggishness, inactivity, and apathy; a state of unconsciousness resembling deep sleep

Leucopenia: an abnormally low number of white blood cells in the circulating blood; also called leukocytopenia

Lignin: a woody fiber found in the stems and seeds of fruits and vegetables and in the bran layer of cereals; because of conjugated double bonds, is an excellent antioxidant

Low-Density Lipoprotein (LDL): a lipoprotein of blood plasma that is composed of a moderate proportion of protein with little triglyceride and a high proportion of cholesterol and that is associated with increased probability of developing atherosclerosis called also bad cholesterol

Lycopene: a red crystalline substance, $C_{40}H_{56}$, which is the main pigment of certain fruits, as the tomato and paprika, and is a precursor to carotene in plant biosynthesis

Macronutrients: macromolecules in plant and animal structures that can be digested, absorbed, and used by another organism as energy sources and as substrates for synthesis of the carbohydrates, fats, and proteins required to maintain cell and system integrity

Maltase: an intestinal enzyme that hydrolyzes maltose into glucose

Metabolic equivalents (METs): the measure of caloric expenditure by the amount of oxygen consumed per minute per kilogram of body weight; 1 MET = ~3.5 ml oxygen consumed per kilogram of body weight per minute in adults

Methylation: the process of replacing a hydrogen atom with a methyl group

Micelle: a complex of primarily free fatty acids, monoglycerides, and bile salts that allows lipids to be absorbed into intestinal mucosal cells

Micronutrient: an essential nutrient, as a trace mineral or vitamin, which is required by an organism in minute amounts

Monoacylglycerols (monoglycerides): lipids with only one fatty acid attached to the glycerol molecule

Monoamine oxidase B (MAO-B): a protein enzyme which in humans is encoded by the MAO-B gene

Monosaccharides: the simplest sugar units with formula $(CH_2O)_n$

Monounsaturated fatty acids (MFAs): fatty acids containing one double bond

Mucilage: a gelatinous substance of various plants that contains protein and polysaccharides and is similar to plant gums

Myoglobin: the oxygen-transporting protein of muscle, resembling blood hemoglobin in function but with only one heme as part of the molecule and with one fourth the molecular weight; also called muscle hemoglobin

Neuropathy: a disease or an abnormality of the nervous system, especially one affecting the cranial or spinal nerves

Neuritis: the inflammation of a nerve or group of nerves that is characterized by pain, loss of reflexes, and atrophy of the affected muscles

Neutropenia: an abnormal decrease in the number of neutrophils in the blood

Night blindness: impaired dark adaptation caused by loss of visual pigments from vitamin A deficiency; also called nyctalopia

Norepinephrine: a substance, both a hormone and neurotransmitter, secreted by the adrenal medulla and the nerve endings of the sympathetic nervous system to cause vasoconstriction and increases in heart rate, blood pressure, and the sugar level of the blood; also called levarterenol, noradrenalin

Numbness: unability or only partially ability to feel sensation or pain

Obligatory thermogenesis: a portion of the thermic effect of food; the energy required to digest, absorb, and metabolize nutrients

Omega-3 fatty acid: a fatty acid with the first double bond located at the third carbon from the methyl end (e.g., eicosapentaenoic acid [C20:5 ω-3])

Omega-6 fatty acid: a fatty acid with the first double bond located at the sixth carbon from the methyl end (e.g., linoleic acid [C18:2 ω-6])

Optimization: the procedure or procedures used to make a system or design as effective or functional as possible, especially the mathematical techniques involved

Osteoarthritis: a form of arthritis, occurring mainly in older persons, that is characterized by chronic degeneration of the cartilage of the joints

Osteoblast: a cell from which bone develops; a bone-forming cell

Osteomalacia: a condition characterized by softening of the bones with resultant pain, weakness, and bone fragility, caused by inadequate deposition of calcium or vitamin D

Osteoporosis: a disease of bone that leads to an increased risk of fracture

Palpitation: perceptible forcible pulsation of the heart, usually with an increase in frequency or force, with or without irregularity in rhythm

Pancreatic lipase: an enzyme in pancreatic juice that hydrolyzes the ester linkages between fatty acid and glycerol

Paresthesia: a skin sensation, such as burning, prickling, itching, or tingling, with no apparent physical cause

Parietal cells: large cells that are scattered along the walls of the stomach and secrete the hydrochloric acid in gastric juice

Passive diffusion: the random movement of particles through openings in cellular membranes according to electrochemical and concentration gradients

Pectin: any of a group of water-soluble colloidal carbohydrates of high molecular weight found in ripe fruits, such as apples, plums, and grapefruit, and used in fruit jellies, pharmaceuticals, and cosmetics for its thickening and emulsifying properties and its ability to solidify to a gel.

Pentose: a monosaccharide $C_5H_{10}O_5$ (as ribose) that contains five carbon atoms in a molecule

Peristalsis: the movement by which the alimentary canal propels its contents

Pernicious: tending to cause death or serious injury; deadly

Peroxidase: any of a class of oxidoreductase enzymes that catalyze the oxidation of a compound by the decomposition of hydrogen peroxide or an organic peroxide

Phospholipid: a lipid molecule used to construct biologic membranes; composed of two fatty acids and one of several polar groups linked to glycerol phosphate

Phosphorylation: the addition of phosphate to an organic compound through the action of a phosphorylase or kinase

Photophobia: an abnormal sensitivity to or intolerance of light, especially by the eyes, as may be caused by eye inflammation, lack of pigmentation in the iris, or various diseases; an abnormal or irrational fear of light

Physical activity level (PAL): the ratio of total energy expenditure (TEE) to basal energy expenditure (BEE)

Phytic acid (phytate): a phosphorus-containing compound that is found in the outer husk of cereal grains; binds with minerals and inhibits absorption

Pneumonitis: inflammation of the lung caused by a virus or exposure to irritating substances

Polyneuropathy: a disease of nerves; especially, a noninflammatory degenerative disease of nerves usually caused by toxins (as of lead)

Polysaccharide: a carbohydrate polymer with more than 10 monosaccharide units

Polyunsaturated fatty acids (PUFAs): fatty acids containing at least two double bonds

Porphyrin: any of various compounds with a structure that consists essentially of four pyrrole rings joined by four =CH– groups; especially, one (as chlorophyll or hemoglobin) containing a central metal atom and usually having biological activity

Psoriasis: a chronic, non-contagious autoimmune disease that affects the skin and joints

Proteins: complex nitrogenous compounds made up of amino acids in peptide linkages

Proteolytic enzymes: the enzymes trysin, chymotrypsin, and carboxypeptidase, all of which break down protein into proteoses, peptides, and amino acids

Pyruvate carboxylase: an enzyme that contains biotin as a prosthetic group and in the presence of acetyl coenzyme A catalyzes the fixation of carbon dioxide by pyruvate to form oxalacetate

Resting energy expenditure (REE): a measurement of the resting metabolic rate; usually expressed as kilocalories per 24 hours (kcal/24 hr)

Resting metabolic rate (RMR): the energy expended for the maintenance of normal body functions and homeostasis; represents the largest portion of total energy expenditure; may be as much as 10% to 20% higher than the basal energy expenditure, allowing for energy spent as a result of the thermic effect of food or excess post exercise oxygen consumption

Rheumatoid arthritis: a chronic and progressive systemic disease, especially common in women, characterized by stiffness and inflammation of the joints and sometimes leading to deformity and disability; also called arthritis deformans

Rickets: a disease of infants and young animals characterized by impaired mineralization of growing bone caused by deficiencies of vitamin D, calcium, or phosphorus

S-adenosylmethionine: the active sulfonium form of methionine$C_{15}H_{22}N_6O_5S$ that acts as a methyl group donor in various biochemical transmethylation reactions (as the formation of epinephrine or creatine), that is formed when methionine reacts with ATP, and that is an intermediate in the formation of homocysteine

Saturated fatty acid (SFA): a fatty acid in which all available carbon binding sites are saturated with hydrogen

Scurvy: a disease characterized by impaired maturation of connective tissues caused by a vitamin C deficiency

Secretin: a hormone released from duodenal wall into the bloodstream that stimulates the pancreas to secrete water and bicarbonate and inhibits gastric secretion

Serotonin: a neurotransmitter, derived from tryptophan, that is involved in sleep, depression, memory, and other neurological processes; also called 5-hydroxytryptamine

Somatostatin: a polypeptide hormone secreted from the stomach, small intestine and pancreas that tends to inhibit other GI secretions and inhibit motility

Sphingolipid: any of a group of lipids, such as sphingomyelins or cerebrosides, which yield sphingosine or its derivatives upon hydrolysis

Sprue: a disease of tropical regions that is of unknown cause and is characterized by fatty diarrhea and malabsorption of nutrients called also tropical-sprue

Steatosis: accumulation of fat in the interstitial tissue of an organ

Stomotitis: inflammation of the mucous membrane of the mouth

Sucrase: the intestinal enzyme that hydrolyzes sucrose into glucose and fructose

Sucrose: a disaccharide composed of one glucose unit and one fructose unit; the major form in which glucose is transported between plant cells; ordinary table sugar

Superoxide dismutase (SOD): a metal-containing antioxidant enzyme that reduces potentially harmful free radicals of oxygen formed during normal metabolic cell processes to oxygen and hydrogen peroxide

Tardive dyskinesia: a chronic disorder of the nervous system characterized by involuntary jerky movements of the face, tongue, jaws, trunk, and limbs, usually developing as a late side effect of prolonged treatment with antipsychotic drugs; also called tardive oral dyskinesia

Thermic effect of food (TEE): the increase in energy expenditure associated with the processes of digestion, absorption, and metabolism of food; represents approximately 10% of the sum of the resting metabolic rate and the energy expended in physical activity and includes facultative thermogensis and obligatory thermogensis; often called diet-induced thermogensis (DIT), specific dynamic action (SDA), or the specific effect of food (SEF)

Thromboplastin: a plasma protein present in tissues, platelets, and white blood cells necessary for the coagulation of blood and, in the presence of calcium ions, necessary for the conversion of prothrombin to thrombin

Thyroglobulin: an iodine-containing protein ofthe thyroid gland that on proteolysis yields thyroxine and triiodothyronine

Thyroxine (T_4): an iodine-containing hormone secreted by the thyroid gland to regulate the rate of cell metabolism

Transcuprein: a macroglobulin regulated by copper and iron availability

Transferrin: a beta globulin in blood serum that combines with and transports iron; also called siderophilin

Tremor: a trembling or shaking usually from physical weakness, emotional stress, or disease

Triglyceride (triacylglycerol): a lipid consisting of three fatty acid chains esterified to a glycerol phosphate molecule

Triiodothyronine (T_3): an iodine-containing thyroid hormone with several times more biologic activity than thyroxine

Trimethylamine: an irritating gaseous orvolatile liquid tertiary amine $(CH_3)_3N$ that has a fishy odor, is only slightly more basic than ammonia, is flammable and forms explosive mixtures with air, is formed as adegradation product of many nitrogenous animal and plant substances, and is used chiefly in making quaternary ammonium compounds (as choline)

Total energy expenditure: the sum of the resting energy expenditure, energy expended in physical activity, and the thermic effect of food; the energy expended by an individual in 24 hours

Xanthine oxidase: a crystallizable flavoprotein enzyme containing iron and molybdenum that promotes the oxidation especially of hypoxanthineand xanthine to uric acid and of many aldehydes to acids called also Schardinger enzyme

Index

Anti-aging, 31
Antioxidants, 30, 45, 89, 316
Anxiety, 53
Appetite loss, 41, 53, 65
Arteriosclerosis, 75
Arthritis, 31, 66, 97
Asbestos, 316
Ascorbic acid, 66. See also Vitamin C
Asthma, 54, 71
Atherosclerosis, 21, 79, 316
ATP. See Adenosine triphosphate

B

Bacteria, 66
Basal energy expenditure (BEE), 105, 316
Basal metabolic rate (BMR), 105, 316
BEE. See Basal energy expenditure
Beriberi, 34, 316
Betacarotene, 27
Beverages, 155. See also Water
    ORAC scores per 100g and per normal portion, 87–88
Biotin. See Vitamin B7
Birth defects, 67
Bleeding gums, 46
Blood, 186
    amount in the human body, 93–94
    composition, 91–92
    effects of common foods on blood pH balance, 99–101
    functions, 92–93
    pH and human health, 91–101
    pH balance in the human body, 98–99
    plasma, 92
    platelets, 92
    red cells, 91
    theory of disease and aging and, 94–98
    weights and volumes of different body weights, 93–94
    white cells, 91
Blood glucose. See also Diabetes
    carbohydrates and, 22
Blood pressure, 48, 57, 59, 60, 65, 74
Blood sugar levels, 74
BMI. See Body Mass Index
BMR. See Basal metabolic rate
Body Mass Index (BMI), 102–103, 176, 189
    body weight classification, 103
Body temperature, 61, 62, 67
    water to regulate, 15
Bones, 65, 66
    chemical composition, 9
Brain
    chemical composition, 9
    oxygen and, 12
Bread
    energy, macronutrients, cholesterol, and ORAC values of selected foods, 203–204
    nutrition values of essential amino acids, EPA, DHA, lutein, and zeaxanthin, 285
    nutrition values of minerals, 231–232
    nutrition values of vitamins, 258–259
British Journal of Nutrition, 184
Buettner, Dan, 175–176
Buffer, 99, 316
Butyrate, 24, 316

C

Triiodothyronine (T3), 69, 327
Trimethylamine, 327
Trolox, 82
TTP. See Thiamin triphosphate

U

Ultratrace minerals, 69–77
Urination, 75
U.S. Department of Agriculture (USDA), 78, 82
U.S. Environmental Protection Agency (EPA), 153
U.S. Food and Drug Administration (FDA), 153
USDA. See U.S. Department of Agriculture

V

Vegetables
  energy, macronutrients, cholesterol, and ORAC values of selected foods, 191–194
  nutrition values of essential amino acids, EPA, DHA, lutein, and zeaxanthin, 274–277
  nutrition values of minerals, 220–223
  nutrition values of vitamins, 246–249
  ORAC scores per 100g and per normal portion, 82–84
Vision, 64, 74
Visual acuity, 35
Vitamin A, 18, 26–28
  values of selected foods, 135–136 (See also Night blindness)
    deficiency symptoms, 28
    functions, 27
    health benefits, 28
Vitamin B1 (Thiamin), 33–34, 52

deficiency symptoms, 34
functions, 33
health benefits, 33–34
values of selected foods, 138
Vitamin B2 (Riboflavin), 34–36
  deficiency symptoms, 35–36
  functions, 34–35
  health benefits, 35
  values of selected foods, 138–139
Vitamin B3 (Niacin), 36–37
  deficiency symptoms, 37
  functions, 36
  health benefits, 36
  values of selected foods, 139
Vitamin B5 (Pantothenic acid), 37–38
  deficiency symptoms, 38
  functions, 38
  health benefits, 38
  values of selected foods, 139–140
Vitamin B6 (Pyridoxine), 39–40
  deficiency symptoms, 40
  functions, 39
  health benefits, 39–40
  values of selected foods, 140
Vitamin B7 (Biotin), 40–41
  deficiency symptoms, 41
  functions, 41
  health benefits, 41
  values of selected foods, 140–141
Vitamin B9 (Folic acid/Folate), 42–43
  deficiency symptoms, 43
  functions, 42
  health benefits, 42–43
  values of selected foods, 141
Vitamin B12 (Cobalamin), 43–45
  deficiency symptoms, 44–45

menopause, 73
pregnancy, 30, 64, 67
premenstrual syndrome, 31
reference heights and weights, 104–105
World Health Organization (WHO), 153, 176, 177, 183, 189
Wound healing, 64, 72

X

Xanthine oxidase (XO), 76, 327
XO. See Xanthine oxidase

Z

Zeaxanthin, 27
nutrition values of food, 274–297
ten foods containing richest, 144–145
values of selected foods, 142–143
Zinc, 63–65
deficiency symptoms, 65
functions, 63–64
health benefits, 64–65
ten foods containing richest, 132